DMU 0350482 01 9

AF784502

Blood Coagulation and Haemostasis

A Practical Guide

For Churchill Livingstone:

Publisher: Mike Parkinson
Project Editor: Jane Starling
Design: Design Resources Unit
Production Controller: Mrs N. G. C. Small
Editorial Co-ordination: Editorial Resources Unit
Sales Promotion Executive: Marion Pollock

Blood Coagulation and Haemostasis

A Practical Guide

Edited by

Jean M. Thomson PhD MRC Path
Honorary Lecturer, University of Manchester; Deputy Director,
UK Reference Laboratory for Anticoagulant Reagents and Control,
Withington Hospital, Manchester, UK

FOURTH EDITION

CHURCHILL LIVINGSTONE
EDINBURGH LONDON MELBOURNE NEW YORK AND TOKYO 1991

CHURCHILL LIVINGSTONE
Medical Division of Longman Group UK Limited

Distributed in the United States of America by Churchill Livingstone Inc., 1560 Broadway, New York, N.Y. 10036, and by associated companies, branches and representatives throughout the world.

© J & A Churchill Ltd 1970
© Longman Group Limited 1980, 1985
© Longman Group UK Limited 1991

All rights reserved. No part of this publication may be reproduced, stored in a retrieval system, or transmitted in any form or by any means, electronic, mechanical, photocopying, recording or otherwise, without either the prior permission of the publishers (Churchill Livingstone, Robert Stevenson House, 1–3 Baxter's Place, Leith Walk, Edinburgh EH1 3AF), or a licence permitting restricted copying in the United Kingdom issued by the Copyright Licensing Agency Ltd, 90 Tottenham Court Road, London, WIP 9ME.

First edition 1970
Second edition 1980
Third edition 1985
Fourth edition 1991

ISBN 0-443-04383-3

A catalogue record for this book is available from the British Library.

Library of Congress Cataloging in Publication Data
Blood coagulation and haemostasis: a practical guide / edited by Jean M. Thomson. — 4th ed.
p. cm.
Includes index.
ISBN 0-443-04383-3
1. Blood—Coagulation, Disorders of—Diagnosis. 2. Blood coagulation tests. 3. Hemostasis. I. Thomson, Jean M.
[DNLM: 1. Blood Coagulation Disorders—diagnosis. 2. Blood Coagulation Factors—analysis. 3. Blood Coagulation Tests. 4. Hemostasis. QY 410 B655]
RC647.C55B56 1991
616.1'57—dc20
DNLM/DLC
for Library of Congress
91-275
CIP

DE MONTFORT UNIVERSITY
LIBRARY
Acc. No.
Date 19/6/97
Loc./Form
Class 616.157075
BLO

Produced by Longman Singapore Publishers Pte. Ltd.
Printed in Singapore

Preface

In the six years which have elapsed since publication of the third edition of this series, considerable advances have been made in the approach to the laboratory investigation of haemostasis and blood coagulation. It is with these recent developments in mind that a group of experts, actively engaged in the relevant areas, have been invited to contribute to the new edition. I am deeply indebted to them for undertaking the task and for the high quality of their chapters as the preparation of a manuscript is so demanding and time consuming. My gratitude and appreciation is warmly extended to all of them for their goodwill and cooperation.

The aim of the series has been to provide assessments and details of clinical and laboratory aspects of a comprehensive range of methods to facilitate and assist in the laboratory diagnosis of abnormalities of the haemostatic and coagulation mechanism; both haemorrhagic and thrombotic. As in previous editions the emphasis has been on the practical approach to the problems. It is stimulating to observe that existing techniques are continually being improved in sensitivity and specificity to the numerous defects and many new approaches are being introduced. The development of monoclonal antibodies and other applications of molecular biology have provided major advances in this field.

Part of the present edition is devoted to the detection and investigation of thrombophilia; the incidence of which has only been appreciated in recent years. The introductory chapter is supported by others concerned with specific, related topics including protein C and S, the serpin inhibitors of blood coagulation and lupus-like anticoagulants. An update on the laboratory investigation of fibrinolysis has also been included, followed by a chapter evaluating the measurement of fibrinogen derivatives.

A comprehensive section, devoted to the occurrence and identification of impaired haemostasis in the infant has been included in the series for the first time. It fulfils a need for the availability of such information to the clinician, as well as being an aid to laboratory diagnosis in this specialized area. The final chapter, which examines the implementation of the INR system, demonstrates the value of the application of prothrombin time standardisation.

Manchester, 1991 J.M.T.

Contributors

Maureen M. Andrew MD FRCP(C)
Associate Professor of Pediatrics and Director, Coagulation Laboratory, McMaster University Medical Center, Hamilton, Ontario, Canada

Linda Barna MT(ASCP) SH
Supervisor, Research Laboratory, Ball Memorial Hospital, Muncie, Indiana, USA

Michael D. Boisclair MSc
Research Assistant, Department of Haematology, Charing Cross & Westminster Medical School, London, UK

Nuala A. Booth PhD
Lecturer in Biochemistry, University of Aberdeen, Marischal College, Aberdeen, UK

Jacqueline Conard PhD MCU-PH
Central Laboratory of Haematology, Hôtel-Dieu Hospital, Paris, France

Marilyn Johnston ART
Chief Technologist, Coagulation Laboratory, McMaster University Medical Center, Hamilton; Regional Technical Director, Hamilton, Ontario, Canada

David A. Lane PhD
Reader, Department of Haematology, Charing Cross & Westminster Medical School, London, UK

Gordon D. O. Lowe MD FRCP(Edin, Glasg & Lond)
Senior Lecturer in Medicine, University of Glasgow; Honorary Consultant Physician, Glasgow Royal Infirmary, Glasgow, UK

Pier M. Mannucci MD
Director, A Bianco Bonomi Haemophilia and Thrombosis Centre, Institute of Internal Medicine, University of Milan and Maggiore Hospital, Milan, Italy

Willem Nieuwenhuizen PhD
Head of Department of Lipid Research and Pathophysiology of Endothelium, Gaubius Institute TNO, Leiden, The Netherlands

Ann Rumley BSc
Biochemist, Royal Infirmary, Glasgow, UK

Jean M. Thomson PhD MRC Path
Honorary Lecturer, University of Manchester; Deputy Director, UK Reference Laboratory for Anticoagulant Reagents & Control, Withington Hospital, Manchester, UK

Douglas A. Triplett MD FACP
Professor of Pathology and Assistant Dean, Indiana School of Medicine, Muncie, Indiana, USA

Armando Tripodi PhD
A Bianchi Bonomi, Haemophilia and Thrombosis Centre, Institute of Internal Medicine, University of Milan and Maggiore Hospital, Milan, Italy

Contents

1. Familial thrombophilia

Jacqueline Conard

The definition of thrombophilia is still unclear. Egeberg was one of the first to use the term thrombophilia to designate a disease associated with a high risk of venous thrombosis, namely congenital deficiency in antithrombin III (Egeberg 1965). This term has become more and more common and it can be defined as a clinical condition characterized by an increased tendency to venous thrombosis and recurrence which cannot be explained by known risk factors, such as pregnancy or surgery.

It has to be clarified whether thrombophilia is familial only, or may be acquired (e.g. a circulating anticoagulant), and whether it is associated with venous and, eventually, arterial thrombosis. The opposite syndrome, haemophilia, is well defined and associated with a high risk of bleeding and concerns a congenital disorder with a specific deficiency (factor VIII or IX).

Familial thrombophilia is considered in this chapter, with the aim of determining its characteristics. The congenital disorders of coagulation and fibrinolysis recognized or suspected of predisposing to thrombosis are described. Finally, a practical scheme for selecting and screening patients is defined, with special attention to the interpretation of biological results.

CHARACTERISTICS

The formation of haemostatic clots as well as the permeability of veins and arteries is maintained because of the existence of the well known balance between primary haemostasis and coagulation on one side and fibrinolysis on the other. (Fig. 1.1).

Consequently, at least theoretically, a number of abnormalities may be responsible for a thrombotic tendency. These are:

1. Increased coagulation due to:
    - Increased platelet number or function
    - Increased levels of clotting factors
    - Decreased activity of physiological inhibitors either due to a deficiency of the inhibitor or to a decrease of its activation (lack or

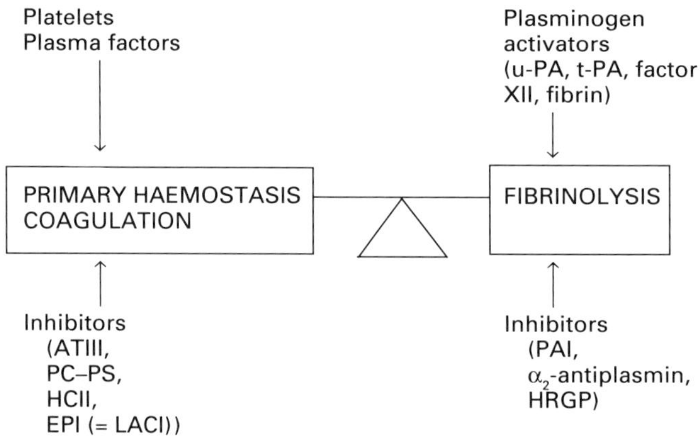

Fig. 1.1 Haemostatic balance. ATIII, antithrombin III; EPI (=LACI), extrinsic pathway inhibitor (=lipoprotein-associated coagulation inhibitor); HCII, heparin cofactor II; HRGP, histidine-rich glycoprotein; PAI, plasminogen activator inhibitor; PC, protein C; PS, protein S; t-PA, tissue-type plasminogen activator; u-PA, urokinase-type plasminogen activator.

decreased availability of thrombomodulin to activate protein C, reduced availability of glycosaminoglycans for antithrombin III).

2. Decreased fibrinolytic activity due to:
   Decreased activation of plasminogen through tissue-type plasminogen activator (t–PA), urokinase–type plasminogen activator (u–PA) or factor XII pathway.
   Elevated levels of fibrinolytic inhibitors
   Abnormal lysability of the fibrin clot related to dysfibrinogenaemia or abnormal fibrin structure.

In addition to blood abnormalities, the vessel wall probably plays an important role but its study is far more difficult.

Each time a test is abnormal, one should wonder if it is the cause or the consequence of thrombosis or if it is only coincidental. To help solve this question:

1. The prevalence of thrombosis is evaluated in patients with a biological abnormality
2. The prevalence of the abnormalities is evaluated in healthy subjects or in patients with thrombosis
3. A family study should be undertaken in order to detect other cases of biological defects and compare them with the occurrence of thrombosis
4. A genetic study may reveal gene defects associated with both the biological alteration and thrombotic episodes.

Consequently, coagulation and fibrinolysis abnormalities, considered as predisposing to thrombosis, can be divided into well-documented or uncertain biological risk factors detected either by routine or specific tests.

Although thrombosis may be atypical or 'spontaneous' and usually denominated idiopathic, in a number of congenital defects one of the following acquired risk factors is often present:

Surgical procedure or various trauma
Pregnancy and puerperium
Treatment with oral contraceptives
Malignancy
Nephrotic syndrome
Obesity
Advanced age, etc.

The above outlines the multifactorial origin of thrombosis and may explain why some affected subjects remain free of thrombosis. However, unknown precipitating factors probably exist and could explain why some patients remain asymptomatic or why, after one thrombotic episode, some have recurrences and others do not. Their identification would be of paramount importance in order to institute or prolong anticoagulant treatment.

DEFICIENCY IN COAGULATION INHIBITORS

Natural coagulation inhibitors include (Figs 1.1 and 1.2):

1. Heparin cofactors:
   Antithrombin III (ATIII)
   Heparin cofactor II (HCII)
2. Inhibitors of the protein C anticoagulant pathway:
   Protein C (PC)
   Protein S (PS)
3. Inhibitor of the factor VIIa–tissue factor complex:
   Extrinsic pathway inhibitor (EPI), also called lipoprotein–associated coagulation inhibitor (LACI).

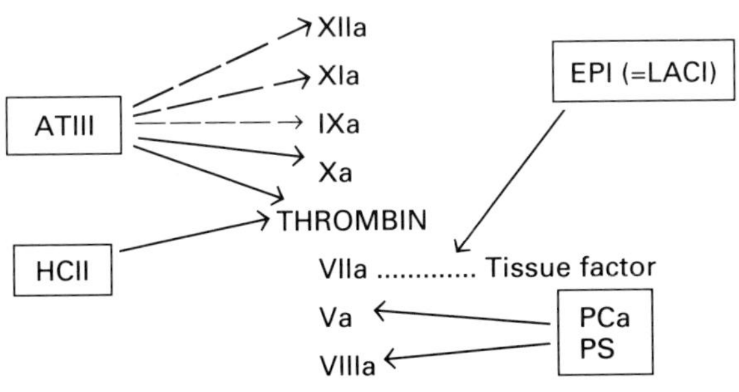

Fig. 1.2 Factors affected by physiological coagulation inhibitors.

Congenital deficiencies of these inhibitors are classically associated with venous thromboembolism and transmitted as an autosomal dominant trait.

1. Antithrombin III

ATIII is a glycoprotein synthesized in the liver. It inhibits thrombin and factor Xa, and to a lesser extent, factors XIIa, XIa and IXa (Fig. 1.2). The rate of inhibition is greatly enhanced by heparin, and by a heparin-like glycosaminoglycan, heparan sulphate, present on the surface of endothelial cells. This might explain the importance of the inhibiting effect of ATIII towards thrombin in vivo.

The gene for ATIII is localized on chromosome 1; exon II has been demonstrated to code for the heparin-binding site and exon VI for the reactive site (Molho-Sabatier et al 1989).

Since the first case of congenital deficiency described in 1965 by Egeberg, many cases have been reported, and reviewed (Thaler & Lechner 1981, Hultin et al 1988, Lane & Caso 1989).

The comparison of immunological assays (electroimmunoassay, radial immunodiffusion or nephelometric assay) and activity assays (heparin cofactor activity or progressive antithrombin activity) leads to the detection of quantitative type I deficiency and functional type II deficiency. In addition, subgroups have been distinguished depending upon the ability to bind heparin, thrombin or both. The following classification has been proposed by Sas et al (1980):

Type I. Low functional and immunological ATIII
- *Ia.* Reduced synthesis and/or turnover of a normal molecule,
- *Ib.* Reduced synthesis and/or turnover of a molecule with abnormal heparin binding as determined by crossed immunoelectrophoresis, e.g. ATIII Oslo (Hultin et al 1988)

Type II. Low functional but normal immunological ATIII.
- *IIa.* Functional abnormalities of both the reactive site and the heparin-binding site
- *IIb.* Functional abnormalities of the reactive site only
- *IIc.* Functional abnormalities of the heparin-binding site only; it has also been denominated type III.

Another classification has been proposed recently by Prochownik (1989), and it may change again in the coming years with the results of genetic studies. It is suggested that type I deficiencies result from genetic mutations producing silent ATIII alleles, while type II deficiencies are caused by point mutations that induce abnormal thrombin or heparin binding. Details on the characterization of ATIII variants are presented in Chapter 3.

Most patients are heterozygotes with a plasma level close to 50% of the normal control value. No homozygotes for type I, IIa or IIb deficiency have been described and this suggests they may not be compatible with life. In contrast, a few homozygous patients with a type IIc defect have been reported.

Table 1.1 Prevalence of ATIII, PC and PS congenital deficiencies in normals and in patients with a history of thrombosis

	ATIII	PC	PS	Total
Normals				
Odegard & Abildgaard (1977)	1 in 5000			
Broekmans et al (1986)		1 in 15 000		
Miletich et al (1987)		1 in 200–300		
Patients with a history of thrombosis (%)				
Juillet et al (1978)	2.3	—	—	—
Gladson et al (1988)	3.0	4.0	5.0	12
Engesser et al (1987a)	3.0	7.8	8.0	18
Conard et al (1988b)	4.3	7.8	1.8	14
Ben-Tal et al (1989)	7.5	5.6	2.8	16
Pabinger et al (1988)	1.8	1.0	0.5	3
Heijboer et al (1989)				6.7
Patients with first episode before 40 years and recurrences (%)				
Gladson et al (1988)	—	12	15	
Broekmans et al (1986)	—	18	14	

The prevalence of congenital ATIII deficiency in normals (Table 1.1) has been found to be one in 5000, i.e. 0.02% (Odegard & Abildgaard 1977), while in patients with a history of venous thrombosis it is about 2–6% (Juillet et al 1978, Thaler & Lechner 1981, Conard et al 1988b, Engesser 1988, Gladson et al 1988, Ben-Tal et al 1989). The true prevalence is difficult to assess because criteria for diagnosis of thrombosis may be different and an overestimation due to bias in the selection of patients is possible. In recent studies (Pabinger et al 1988, Heijboer et al 1989), a total prevalence of 3.1 and 6.7% has been found for congenital deficiencies in ATIII, PC and PS in groups of 380 and 279 patients respectively.

Clinical manifestations of thrombosis were present in 55% of the patients reported by Thaler and Lechner (1981), but this type of estimation greatly depends on the number of young patients included in the studies. It is more appropriate to construct the thrombosis-free survival curves according to the Kaplan–Meier method: more than 85% of the patients older than 50 years had suffered at least one thrombotic episode (Thaler & Lechner 1981). In addition, it has been suggested that, if a deficient patient was still free of thrombosis at the age of 40 years, the risk of developing a thrombosis was very low (Hirsh et al 1989).

The prevalence of thrombosis has been shown to be dependent upon the type of deficiency (Finazzi et al 1987, Hultin et al 1988). Indeed, in types I, IIa and IIb, about 50% of the patients with the deficiency had experienced thrombosis whereas in type IIc, also called type III, only 6% had thrombotic episodes and they were homozygotes.

These findings are important for the consideration of the need, the choice and the duration of prophylactic anticoagulant treatment. They also emphasize that ATIII deficiencies must be precisely classified.

Table 1.2 Thrombotic manifestations in patients with congenital ATIII, PC and PS deficiencies

	ATIII[a)]	PC[b)]	PS[c)]
Number of patients	120	116	39
Thrombosis before 40 years of age (%)	75	80	75
Type of thrombosis (%)			
Deep vein thrombosis	88	82	74
Superficial vein thrombosis	8	47	72
Pulmonary embolism	40	49	38
Arterial thrombosis	?	6	?
Recurrences (%)	60	70	77

[a)] Thaler & Lechner (1981),
[b)] Broekmans & Conard (1988),
[c)] Engesser et al (1987a).

Thromboses are essentially venous: deep vein thrombosis, pulmonary embolism and, less often, superficial vein thrombosis (Table 1.2). They may also occur at unusual sites (mesenteric, cerebral, portal, renal veins) and are often recurrent. Arterial thromboses are uncommon and the relationship with ATIII deficiency is unclear (Conard & Samama 1986, Coller et al 1987, Johnson et al 1990).

Asymptomatic patients are not given anticoagulant treatment unless they are in high-risk situations such as surgery, pregnancy and immobilisation. Oestroprogestogens are contraindicated in the affected women.

Patients with established thrombosis may receive heparin associated with ATIII concentrates followed by long-term oral anticoagulants, or heparin and oral anticoagulants started together to avoid the heparin-induced ATIII decrease (Marciniak & Gockerman 1977). Low-molecular-weight heparins may not be associated with ATIII decrease (Holm et al 1986).

2. Protein C

PC is a glycoprotein dependent on vitamin K with nine γ-carboxyglutamic acid residues, synthesized by the liver. It is a zymogen of a serine protease that is activated by the thrombin–thrombomodulin complex at the

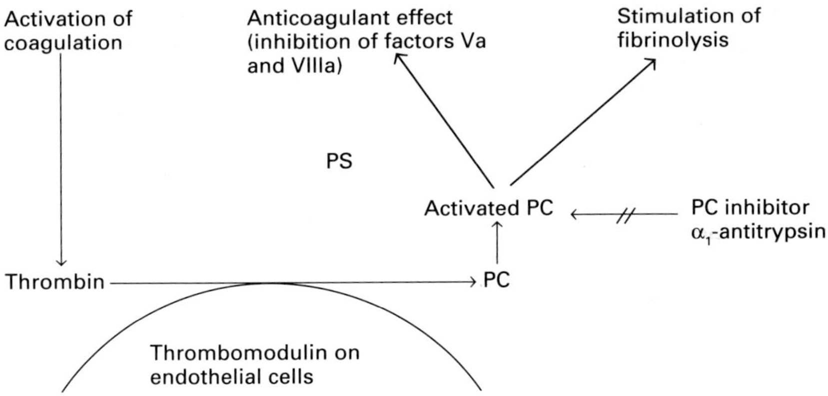

Fig. 1.3 Mechanism of action of PC.

endothelial surface. Activated PC inhibits activated factors V and VIII in the presence of phospholipids and of a plasma cofactor, PS. It may also stimulate fibrinolysis (Fig. 1.3). The PC gene is located on chromosome 2.

Different immunoassays are used for its measurement: electroimmunoassay (EIA), enzyme-linked immunosorbent assay (ELISA) and radioimmunoassay (RIA). Kits for EIA and ELISA are commercially available (see also Chapter 2).

Activity assays (Fig. 1.4) require activation of PC followed by measure-

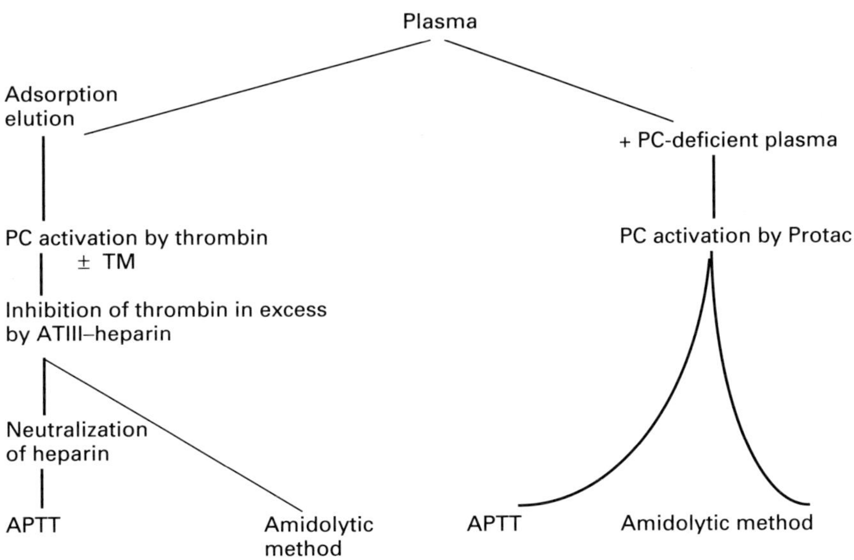

Fig. 1.4 PC activity assays. Activation by thrombin ± thrombomodulin (TM) or by Protac.

ment of activated PC (Bertina 1988). The natural activator of PC is thrombin but it is not the only property of this serine protease. For this reason, activity assays were for a long time both complicated and time consuming. Carboxylated PC had first to be separated from non-carboxylated forms and from its inhibitor, by barium citrate or aluminium hydroxide adsorption, and eluted. PC was then activated by thrombin with or without thrombomodulin and thrombin was later neutralized by ATIII and heparin.

The discovery of a specific PC activator in a snake venom (Protac) led to a simplification of activity assays with the suppression of the adsorption, elution and neutralization steps.

Quantification of the activated PC may be achieved by coagulation (Francis & Patch 1983, Francis 1985, Martinoli & Stocker 1986) or by amidolytic (Bertina et al 1984, Sala et al 1984) methods. Different functional and immunological PC assays have been compared (Espana et al 1986, Mannucci et al 1987, Vinazzer & Pangraz 1987). (See also Chapter 2.)

Type I congenital deficiency is the most frequent but type II has been described (Barbui et al 1984, Bertina et al 1984, Conard et al 1985, Tirindelli et al 1986, Sala et al 1987, Matsuda et al 1988, Faioni et al 1988). A subgroup of type II could be predicted with normal amidolytic activity and decreased anticoagulant activity. Two cases have been reported (Vigano d'Angelo et al 1986, Vasse et al 1989). Newborns (Marlar et al 1988) and a few adults (Samama et al 1984, Melissari et al 1989, Tripodi et al 1990) with severe and homozygous deficiencies have been found.

The prevalence of congenital PC deficiency in the normal population has been controversial (Table 1.1). It was first suspected to be 1 in 15000 (Broekmans et al 1986) but it was then reported to be one in 200–300 (Miletich et al 1987). In addition, four families with asymptomatic deficient subjects were found by these authors. They conclude that this prevalence is consistent with the relatively important number of homozygous patients identified. However, even when considering a prevalence of one in 300 (i.e. 0.3%) it is lower than that in patients with a history of venous thrombosis at a young age (7–8%) (Broekmans et al 1986, Conard et al 1988b, Gladson et al 1988). In a study of a very large family including 46 PC-deficient patients and 138 non-deficient family members, a history of thrombosis was present in 13 and five patients respectively. The Kaplan–Meier analysis and the comparison of thrombosis-free survival curves in heterozygotes and in unaffected family members demonstrated that heterozygous PC deficiency is an important independent risk factor for thrombosis (Bovill et al 1989). However, it cannot be excluded that some other factors may play a role in the clinical expression of PC deficiency.

Transmission of the deficiency is classically autosomal dominant. An autosomal recessive transmission has been suspected in a few families where homozygous patients only experienced thrombosis (Seligsohn et al 1984).

Clinical manifestations of congenital PC deficiency are very similar to those of ATIII deficiency (Griffin et al 1981, Horellou et al 1984, Broekmans & Conard 1988) (Table 1.2) but superficial vein thrombosis seems more frequent and purpura fulminans has been observed in homozygous newborns (Marlar et al 1988). In addition, skin necrosis may develop at the initiation of oral anticoagulant treatment but this manifestation seems infrequent (Broekmans & Conard 1988). Arterial thrombosis might be more frequent than in ATIII deficiency (Conard & Samama 1986, Coller et al 1987).

So far, there is no established difference in clinical manifestations between patients with type I and type II deficiencies. Concerning homozygous patients, they can be divided into two groups: newborns with severe purpura fulminans and less than 1% PC and homozygous adults with a severe or mild defect (less than 10%) who had the first thrombotic episode after the age of 10 years (Samama et al 1984, Melissari & Kakkar 1989). In this last group, the absence of neonatal purpura or thrombosis is surprising since the patients probably had a very low PC level at birth, due to the addition of the physiological deficiency observed at this time of life. Moreover, recently, a case of homozygous deficiency without thrombosis has been reported (Tripodi et al 1990).

Management of asymptomatic patients is similar to ATIII-deficient patients.

Treatment of established thrombosis in heterozygous patients is not different from the treatment of patients without PC deficiency but no loading dose of oral anticoagulants should be given at the initiation of therapy. We continue heparin therapy for 2–3 days after the oral anticoagulant treatment has induced the required therapeutic hypocoagulability. Thrombotic episodes have been observed when heparin was discontinued too early.

3. Protein S

PS is a vitamin K-dependent protein with 11 γ-carboxyglutamic acid residues. It is synthesized by the liver and also by endothelial cells and megakaryocytes. It is a cofactor required for the inhibitory effect of activated PC (Fig. 1.3). PS circulates either free (40%) or bound to the C_4b-binding protein (C_4bBP) (60%) but the free form only has PC cofactor activity. The PS gene is located on chromosome 3.

Total PS antigen assays are widely used. These are immunoradiometric assays, RIA, EIA and ELISA (Bouma 1988) (see Fig. 1.5). Free PS antigen may be measured using the above methods after precipitation of the complex with C_4bBP by PEG (polyethylene glycol) 6000 (Comp et al 1986a), or calculated from levels of total PS and C_4bBP determined by EIA,

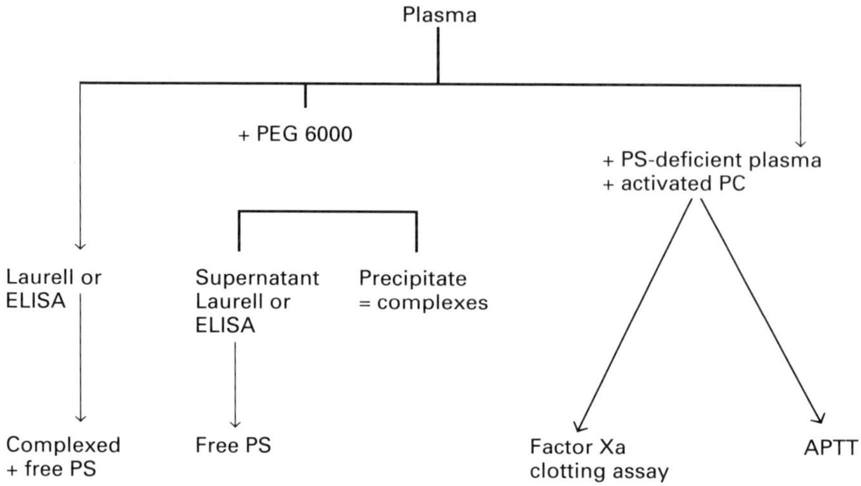

Fig. 1.5 Principle of the determination of PS by immunological or functional assays.

assuming a dissociation constant of 7×10^{-8} m/mol for the complex (Dahlback & Stenflo 1981, Bertina et al 1985). It should be noted that this calculation is based on results obtained in purified proteins systems. Kits for the determination of PS antigen are commercially available (see Chapter 2).

Monoclonal antibodies against PS have been proposed to quantitate this protein but their routine use for the detection of congenital deficiencies may give misleading results. Indeed, in a Dutch family with an abnormal PS molecule (PS Heerlen) it was shown that, due to the frequency of the same genetic abnormality in 1182 patients with unexplained thrombosis, the Heerlen allele was not linked with increased risk for thrombosis (Bertina et al 1989).

Crossed immunoelectrophoresis can be very useful to show the proportions of the slow migrating PS–C_4bBP complex and the faster free PS.

PS activity assays solely reflect free PS, but they are still performed only in a few specialized laboratories because they require reagents which are not easily available, such as activated PC– and PS–deficient plasmas. These assays are based on the ability of PS to function as a cofactor of the anticoagulant effect of activated PC, i.e. factor Xa clotting assay (Comp et al 1984) or prolongation of the partial thromboplastin time (Kamiya et al 1986, Suzuki & Nishioka 1988). More recently, bovine serum was used as a source of activated factor V to measure the anticoagulant effect of activated PC (Wolf et al 1989).

A classification of congenital PS deficiencies was proposed by Comp et al (1986a): type I with decreased free PS but normal total PS (and increased level of C_4bBP) and type II with low levels of both free and total PS antigen. However, this nomenclature is probably not definite because it may be confused with deficiencies of other proteins where type I is a quantitative deficiency and type II corresponds to a normal antigen associated with a decreased activity.

The prevalence of congenital PS deficiency in healthy individuals is still unknown. In patients with a history of venous thrombosis it has been estimated to be 0.5–8% (Gladson et al 1988, Engesser et al 1987a, 1988b, Pabinger et al 1988, Conard et al 1988b).

Clinical manifestations are very similar to those observed in PC congenital deficiencies (Schwartz et al 1984, Engesser et al 1987a, Engesser, 1988), including the relatively high risk of superficial vein thrombosis (Table 1.2). Surprisingly, skin necrosis at the initiation of oral anticoagulants has been reported (Friedman et al 1986) although PS has a much longer half-life than PC (60 h versus 8 h). Anecdotal arterial occlusions of the limbs have also been noted (Coller et al 1987) and arterial and cerebral thromboses appear to be frequently observed (von Felten & Schaeffer 1989, Girolami et al 1989, Sacco et al 1989, Thommen et al 1989).

A homozygous PS deficiency associated with neonatal purpura fulminans has been recently reported (Mahasandana et al 1990).

The association between PS deficiency and thromboembolic disease has been confirmed by the genetic study of a Dutch family (Ploos van Amstel et al 1989). A partial deletion of the PS gene was observed and co-segregated with heterozygosity for PS deficiency. In addition, thrombosis occurred only in members with a PS gene defect.

4. Heparin cofactor II

Heparin cofactor II (HCII) is a glycoprotein synthesized in the liver that inhibits thrombin but not factor Xa. Its rate of inhibition is accelerated by heparin and also by heparan sulphate and dermatan sulphate. For this reason, it was also named dermatan sulfate cofactor (Abildgaard & Larsen 1984).

HCII can be measured by an immunological assay (Sié et al 1985, Tran et al 1985) or by a functional assay (Abildgaard & Larsen 1984, Tollefsen et al 1983, Sié et al 1985, Andersson et al 1986) (see also Chapter 3).

Two inherited HCII deficiencies associated with thrombosis were independently reported (Sié et al 1985, Tran et al 1985) and families with functionally abnormal molecules were then described (Andersson et al 1987). However, the prevalence of HCII deficiency has been found to be very similar (less than 1%) in normals and in patients with a history of venous thrombosis and the deficiency has been denied as a risk factor for thrombosis (Bertina et al 1987).

5. EPI or LACI

The extrinsic pathway inhibitor (EPI) (Rao & Rapaport 1987) and the lipoprotein-associated coagulation inhibitor (LACI) (Broze et al 1988) correspond to the same inhibitor which is directed against the factor VIIa–tissue factor complex in the presence of factor Xa.

Time-consuming assays have been reported for its measurement in plasma (Sandset et al 1987). No case of congenital deficiency in this inhibitor has yet been reported.

HYPOFIBRINOLYSIS

Hypofibrinolysis may result from an alteration of the plasminogen molecule or of its activation by t-PA or the factor XII-dependent pathway from an increase in inhibitors (such as histidine–rich glycoprotein), or from an abnormal structure of fibrin (Fig. 1.6).

Plasminogen alteration

Plasminogen is synthesized in the liver and is converted into plasmin in the presence of a physiological activator, t-PA, or by the coagulation factor XII-dependent pathway.

It can be measured by radial immunodiffusion or by a functional method using chromogenic or fluorogenic substrates, allowing the detection of quantitative (hypoplasminogenaemia) or functional defects (dysplasminogenaemia) (see also Chapter 5).

Hypo- and dysplasminogenaemias associated with venous thrombosis

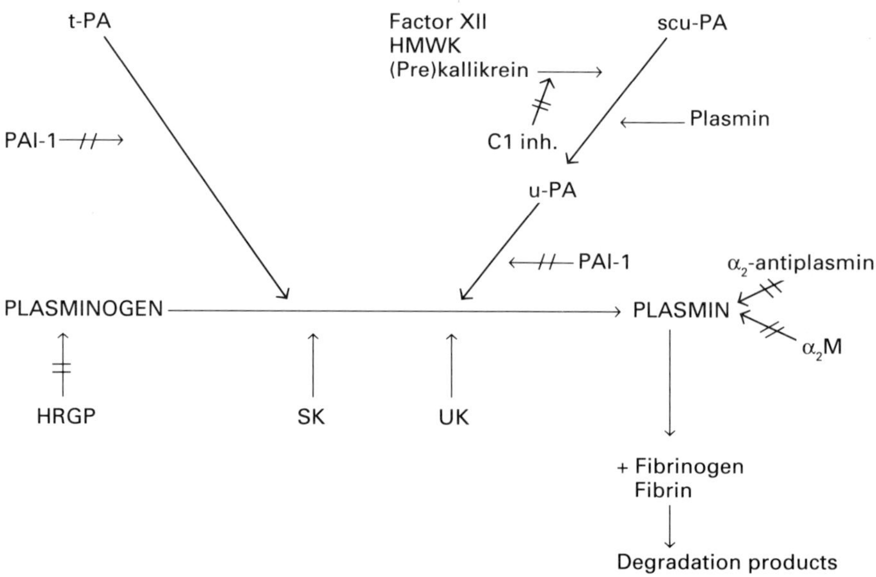

Fig. 1.6 Simplified scheme for fibrinolysis. α_2M, α_2-macroglobulin; scu-PA, single-chain plasminogen activator; SK, streptokinase; UK, urokinase.

have been reviewed (Dolan and Preston 1988). It appears that although the association is present in the proband, thrombosis may not be observed in the family members with the plasminogen alteration.

The molecular defect has been identified in one family (Miyata et al 1982) and the gene frequency distribution of the abnormal molecule was found to be 0.018 in the Japanese population but was absent in a US population (Aoki et al 1984).

Since the frequency of thrombosis is low in patients with plasminogen deficiency and since such a deficiency is present in 3% of normals (Kazama et al 1983) and less than 3% of patients with a history of thrombosis (Conard et al 1988b, Gladson et al 1988), this alteration is probably a weak (if any) risk factor for thrombosis.

Alterations of the t-PA pathway

Hypofibrinolysis may result from defective synthesis or release of t-PA from the vascular wall or from increased plasma levels of the natural inhibitor, PAI-1 (plasminogen activator inhibitor 1).

An impaired fibrinolytic activity after stimulation (venous occlusion or administration of desmopressin (DDAVP)) is a frequent finding in patients with a history of thrombosis and is present in 25–30% (Conard et al 1982, Juhan-Vague et al 1987). In our experience, only 48 of the 105 thrombotic patients with this abnormality had a positive family history of thrombosis. Thus, in most cases, it is probably acquired.

The measurement of t-PA and PAI-1 in the most recent studies shows that an abnormal response to venous occlusion is frequently associated with an elevated level of PAI-1, possibly related to obesity or hypertriglyceridaemia, and is usually acquired. However, few families with reduced plasminogen activator activity have been reported (Johansson et al 1978, Jorgensen et al 1982, Stead et al 1983, Petaja et al 1989), and in one of them a genetic defect was found (Phillips et al 1987).

It is now clear that many fibrinolytic abnormalities are transient and associated with the acute phase of thrombotic episodes. In addition, the criteria for good and bad responders to stimulation are still unclear but the methodological progress with specific assays for t-PA and PAI-1 should help in this respect.

Deficiency in contact factors

Alteration of the factor XII-dependent fibrinolytic pathway may explain venous thrombotic accidents observed in severe congenital deficiencies of this factor, including the index patient, Mr Hageman.

An incidence of 8–11% of thrombosis was reported in factor XII-deficient patients (Goodnough et al 1983) and of 8.6% in patients with prekallikrein deficiency (Goodnough et al 1983).

These data indicate that deficiencies in contact factors do not protect against thromboembolism but they do not seem to suggest a high risk factor.

Increase in histidine-rich glycoprotein

It has been suggested that elevated levels of histidine-rich glycoprotein (HRGP) might be a risk factor for thrombosis because of the subsequent low levels of free plasminogen. Such an abnormality was reported in 4–9% of patients with thrombophilia (Samama et al 1983, Engesser et al 1987b), but there is not yet sufficient evidence to establish a causal relationship between elevated levels of HRGP and thrombosis. It is possible that an increase of HRGP is related to an abnormality of the regulation of the synthesis of this inhibitor and genetic analysis may provide some valuable information in the near future.

A recent finding must be taken into account for the interpretation of the results of HRGP. It is a negative acute-phase reactant (Saigo et al 1990).

Alterations of the fibrinogen molecule

Functional alterations of the fibrinogen molecule are usually asymptomatic although venous or arterial thromboses have been observed in about 10% of the reported dysfibrinogenaemias (Samama et al 1988). It should be pointed out that in many cases the propositus was the only member with thrombosis and thrombosis was often present in patients with or without the fibrinogen defect. Moreover, another risk factor for thrombosis was associated with dysfibrinogenaemia in five patients; PC deficiency in two (Gandrille et al 1987); lupus-like anticoagulant or anticardiolipin in another two cases (Al-Mondhiry & Galanakis 1986, Yoshida et al 1987) and hypercholesterolaemia in one (Engesser 1988).

A structure–function relationship could not be clearly documented (Haverkate & Samama 1990). The cause of thrombosis may be related to (a) a defective cofactor function of abnormal fibrin in t-PA-mediated fibrinolysis as in fibrinogen Dusard and Nijmegen, (b) a defective thrombin binding of the fibrin as in fibrinogens Malmo or Naples (Milano II) or (c) an increased activity of platelet aggregation cofactor as in fibrinogen Oslo I (Samama et al 1988).

COMBINED ABNORMALITIES

Different abnormalities may be present in some patients:

1. Deficiency of PC associated with a deficiency in ATIII, PS (in Broekmans & Conard 1988), a dysplasminogenaemia (Manabe & Matsuda 1985) or a dysfibrinogenaemia (Gandrille et al 1987)

2. Deficiency of PS associated with a deficiency of HCII (Bertina et al 1987)
3. Type II deficiency in ATIII associated with hypoplasminogenaemia (Bauer et al 1983) or with PC deficiency (Wolf et al 1990).

In addition, congenital deficiencies in coagulation inhibitors may be associated with hypofibrinolysis.

Consequently, any patient with a deficiency in a given protein must have a complete study of the different proteins possibly involved in thrombosis.

OTHER DEFICIENCIES ASSOCIATED WITH VENOUS THROMBOSIS

Patients with factor V deficiency and a history of venous thrombosis have been observed (Goodnough et al 1983) and the estimated prevalence of thromboembolism in factor V deficiency was 0.7%.

Some cases of factor VII deficiency (undetectable levels to levels of 10%) and thrombophlebitis or pulmonary embolism have also been reported (in Goodnough et al 1983).

Conversely, no case of thrombosis has been reported in patients with factor X, II or XIII deficiencies but myocardial infarction has been observed in factor XI-deficient patients (Goodnough et al 1983).

SCREENING FOR THROMBOPHILIA

As reported above, a number of coagulation and fibrinolytic abnormalities are or may be risk factors for thrombosis but their relatively low prevalence shows the importance of selecting patients to be studied and the tests to be performed.

1. Selection of patients (Table 1.3)

Patients with a history of venous thrombosis

Patients to be selected should have had at least one episode of thrombosis documented by an objective procedure such as venography, lung scan or angiography, and preferably recurrences. Thrombosis at unusual sites (mesenteric, portal, cerebral veins) should also be included since, although infrequent in the general population, they have been reported in congenital deficiencies of inhibitors at an unexpected frequency.

The existence of PC deficiency may also be suspected in purpura fulminans or massive thromboses in a newborn, or in skin necrosis at the initiation of oral anticoagulant treatment. A warfarin-induced skin necrosis has also been reported in a single patient with PS.

Superficial vein thrombosis seems common in patients with PC or PS

Table 1.3 Selection of patients for inherited thrombotic disorders

1. Venous thrombosis
Exclusion of common acquired aetiologies: malignancy, lupus anticoagulant, myeloproliferative disorders
First episode before the age of 40 years, preferably recurrent
Documented deep vein thrombosis or pulmonary embolism (venography, lung scan, angiography)
Unusual site of thrombosis (mesenteric, renal, portal or cerebral veins)
Repeated superficial vein thrombosis
With or without triggering factors
With a positive family history of thrombosis (or without family history but recurrent episodes before the age of 40 years)
2. Arterial thrombosis
Before the age of 40–50 years: cerebral arterial thrombosis, myocardial infarction, peripheral artery occlusion
Recurrent peripheral artery occlusion despite satisfactory surgical procedure at any age

deficiency so that, in the absence of underlying disease, patients with repeated superficial vein thromboses at a young age should be screened.

The age of the patients at the time of the first episode of thrombosis is of paramount importance. Most of the patients with congenital deficiencies of inhibitors have experienced thrombosis before the age of 40 years: 80% of ATIII (Thaler & Lechner 1981), 80% of PC (Broekmans & Conard 1988) and 75% of PS (Briet et al 1988) deficiencies. The association of the two following criteria, thrombosis before the age of 40 years and recurrences, leads to a prevalence of 11–18% PC deficiencies and of 13–14% PS deficiencies respectively (Broekmans et al 1986, Gladson et al 1988).

Special attention should be drawn to spontaneous thromboses but, according to our experience, thromboses with triggering factors must also be included in screening studies. Indeed, a thrombosis considered as spontaneous may be the result of too rapid, non-oriented report of the medical history. It is then recorded as a thrombosis without known cause by the investigator. In patients with congenital deficiencies detected in our laboratory, a triggering factor was found in 50% of them after an accurate history.

Resistance to anticoagulant treatment, and especially to heparin, may suggest ATIII deficiency. However, it is often difficult to distinguish between a thrombosis recurring in a well-anticoagulated patient from a thrombosis due to insufficient treatment.

Since the transmission of an alteration in coagulation is usually autosomal and dominant, patients with a positive family history of thrombosis should be studied with priority. However, the value of the information provided by the family must be considered. In five of 36 patients with congenital deficiencies studied by our group, there was no positive family history. Either the family was small and not informative or the patient had no information on members of his or her family. For these reasons, patients who have had repeated and objectively diagnosed episodes of thrombosis should probably be studied even if they have no positive history of thrombosis.

Patients with arterial thrombosis

Arterial thrombosis has been observed in less than 10% of the larger series of patients with congenital deficiencies in ATIII (Thaler & Lechner 1981), PC (Broekmans & Conard 1988) or PS (Briet et al 1988) and also in dysfibrinogenaemias (Samama et al 1988). We have seen anecdotal cases of peripheral occlusions of the limbs in PC-deficient patients referred to us because of recurrence of occlusions shortly after surgical procedures which were considered as technically satisfactory.

Recent papers have focused on the association of PS deficiency and cerebral arterial disease (Sacco et al 1988, von Felten & Shaeffer 1989, Thommen et al 1989).

Thus, it is our feeling that screening for congenital thrombophilia should be extended to patients with a history of unexpected arterial thrombosis before the age of 50 years, when thromboses are recurrent despite appropriate treatments and especially when there is also a personal or family history of venous thrombosis.

In summary, the selection of patients is highly dependent on the clinical history of the patients and the records must be oriented and as precise as possible.

2. **Selection of the tests** (Table 1.4)

Biological risk factors may be divided into three groups:

1. Well-documented risk factors, not detected by routine tests and requiring specific tests, i.e. congenital deficiency in ATIII, PC or PS
2. Not well-documented risk factors but easy to detect by routine tests, i.e. congenital deficiency of contact factors or dysfibrinogenaemia and also a well-documented acquired risk factor easy to detect, lupus anticoagulant
3. Still uncertain risk factors requiring specific tests for their detection, i.e. plasminogen or HCII deficiency, hypofibrinolysis.

Consequently, the detection of risk factors in selected patients with a history of thrombosis may be achieved in two steps.

Table 1.4 Recommended tests to be performed on selected patients with thrombosis

Step 1
PT, APTT, fibrinogen (Clauss method)
ATIII (heparin cofactor) activity
PC activity
PS antigen (or activity)
PAI-1 activity (if possible)
Step 2
Venous occlusion test with clot lysis times, t-PA and PAI-1 before and after occlusion
Plasminogen activity
HCII activity
HRGP
Other tests? (Keep frozen plasma aliquots)

Step 1

All tests are performed on citrated plasma.

Prothrombin time (PT) and *activated partial thromboplastin time (APTT)* by conventional methods.

If there is a prolongation of the APTT the test must be repeated on a mixture of patient and normal plasma to distinguish between a deficiency and a circulating anticoagulant: a lupus anticoagulant is frequently associated with thrombosis.

Fibrinogen measurement by the clotting method of Clauss.

ATIII determination by the amidolytic method using an automatic instrument. Several kits are commercially available. They measure the heparin cofactor activity of ATIII and the principle of the test is as follows:

plasma (ATIII) + Heparin → [ATIII–heparin]

[ATIII–heparin] + Thrombin in excess
↓ incubation
[ATIII–heparin–thrombin] + Residual thrombin +
Chromogenic substrate
↓ incubation
Release of para-Nitro-Analine (pNA)
(yellow colour measured at 405 nm)

The recommendations of the manufacturers must be strictly followed. The nature of the thrombin used in the test may influence the specificity of the test. With human thrombin, HCII may interfere with ATIII. Thus, bovine thrombin is generally preferred.

An amidolytic method in the presence of heparin has the advantage of detecting all types of congenital deficiencies. However, since deficient patients usually have levels of ATIII close to 50%, the method must be well standardized, and give accurate results. For this reason, we feel it has to be automated. If it is not possible, an immunological technique using commercially available Mancini plates is probably to be preferred since technologists are generally familiar with this method although type II deficiencies will not be detected.

When a deficiency in ATIII (heparin cofactor activity) is detected, an immunological assay has to be performed (antigen ATIII concentration) as well as crossed immunoelectrophoresis in the presence and absence of heparin. It will help to classify the deficiency.

PC determination (see also Chapter 2). Activity methods are preferred and kits are commercially available.

Clotting methods using Protac as an activator are appropriate for short series and have the advantage of an apparent simplicity, i.e. determination of a cephalin clotting time in the presence of Protac and of PC-deficient plasma. However, their reproducibility must be verified and a false diagnosis of deficiency is possible (see below).

Amidolytic methods are widely used on automatic instruments. Kits either contain thrombin or Protac as the activator. Protac methods are simpler and, in our experience, they give very reliable results.

PS determination (see also Chapter 2). At present, only immunological methods are commercially available. The Laurell method is more adapted to short series of tests than an ELISA method. Owing to the existence of free and complexed PS, the following procedure may be recommended:

Determination of total PS
Precipitation of the complex by treating the plasma with 3.75% PEG 6000
Determination of free PS in the supernatant; the results of free PS are either expressed as compared to untreated or PEG-treated control plasma.

Basal PAI-1 activity can be performed at this stage if possible.

Step 2

When tests in step 1 are normal and, especially when patients have had repeated thromboses together with a heavy strong history of thrombosis in the family, uncertain risk factors are investigated.

Plasminogen determination by amidolytic assay (see also Chapter 5). The level may be overestimated in samples with high levels of fibrin degradation products but methods recommended by manufacturers usually avoid this source of error.

HCII determination by amidolytic assay. A commercial kit is now available. (See also Chapter 3.)

Venous occlusion test. A study of fibrinolysis must be performed at a distance between thrombotic episodes (more than 3 months), after fasting overnight and a 15 min rest in the morning and before 10 a.m. because fibrinolytic activity shows circadian variations. We perform a 10 min venous occlusion with a cuff pressure midway between systolic and diastolic pressure but a 20 min occlusion might be preferable.

Overall tests such as euglobulin lysis time and/or dilute whole blood lysis time, as well as the fibrin plate method, are still commonly used.

Special blood collection is required for measurement of t-PA and PAI-1, i.e. on EDTA or citrate in an ice bath or in a special anticoagulant at room temperature (Biopool Stabilyte tubes).

Measurement of t-PA by specific but expensive amidolytic methods can be done with commercially available kits. The conversion of plasminogen to plasmin is catalysed by fibrin fragments and the amount of plasmin formed which reacts with the chromogenic substrate is dependent on the t-PA present in the plasma.

The determination of PAI-1 activity may be more important. Methods are derived from those measuring t-PA. Fixed amounts of t-PA are added to the plasma so that the amidolytic activity reflects the plasma PAI-1 content. (See also Chapter 5).

HRGP can be measured by the Laurell method.

By performing all the above-mentioned tests, a congenital abnormality may be found in only 20–25% of patients with a history of thrombosis starting before the age of 40 years and associated with a positive family history (Conard et al 1988). Consequently, it is recommended that frozen plasma aliquots from these selected patients are kept frozen in order to be able to perform new tests which may become available in the near future.

3. Interpretation of the results

Results must be interpreted as normal or abnormal and abnormalities as acquired or congenital (Table 1.5).

Normal values

Each laboratory should determine its normal values. The following are frequent in adults:

ATIII, 80–120%
PC, 70–130%
PS, 65–130% total or free antigen as compared with a control treated in the same way as the patient plasma
HCII, normal range wide and age dependent (Bertina et al 1987)
Plasminogen, 80–120%

Table 1.5 Acquired deficiencies of ATIII, PC and PS, according to Thaler & Lechner (1981) and Pabinger & Lechner (1988)[a]

ATIII	PC	PS
Neonatal period	Neonatal period	Neonatal period
Pregnancy (±)		Pregnancy
Liver disease	Liver disease	Liver disease
Disseminated intravascular coagulation (±)	Disseminated intravascular coagulation (±)	Disseminated intravascular coagulation (±)
Nephrotic syndrome	Obesity (±)	Lupus
Treatment:		
Heparin	Vitamin K antagonists	Vitamin K antagonists
L-Asparaginase	L-Asparaginase	L-Asparaginase
Oestroprogestogens		Oestroprogestogens

[a] (±) indicates that controversial results have been published.

PAI-1, normal values depend on the method used. Basal values are considered but also values after venous occlusion. In our experience, using the Verheijen method, good responders have practically no residual PAI-1 after venous occlusion (Nguyen et al 1988).

Euglobulin or whole blood lysis times after venous occlusion depend on the duration of occlusion: less than 80–90 min after a 10 min venous occlusion in our experience.

In newborns, most proteins are lower than in adults (see Chapter 8).

Influence of different physiological or pathological conditions

Causes of acquired deficiencies in inhibitors are summarized in Table 1.5.

Pregnancy may induce a slight decrease in ATIII (Gjonnaess & Fagerhol 1975) and also a decrease in PS levels (Comp et al 1986) and in HRGP (Omri et al 1988). In contrast, plasminogen and PAI-1 are increased and there is a constant decrease in fibrinolytic activity after venous occlusion.

Liver disease is associated with a decrease in most coagulation and fibrinolytic components. They may reach very low levels except for PS (possibly because it is not synthesized exclusively in the liver).

Inflammatory syndrome is responsible for an increase in PAI-1 leading to an abnormal response to venous occlusion and elevated levels of PC. In addition, it has been demonstrated that increased factor VIII levels may be responsible for the false diagnosis of a congenital deficiency in PC when the coagulant method using Protac as an activator is performed (de Moerloose et al 1988). For this reason, any deficiency detected by this method has to be confirmed by another method (immunological or amidolytic).

Influence of the treatment

Heparin, administered intravenously or subcutaneously, may be associated with normal or often low levels of ATIII (Marciniak & Gockerman 1977). The assay can be performed in heparin-treated patients and if the level is above 80%, a congenital deficiency can be excluded but if it is lower than 60% a congenital deficiency is likely although not certain. Low-molecular-weight heparins do not modify ATIII levels (Holm et al 1986).

Oral anticoagulants induce a decrease in PC and PS. The simultaneous measurements of other vitamin K-dependent proteins, factor II, X or VII antigen, are useful for the diagnosis of congenital deficiencies in PC or PS, during oral anticoagulant treatment. The ratios of PC antigen with other vitamin K-dependent factor antigens must take into account the intensity of the anticoagulant treatment expressed as international normalized ratios in (INR) (Bertina 1988), and they may also depend on the method used for PC antigen. An ELISA method generally gives lower values than the Laurell method.

For PS, in addition to the comparison with vitamin K-dependent factors, it has been proposed to use the lower limit of PS antigen observed in a reference group of anticoagulant-treated patients who are free of a congenital deficiency. A level below 33% would be indicative of a congenital deficiency (Engesser et al 1987a).

Oral anticoagulants have also been reported to increase the ATIII level in congenital deficiencies, or at least some of them (Thaler & Lechner 1981). Thus, a normal level of ATIII in an anticoagulated patient cannot completely rule out the possibility of a congenital deficiency.

Oestroprogestogen preparations are contraindicated in patients with a history of venous thrombosis and consequently do not interfere with the detection of congenital abnormalities in the probands. In contrast, the search for congenital defects in the family members must take into account the variations induced by oestroprogestogens, particularly a decrease in ATIII and PS and an increase in PC and in plasminogen.

4. Precise characterization of abnormalities

Each time an anomaly is detected, it has to be confirmed by different methods; activity and immunological, amidolytic and coagulant. In addition, crossed immunoelectrophoresis may be useful in confirming the diagnosis (e.g. PS) or in defining the subgroup of the deficiency (e.g. ATIII with abnormal heparin binding).

5. Diagnosis of the congenital origin of the anomaly

When the permanent character of the anomaly has been established by repeated measurements on different blood samples (at least two), the familial study is necessary to confirm the congenital deficiency in the proband and detect other family members who may be at risk of thrombosis. The comparison between the presence of the anomaly and the occurrence of thrombosis helps to determine if the anomaly is the cause of thrombosis, its consequence or a coincidence; it might also be useful for subjects with borderline levels. In the last-mentioned situation, a genetic study is sometimes the only way to give a reliable diagnosis. Thus, although gene analysis is often essentially of scientific interest, it may also be important in confirming a diagnosis (borderline results) or in identifying the type of diagnosis (e.g. ATIII type IIc) which may be associated with a lower risk of thrombosis that does not require anticoagulant therapy.

All of these steps finally lead to the delivery of medical certificates to all affected members, symptomatic or not, with general recommendations in high-risk situations. These certificates should be renewed every year since our knowledge concerning the diagnosis and treatment of the defects may improve in the future.

REFERENCES

Abildgaard U, Larsen M L 1984 Assay of dermatan sulfate cofactor (heparin cofactor II) activity in human plasma. Thrombosis Research 35: 257

Al-Mondhiry H, Galanakis D 1986 Fibrinogen Hershey, an abnormal fibrinogen associated with thrombosis and lupus anticoagulant. Blood 68 (suppl 1): 328

Andersson T R, Larsen M L, Handeland G F, Abildgaard U 1986 Heparin cofactor II activity in plasma: application of an automated assay method to the study of a normal adult population. Scandinavian Journal of Haematology 36: 96.

Andersson T R, Larsen M L, Abildgaard U 1987 Low heparin cofactor II associated with abnormal cross immunoelectrophoresis pattern in two Norwegian families. Thrombososis Research 47: 243

Aoki N, Tateno K, Sakata Y 1984 Differences of frequency distributions of plasminogen phenotypes between Japanese and American populations: new method for the detection of plasminogen variants. Biochemical Genetics 22: 871

Barbui T, Finazzi G, Mussoni L, Riganti M, Donati M B, Colucci M, Collen D 1984 Hereditary dysfunctional protein C (protein C Bergamo) and thrombosis. Lancet ii: 819

Bauer K A, Ashenhurst J B, Chediak J, Rosenberg R D 1983 Antithrombin 'Chicago': a functionally abnormal molecule with increased heparin affinity causing familial thrombophilia. Blood 62: 1242

Ben-tal O, Zivelin A, Seligsohn U 1989 The relative frequency of hereditary thrombotic disorders among 107 patients with thrombophilia in Israel. Thrombosis and Haemostasis 61: 50.

Bertina R M, 1988 Assays for protein C. In: Bertina R M (ed) Protein C and related proteins. Churchill Livingstone, London, p 130

Bertina R M, Broekmans A W, Krommenhoek Van E S C, Van Wijngaarden A 1984 The use of a functional and immunologic assay for plasma protein C in the study of the heterogeneity of congenital protein C deficiency. Thrombosis and Haemostasis 51: 1

Bertina R M, Van Wijngaarden A, Reinalda-Poot J, Poort S R, Bom V J J 1985 Determination of plasma protein S — The protein cofactor of activated protein C. Thrombosis and Haemostasis 53: 268

Bertina R M, Van der Linden I K, Engesser L, Muller H P, Brommer E J P 1987 Hereditary heparin cofactor II deficiency and the risk of development of thrombosis. Thrombosis and Haemostasis 57: 196

Bertina R M, Ploos Van Amstel H K, Van Wijngaarden A, Coenen J, Deutz-Terlouw P P, Reitsma P H, Van der Linden I K 1989 The Heerlen polymorphism of protein S, an immunologic polymorphism due to dimorphism of residue 460. Thrombosis and Haemostasis 62: 303
Bouma B N 1988 Assays for protein S. In: Bertina R M (ed) Protein C and related proteins. Churchill Livingstone, London, p 151
Bovill E G, Bauer K A, Dickerman J D, Callas P, West B 1989 The clinical spectrum of heterozygous protein C deficiency in a large New England kindred. Blood 73: 712
Briet E, Broekmans A W, Engesser L 1988 Hereditary protein S deficiency. In: Bertina R M (ed.) Protein C and related proteins. Churchill Livingstone, London, p 203
Broekmans A W, Van der Linden I K, Jansen-Koeter Y, Bertina R M 1986 Prevalence of protein C (PC) and protein S (PS) deficiency in patients with thrombotic disease. Thrombosis Research suppl VI: 135.
Broekmans A W, Conard J 1988 Hereditary protein C deficiency. In: Bertina R M (ed) Protein C and related proteins. Churchill Livingstone, Edinburgh p 160
Broze G J, Warren L A, Novotny W F, Higuchi D A, Girard J J, Miletich J P 1988 The lipoprotein-associated coagulation inhibitor that inhibits the factor VII–tissue factor complex also inhibits factor Xa: insight into its possible mechanism of action. Blood 71: 335
Coller B S, Owen J, Jesty J et al 1987 Deficiency of plasma protein S, protein C, or antithrombin III and arterial thrombosis. Arteriosclerosis 7: 456
Comp P C, Nixon R R, Cooper M R, Esmon C T 1984 Familial protein S deficiency is associated with recurrent thrombosis. Journal of Clinical Investigation 74: 2082
Comp P C, Doray D, Patton D, Esmon C T 1986 An abnormal plasma distribution of protein S occurs in functional protein S deficiency. Blood 67: 504
Comp P C, Thurnau G R, Welsh J, Esmon C T 1986b Functional and immunologic protein S are decreasing during pregnancy. Blood 68: 881
Conard J, Samama M 1986 Inhibitors of coagulation atherosclerosis and arterial thrombosis. Seminars Thrombosis Hemostasis 12: 87
Conard J, Veuillet-Duval A, Horellou M H, Samama M 1982 Etude de la coagulation et de la fibrinolyse dans 131 cas de thromboses veineuses récidivantes. Nouvelle Revue Française d'Hématologie 24: 205
Conard J, Horellou M H, Van Dreden P, Doco-Lecompte T, Valeyre D, Samama M 1985 Deficit qualitatif en protéine C associé à des thromboses veineuses profondes récidivantes. Nouvelle Revue Française d'Hématologie 27: 106
Conard J, Horellou M H, Samama M 1988a Incidence of thromboembolism in association with congenital disorders in coagulation and fibrinolysis. Acta Chirurgica Scandinavica suppl 543: 15
Conard J, Horellou M H, Van Dreden P, Samama M 1988b Prevalence of hereditary hypercoagulable states. Xth International Congress on Thrombosis of the Mediterranean League against Thromboembolic Diseases, Athens, p 68
Dahlback B, Stenflo J 1981 High molecular weight complex in human plasma between vitamine K-dependent protein S and complement component C4bp-binding protein. Proceedings of the National Academy of Sciences USA 78: 2512
de Moerloose P, Reber G, Bouvier C A 1988 Spuriously low levels of protein C with a Protac activation clotting assay. Thrombosis and Haemostasis 59: 543
Dolan G, Preston F. 1988 Familial plasminogen deficiency and thromboembolism. Fibrinolysis 2(suppl 2): 26
Egeberg O 1965 Inherited antithrombin III deficiency causing thrombophilia. Thrombosis Diathesis Haemorrhagica 13: 516
Engesser L 1988 Thrombophilia. Thesis, p 91
Engesser L, Broekmans A W, Briet E E, Brommer E J P, Bertina R M 1987a Hereditary protein S deficiency. Clinical manifestations. Annals of Internal Medicine 106: 677
Engesser L, Kluft C, Briet E, Brommer E J P 1987b Familial elevation of plasma-histidine-rich glycoprotein in a family with thrombophilia. British Journal of Haematology 67: 355
Espana F, Estelles A, Aznar J, Gilabert J 1986 Assay of protein C in human plasma: comparison of amidolytic, coagulation, and immunochemical assays. Thrombosis Research 44: 771
Faioni E M, Esmon C T, Esmon N L, Mannucci P M 1988 Isolation of an abnormal protein

C molecule from the plasma of a patient with thrombotic diathesis. Blood 71: 940
Finazzi G, Caccia R, Barbui T 1987 Different prevalence of thromboembolism in the subtypes of congenital antithrombin III deficiency: review of 404 cases. Thrombosis and Haemostasis 58: 1094
Francis R B 1985 A simplified PTT-based protein C activity assay using the thrombin–thrombomodulin complex. Thrombosis Research 41: 337
Francis Jr R B, Patch M J 1983 A functional assay for protein C in human plasma. Thrombosis Research 32: 605
Friedman K D, Marlar R A, Houston J G, Montgomery R R 1986 Warfarin-induced skin necrosis in a patient with protein S deficiency. Blood 68, abstract 333a
Gandrille S, Priollet P, Capron L, Roncato M, Fiessinger N, Aiach M 1987 Association of hereditary dysfibrinogenemia with protein C deficiency in two patients with thrombotic tendency. Thrombosis and Haemostasis 58: 411
Girolami A, Simioni P, Lazzaro A R and Cordiano I 1989 Severe arterial cerebral thrombosis in a patient with protein S deficiency (moderately reduced total and markedly reduced free protein S): a family study. Thrombosis and Haemostasis 61: 144
Gjonnaess M, Fagerhol M K 1975 Studies on coagulation and fibrinolysis n pregnancy. Acta Obstetricia et Gynecologica Scandinavica 54: 363
Gladson C L, Scharrer J, Hach V, Beck K H, Griffin J H 1988 The frequency of type I heterozygous protein S and protein C deficiency in 141 unrelated young patients with venous thrombosis. Thrombosis and Haemostasis 59: 18
Goodnough L T, Saito H, Ratnoff O D 1983 Thrombosis or myocardial infarction in congenital clotting factor abnormalities and chronic thrombocytopenias: a report of 21 patients and a review of 50 previously reported cases. Medicine 62: 248
Griffin J H, Evatt B, Zimmerman T S, Kleiss A J, Widemann C 1981: Deficiency of protein C in congenital thrombotic disease. Journal of Clinical Investigation 68: 1370
Haverkate F, Samama M 1990 Personal communication
Heijboer H, Brandjes D P M, Rutten G C F M, Bluer H R, ten Cate J W 1989 Prevalence of hereditary thrombophilia in consecutive out patients with deep vein thrombosis (DVT). Thrombosis and Haemostasis 62: 440
Hirsh J, Piovella F, Pini M 1989 Congenital antithrombin III deficiency. American Journal of Medicine 87: 3B–34S.
Holm H A, Ly B, Handeland G H, Abildgaard U, Arnesen K E, Gottschalk P, Hoeg V et al 1986 Subcutaneous heparin treatment of deep venous thrombosis: a comparison of unfractionated and low weight heparin. Haemostasis 16(suppl 2): 30
Horellou M H, Conard J, Bertina R M, Samama M 1984 Congenital protein C deficiency and thrombotic disease in nine French families. British Medical Journal 289: 1285
Hultin M B, McKay J, Abildgaard U 1988 Antithrombin Oslo: type Ib classification of the first reported antithrombin-deficient family, with a review of hereditary antithrombin variants. Thrombosis and Haemostasis 59: 468
Johansson L, Hedner U, Nilsson I M 1978 A family with thromboembolism disease associated with deficient fibrinolytic activity in vessel wall. Acta Medica Scandinavica 203: 477
Johnson E J, Prentice C R M, Parapia L A 1990 Premature arterial disease associated with familial antithrombin III deficiency. Thrombosis and Haemostasis 63: 13
Jorgensen M, Mortensen J Z, Madsen A G, Thorsen S, Jacobsen B 1982 A family with reduced plasminogen activator activity in blood associated with recurrent venous thrombosis. Scandinavian Journal of Haematology 29: 217
Juhan-Vague I, Valadier J, Alessi M C, Aillaud M F, Ansaldi J, Philip-Joet C, Holvoet P, Serradimigni A, Collen D 1987 Deficient t-PA release and elevated PA inhibitor levels in patients with spontaneous or recurrent deep venous thrombosis. Thrombosis and Haemostasis 57: 67
Juillet Y, Aiach M, Fiessinger J N, Leclerc M, Housset E 1978 Antithrombine III et thromboses veineuses. Sem. Hop. Paris 37: 1126
Kamiya T, Sugihara T, Ogata K et al 1986 Inherited deficiency of protein S in a Japanese family with recurrent venous thrombosis: a study of three generations. Blood 67: 406
Kazama M, Tahara C, Naito I, Nakamura K, Matsuda J, Abe T 1983 Incidence of congenital abnormality of plasminogen in healthy adults and in several diseases. Fibrinolysis VIII: 258

Lane D A, Caso R 1989 Antithrombin: structure, genomic organization , function and inherited deficiency. Baillière's Clinical Haematology 2: 961.
Mahasandana 1990 Neonatal purpura fulminans associated with homozygous protein S deficiency. Lancet i: 61
Manabe S, Matsuda M 1985 Homozygous protein C deficiency combined with heterozygous dysplasminogenemia found in a 21-year-old thrombophilic male. Thrombosis Research 39: 333
Mannucci P M, Tripodi A 1987 Laboratory screening of inherited thrombotic syndromes. Thrombosis and Haemostasis 5: 247
Mannucci P M, Boyer C, Tripodi A et al 1987 Multicenter comparison of five functional and two immunological assays for protein C. Thrombosis and Haemostasis 57: 44
Marciniak E, Gockerman J P 1977 Heparin-induced decrease in circulating antithrombin III. Lancet ii: 581
Marlar R A, Montgomery R R, Madden R M 1988 Homozygous protein C deficiency. In: Bertina R M (ed) Protein C and related proteins. Churchill Livingstone, London, p 182
Martinoli J L, Stocker K 1986 Fast functional protein C assay using Protac®, a novel protein C activator. Thrombosis Research 43: 253
Matsuda M, Sugo T, Sakata Y, Murayama H, Mimuro J, Tanabe S, Yoshitaake S 1988 A thrombotic state due to an abnormal protein C. New England Journal of Medicine 319: 1265
Melissari E, Kakkar V V 1989 Congenital severe protein C deficiency in adults. British Journal of Haematology 72: 222
Miletich J, Sherman L, Broze Jr G 1987 Absence of thrombosis in subjects with heterozygous protein C deficiency. New England Journal of Medicine 317: 991
Miyata T, Iwanaga S, Skata Y, Aoki N 1982 Plasminogen Tochigi: inactive plasmin resulting from replacement of alanine-600 by threonine in the active site. Proceedings of the National Academy of Sciences, USA 79: 6132
Molho-Sabatier P, Aiach M, Gaillard I, Fiessinger J N, Fischer A M, Chadeuf G, Clauser E 1989 Molecular characterization of antithrombin III (ATIII). Variants using polymerase chain reaction. Identification of the ATIII Charleville as an Ala 384 Pro mutation. Journal of Clinical Investigation 84: 1236
Nguyen G, Horellou M H, Kruithof E K O, Conard J, Samama M 1988 Residual plasminogen activator inhibitor after venous stasis as a criterion for hypofibrinolysis study in 83 patients with confirmed deep vein thrombosis. Blood 72: 601
Odegard O R, Abildgaard U 1977 Antithrombin III: critical review of assay methods. Significance of variations in health and disease. Haemostasis 127: 7
Omri A, Kruithof E K O, Bachmann F 1988 Histidine-rich glycoprotein during pregnancy. Thrombosis and Haemostasis 59: 341
Pabinger I, Lechner K 1988 Acquired protein C and protein S deficiency. In: Bertina R M (ed) Protein C and related proteins. Churchill Livingstone, Edinburgh, p 213
Pabinger I, Korninger C H, Lechner K 1988 Prevalence of hypercoagulable states in 380 Austrian patients with a history of venous thrombosis. Xth International Congress on Thrombosis of the Mediterranean League Against Thromboembolic Diseases, Athens, p 70
Petaja J, Rasi V, Myllyla G, Vahtera E, Hallman H 1989 Familial hypofibrinolysis and venous thrombosis. British Journal of Haematology 71: 393
Phillips G, Kaufman R E, Pizzo S V 1987 Tissue plasminogen activator deficiency: a molecular analysis. In: Lowe G D O, Douglas J T, Forbes C D, Henschen A, (eds) Fibrinogen 2. Biochemistry, physiology and clinical relevance. Excerpta Medica, pp 281–284
Ploos van Amstel H K, Huisman M V, Reitsma P H, ten Cate J W, Bertina R M 1989 Partial protein S gene deletion in a family with hereditary thrombophilia. Blood 73: 479
Prochownik E V 1989 Molecular genetics of inherited antithrombin III deficiencies. American Journal of Medicine 87: 3B–15S
Rao L V M, Rapaport S I 1987 Studies of a mechanism inhibiting the initiation of the extrinsic pathway of coagulation. Blood 69: 645
Sacco R L, Owen J, Mohr J P, Tatemichi T K, Grossman B A 1989 Free protein S deficiency: a possible association with cerebrovascular occlusion. Stroke 20: 1657
Saigo K, Yoshida A, Ryo R, Yamaguchi N, Leung L L K 1990 Histidine-rich glycoprotein as

a negative acute phase reactant. American Journal of Hematology 34: 149
Sala N, Owen W G, Collen D 1984 Functional assay of protein C in human plasma. Blood 63: 671
Sala N, Borrell M, Bauer K A, Vigano-D'Angelo S, Fontcuberta J, Felez J, Rutllant M L 1987 Dysfunctional activated protein C (PC cadiz) in a patient with thrombotic disease. Thrombosis and Haemostasis 57: 183
Samama M, Conard J, Castel-Gatey M, Horellou M H 1983 Histidine-rich glycoprotein and deep venous thrombosis. In: Jespersen J, Kluft C, Korsgaard O (eds) Clinical Aspects of fibrinolysis and thrombolysis. South Jutland University Press, Esbjerg, pp 163–173
Samama M, Horellou M H, Soria J, Conard J, Nicolas G 1984 Successful progressive anticoagulation in a severe protein C deficiency and previous skin necrosis at the initiation of oral anticoagulant treatment. Thrombosis and Haemostasis 51: 132
Samama M, Conard J, Soria J 1988 Congenital dysfibrinogenemia and thrombosis. Fibrinolysis 2(suppl 2), 18
Sandset P M, Abildgaard U A, Pettersen M 1987 A sensitive assay of extrinsic coagulation pathway inhibitor (EPI) in plasma and plasma fractions. Thrombosis Research 47: 389
Sas G, Peto I, Banhegyi D, Blasko G, Domjan G 1980 Heterogeneity of the 'classical' antithrombin III deficiency. Thrombosis and Haemostasis 43: 133
Schwarz H P, Fischer M, Hopmeier P, Batard M A, Griffin J D 1984 Plasma protein S deficiency in familial thrombotic disease. Blood 64: 1297
Seligsohn U, Berger A, Abend M, Rubin L, Attias D, Zivelin A, Rapaport S I 1984 Homozygous protein C deficiency manifested by massive venous thrombosis in the newborn. New England Journal of Medicine 310: 559—562
Sié P, Dupouy D, Pichon J, Boneu B 1985 Constitutional heparin cofactor II deficiency associated with recurrent thrombosis. Lancet ii: 414
Soria J, Soria C, Caen J P 1983 A new type of dysfibrinogenemia with defective fibrinolysis: Dusard syndrome. Possible relation with thrombosis. British Journal of Haematology 53: 575
Stead N W, Bauer K A, Kinney T R, Lewis J G, Campbell E E, Shifman M A, Rosenberg R D, Pizzo S V 1983 Venous thrombosis in a family with defective release of vascular plasminogen activator and elevated plasma factor VIII/von Willebrand factor. American Journal of Medicine 74: 33
Suzuki K, Nishioka J 1988 Plasma protein S activity measured using protac. A snake venom derived activator of protein C. Thrombosis Research 49: 241
Thaler E, Lechner K 1981 Antithrombin III deficiency and thromboembolism. In: Prentice C R M (ed) Clinics in haematology. W B Saunders, London, p 369
Thommen D, Buhrfeind E, Felix R, Sulzer I, Furlan M, Lammle B 1989 Hemostasis parameters in 55 patients with venous and/or arterial thromboembolism. Thrombosis and Haemostasis 62: 480
Tirindelli M C, Franchi F, Tripodi A, Mariani G, Mannucci P M 1986 Familial dysfunctional protein C. Thrombosis Research 44: 893
Tollefsen D M, Pestka C A, Monafo W J 1983 Activation of heparin cofactor II by dermatan sulfate. Journal Biology Chemistry 258: 6713
Tran T H, Marbet G A, Duckert F 1985 Association of hereditary heparin cofactor II deficiency with thrombosis. Lancet ii: 413
Tripodi A, Franchi F, Krachmalnicoff A, Mannucci P M 1990 Asymptomatic homozygous protein C deficiency. Acta Haematologica 83: 152
Vasse M, Borg J Y, Monconduit M 1989 Protein C: Rouen, a new hereditary protein C abnormality with low anticoagulant but normal amidolytic activities. Thrombosis Research 56: 387
Vigano D'Angelo S, Comp P C, Esmon C T, D'Angelo A 1986 Relationship between protein C antigen and anticoagulant activity during oral anticoagulation and in selected disease states. Journal of Clinical Investigation 77: 416
Vinazzer H, Pangraz U 1987 Protein C: comparison of different assays in normal and abnormal plasma samples. Thrombosis Research 46: 1
Von Felten A, Schaefer H P 1989 Protein S deficiency in young patients with cerebral arterial thrombosis. Thrombosis and Haemostasis 62: 12
Wolf M, Boyer-Neumannn C, Martinoli J L, Leroy-Matheron C, Amiral J, Meyer D,

Larrieu M J 1989 A new functional assay for human protein S activity using activated factor V as substrate. Thrombosis and Haemostasis 62: 1144
Wolf M, Boyer-Neumann C, Molho-Sabatier P, Neumann C, Meyer D, Larrieu M J 1990 Familial variant of antithrombin III (ATIII Bligny, 47 Arg to His) associated with protein C deficiency. Thrombosis and Haemostasis 63: 215
Yoshida N, Terukina S, Matsuda M, Moroi M, Okuma M, Aoki N 1987 Fibrinogens Kyoto and Tochigi, each with an apparent abnormal mol. wt. Asn-308 by Lys and Arg-275 by Cys, respectively. Thrombosis and Haemostasis 57 (suppl 1): 215

[a] Thaler & Lechner (1981),
[b] Broekmans & Conard (1988),
[c] Engesser et al (1987a).

2. Laboratory diagnosis of proteins C and S

Armando Tripodi   Pier Mannuccio Mannucci

INTRODUCTION

There is strong evidence that the system protein C/protein S (PC/PS) plays a major role in maintaining homeostasis of the coagulation system. Evidence stems from the increasing number of patients who have a congenital deficiency of either PC or PS associated with an increased risk of thromboembolic diseases (Griffin et al 1981, Broekmans et al 1983, 1985, Comp et al 1984). Congenital deficiency of either protein seems to be responsible for 8–10% of the unexplained venous thrombosis seen in young patients (Broekmans et al 1986, Gladson et al 1988). The prevalence of both heterozygous defects in the general population has been estimated to be 1:16 000 in The Netherlands (Bertina 1988). Hence, the measurement of PC and PS is now included in the laboratory screening of thrombophilic patients (Mannucci & Tripodi 1987). Even though several assays methods have been described, their measurement remains a relatively demanding task for clinical laboratories. The aim of this chapter is to review the present state of the art and to give technical details about their measurements.

PROTEIN C

Pathophysiology

PC, a vitamin K-dependent plasma glycoprotein, is the zymogen of the serine protease-activated PC (Kisiel et al 1977). Activation of PC is slowly catalysed by thrombin and markedly accelerated by a cofactor from the endothelial cell (thrombomodulin) (Esmon & Owen 1981). Once activated, PC becomes a potent anticoagulant that selectively inactivates factors V and VIII (Walker et al 1979), generates a potent fibrinolytic activity by decreasing the activity of the inhibitor of tissue plasminogen activator (Van Hinsberg et al 1985, Sakata et al 1985), and inactivates the platelet prothrombinase activity by cleavage of platelet-bound factor V, the receptor for factor Xa on the platelet membrane (Comp & Esmon 1979). The anticoagulant properties of activated PC are greatly enhanced by PS (see below).

Inherited deficiency of PC associated with venous thrombosis (more rarely arterial thrombosis) has been described since 1981 (Griffin et al 1981). The majority of patients have half-normal levels of PC and the defect is transmitted from parents to children of both sexes, suggesting heterozygosity for an autosomal dominant gene with variable penetrance (Clouse & Comp 1986). Homozygous PC deficiency has also been described in several families (for a review see Tripodi et al 1990). The phenotypic expression of those patients is variable. Homozygotes with extremely low levels of PC may develop symptoms, such as life-threatening thrombosis of the visceral vessels or purpura fulminans, as early as in the neonatal period (Seligsohn et al 1984). There are, however, homozygotes who survive the neonatal period without thrombotic events and later may develop moderately severe clinical symptoms (Sharon et al 1986, Tripodi et al 1990).

Laboratory diagnosis

The majority of PC-deficient patients have a parallel reduction of PC activity and concentration (type I), but there are cases with low activity and normal concentration (type II). Hence, functional assays are preferred for screening because type II deficiency would remain undetected if only immunoassays were employed (Table 2.1). A problem commonly encountered in the diagnosis of PC congenital deficiency (and also of PS, see below)

Table 2.1 Criteria for the laboratory diagnosis of PC deficiency

	Type I	Type II
PC activity	Reduced	Reduced
PC antigen	Reduced	Normal
Activity/antigen ratio	Normal	Reduced
All other vitamin K-dependent clotting factors	Normal	Normal
Disseminated intravascular coagulation	Absent	Absent
Chronic liver diseases	Absent	Absent
Oral anticoagulant treatment	Stable	Stable

is that PC is lowered by vitamin K antagonists and most patients with recurrent deep vein thrombosis are on long-term oral anticoagulant therapy. PC, however, is on the average lower than factors II or X (taken as examples of vitamin K-dependent procoagulants) in congenitally deficient patients on stabilized treatment with vitamin K antagonists. Conversely, all vitamin K-dependent proteins (including PC) are equally low in non-congenitally deficient patients on vitamin K antagonists. In practice, the finding of a lowered ratio of PC to factor II or X is considered diagnostic for PC deficiency in patients undergoing vitamin K antagonist treatment

(Bertina et al 1982). However, it should be realized that this problem is far from being resolved because different methods for PC measurement give different results in patients on oral anticoagulant therapy (see below), therefore each laboratory should establish its own range of PC antigen or activity in patients treated with different intensity. In addition, this range of PC values is only valid when the patients to be studied are on stabilized treatment because during the early phase of treatment considerable variations of PC and factors X and II may occur due to their different half-lives.

Recently an international standard preparation for PC has been established (Hubbard 1988) and is now distributed by the National Institute for Biological Standards and Control UK. Home-made pooled normal plasmas used for preparing calibration curves can be calibrated against that material, thus easing the problem of interlaboratory comparability of PC results for normal and patient populations.

Antigen assay

Different immunological techniques are available for this measurement; they are based on electroimmunoassay (Griffin et al 1981, Bertina et al 1982), enzyme-linked immunosorbent assay (ELISA) (Boyer et al 1984) and radioimmunoassay (Epstein et al 1984). Laurell plates ready for use and ELISA kits are also commercially available. For normal and congenitally deficient patients there is usually a fair agreement between results obtained with different techniques calibrated against the same standard preparation. However, this does not hold true for patients treated with oral anticoagulants in which the extent of PC carboxylation is variable, depending on the intensity of the treatment. In such cases the electroimmunoassay may give higher PC antigen than ELISA (Tripodi et al 1985, Mannucci et al 1987, Bertina 1987) because of the increased electrophoretic mobility of non-carboxylated PC (Mikami & Tuddenham 1986). The presence of EDTA in the electrophoretic buffer as well as in the gel may contribute to solve this problem. Finally, it must be mentioned that in some conditions, such as disseminated intravascular coagulation (DIC), where there is an increased turnover of coagulation factors, PC may be variably complexed with its physiological inhibitor(s). A collaborative study designed to address the extent to which the various immunological assays recognize this complex, demonstrated a highly variable behaviour, ranging from complete recognition by the electroimmunoassays, to partial recognition by ELISA to no recognition at all by immunological assays using monoclonal antibodies (Bertina 1987).

Functional assays

On the basis of their properties, functional assays for PC can be subdivided into two groups: those which measure the inhibitory activity of activated PC against the natural substrates factors V and VIII through activated partial thromboplastin time (APTT)-derived or factor Xa clotting time-derived methods (Francis 1986, Vigano'-D'Angelo et al 1986) and those which measure the amidolytic activity of activated PC against a synthetic substrate (Sala et al 1984, Bertina et al 1984, Vigano'-D'Angelo et al 1986). Both groups of methods require activation of native PC, which can be achieved by thrombin alone (Bertina et al 1984), by the complex thrombin–thrombomodulin (Sala et al 1984, Francis 1986, Vigano'-D'Angelo et al 1986), or by the snake venom Protac (Loberman et al 1986, Martinoli & Stocker 1986) (Table 2.2). With the exception of the snake venom method, all the other methods require isolation of PC from plasma, achieved by its adsorption on insoluble salts (Sala et al 1984, Bertina et al 1984, Francis 1986), or calcium-dependent monoclonal antibody (Vigano'-D'Angelo et al 1986) (Fig 2.1). Studies have been designed to compare the results of the principal functional assays for a large number of clinical samples taken from patients with conditions known to be associated with alterations of PC levels (Mannucci et al 1987, Franchi et al 1988). They demonstrated that in patients undergoing treatment with oral anticoagulants there were significant between-assay differences, probably related to the various extents to which different assay systems recognize a carboxylated PC. For patients with liver diseases and DIC all functional assays gave similar

Table 2.2 Main characteristics of the functional PC assays

Assay	PC separation	PC activation	Measurement of activated PC
Bertina et al (1984)	Aluminium hydroxide	Human thrombin	Amidolytic method
Sala et al (1984)	Barium citrate	Human thrombin + rabbit thrombomodulin	Amidolytic method
Francis (1986)	Barium citrate	Human thrombin + rabbit thrombomodulin	Clotting method (APTT prolongation)
Vigano'-D'Angelo et al (1986)	Calcium-dependent monoclonal antibody	Bovine thrombin + rabbit thrombomodulin	Amidolytic method
Vigano'-D'Angelo et al (1986)	As above	As above	Clotting method (factor Xa clotting time prolongation)
Loberman et al (1986)	No	Snake venom (Protac)	Amidolytic method
Loberman et al (1986)	No	As above	Clotting method (APTT prolongation)
Martinoli & Stocker (1986)	No	As above	As above

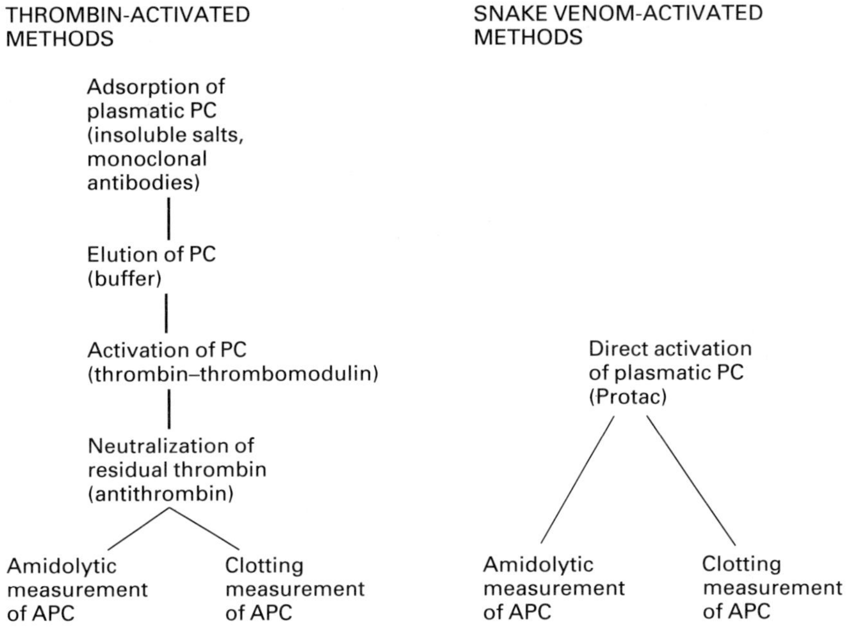

Fig. 2.1 Diagramatic representation of the analytical steps in PC functional assays. APC, activated PC.

results. In patients with established congenital PC defects, all the functional assays gave no significant between-assay difference, although there was an overlap of PC levels between normal and heterozygous deficient populations, so that some symptomatic patients were misclassified as normals and some healthy subjects as abnormals. These findings indicate that whatever the assay used, there is the possibility of incorrect classification of normals and patients. Such dubious diagnostic situations, which are also relatively frequent because of the large biological variation of PC (and PS, see below), may be solved by measuring PC activity in other family members.

In conclusion, even though no PC functional assay is entirely satisfactory for the detection of patients with congenital deficiency, a few widely employed assays, for which there are also commercial kits, appear to be equivalent in terms of diagnostic accuracy. For the final choice of method the following considerations can be made. We first recommend the method proposed by Francis (1986) because, being a clotting method activated with thrombin–thrombomodulin, its principle is the closest to what presumably happens in vivo; of the necessary reagents only thrombomodulin is rather sophisticated, but is now commercially available. However, considerable experience with clotting assays is required. For those laboratories which are not particularly expert in coagulation, an attractive alternative could be the snake venom method which is easy to perform, requires neither sophisticated reagents nor considerable expertise, or separation of PC from plasma (a potential source of methodological variability) and is amenable to automation (Franchi et al 1988). The existence of variant PC molecules which are activated by the snake venom, but not by thrombin–thrombomodulin, though theoretical up to now, should be taken into account.

PROTEIN S

Pathophysiology

PS is a vitamin K-dependent glycoprotein which functions as a cofactor of activated PC in the inactivation of factors V and VIII by enhancing the binding of activated PC to negatively charged phospholipids and platelets (Walker 1980, 1984). PS circulates in plasma in two forms. Approximately 60% of the total antigen is complexed with the complement component C_4b binding protein (C_4bBP) and the remaining 40% is free. The two forms are in dynamic equilibrium and only the free form possesses biological activity (Dahlback & Stenflo 1981, Dahlback 1983, Bertina et al 1985). The assumption that congenitally low levels of plasmatic PS would favour a thrombotic tendency is now clearly proven by the fact that many families have been reported in which individuals deficient in PS are at high risk of developing venous thromboembolic events (Comp et al 1984, Broekmans et al 1985). The prevalence of the deficiency in the general population (1:16 000) (Bertina 1988) and its incidence in patients with juvenile recurrent venous thrombosis (8–10%) (Broekmans et al 1986, Gladson et al 1988) are similar to those for PC. The pattern of inheritance (autosomal dominant) and the clinical presentation of heterozygous deficiency are also similar. Homozygous PS deficiency with unmeasurable levels first reported by Comp et al (1984) was not associated with the dramatic clinical picture of homozygous PC deficiency. However, more recently, a neonate born to heterozygous PS-deficient parents has been reported in whom extremely low PS levels were associated with purpura fulminans (Mahasandana et al 1989).

Laboratory diagnosis

As with PC, PS can be measured as an antigen with immunological methods and as an activity with functional methods. At present, there is no international standard for PS and, therefore, results are expressed in terms of pooled normal plasmas to which an arbitrary potency of 100 U/dl is assigned. This may lead to important variations in the measurements made in different laboratories. In fact, due to the large biological variability of vitamin K-dependent proteins, the adequacy of a pooled normal plasma in reflecting the average normal content of PS is largely dependent on the number of normal donors selected for the preparation. A seemingly adequate number of normal donors is 40–50 or more.

Antigen assay

Different immunological techniques are available for this measurement. They are based on electroimmunoassay (Schwarz et al 1984), ELISA (Boyer-Neumann et al 1988, Krachmalnicoff et al 1990), radioimmunoassay (Fair & Revak 1984) and immunoradiometric assay (IRMA) (Bertina et al 1985). Whatever the method used it is important to realize that even the measurement of total PS antigen presents some problems. Heterologous anti-PS antibodies react with both the free and bound PS and, therefore, the assays may be influenced by the level of C_4bBP. The use of special conditions, such as prolonged electrophoretic migration at 25°C, high sample dilutions and prolonged incubation times which are characteristic of ELISA and IRMA favour the dissociation of the complex and hence the measurement of total PS antigen (Schwarz et al 1984, Bertina et al 1985). Even with this problem resolved, the measurement of total antigen may not be, in principle, sufficient to reflect the anticoagulant property of the patient plasma. According to many investigators the free PS antigen may be a more informative parameter. This measurement is based on the treatment of plasma with polyethylene glycol (PEG), which precipitates the complex PS–C_4bBP and leaves free PS in the supernatant where it can be easily quantitated by electroimmunoassay or ELISA (Malm et al 1988). This technique must be carefully standardized to avoid variable amounts of free PS being precipitated with the complexed form or complexed PS remaining in the supernatant. Another approach to the immunological diagnosis of PS deficiency is two-dimensional immunoelectrophoresis, which gives semiquantitative information about the relative proportions of free and bound PS. Since the free and bound PS have differences in charge density, electrophoresis in the first dimension resolves the two components which are then immunoidentified in the second dimension by using specific antibodies (Comp et al 1986) (Fig. 2.2). With this method two groups of PS deficiencies have been identified. In one, the free PS peak is greatly reduced or absent, whereas the peak of the bound protein is normal; in the other, there is usually no free PS and the peak of the bound PS is also greatly reduced (Comp et al 1986).

Functional assay

Since congenital PS deficiency may be due to low levels of total protein (free and complexed), low levels of free protein (Comp et al 1986) or to dysfunctional protein (Mannucci et al 1989), the obvious candidate for the detection of all these types of congenital deficiency is a functional assay.

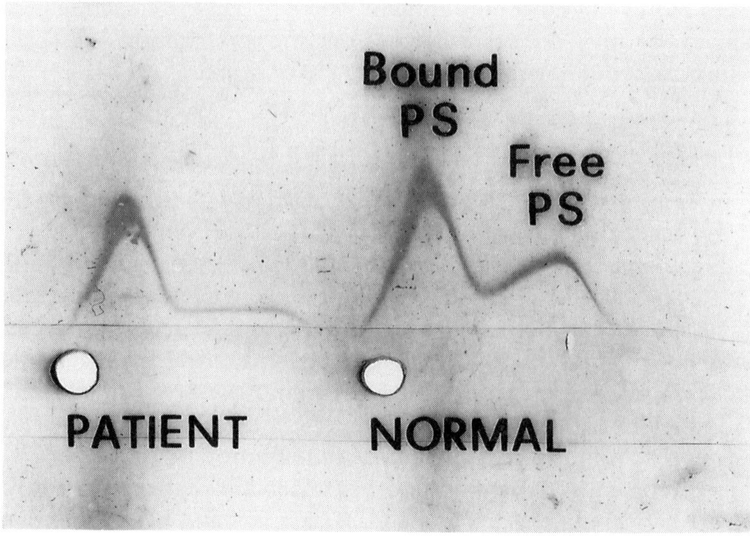

Fig. 2.2 Two-dimensional immunoelectrophoresis of PS: normal pooled plasma (right) and a patient with considerable reduction of the free PS antigen (left). The cathode is on the left of each plate. The cathodic peak represents the complex PS–C4b-binding protein; the anodic peak the free PS antigen.

Several efforts have been made in the last few years to set up functional assays for PS (Comp et al 1984, Kamiya et al 1986, van de Waart et al 1987, Suzuki & Nishioka 1988, D'Angelo et al 1988, Wolf et al 1989). In general they are based on the ability of PS to enhance the anticoagulant activity of activated PC. They essentially rest on two basic principles. The factor Xa assay is based on the one-stage factor Xa clotting time. When native test plasma (Comp et al 1984) or immunoadsorbed test plasma (D'Angelo et al 1988) are mixed with PS-depleted plasma, purified bovine factor Xa, cephalin and activated PC, the prolongation of the clotting time is linearly related to the amount of PS. The assay described by Kamiya et al (1986) is based on the APTT. When test plasma is mixed with PS-depleted plasma, APTT reagent and activated PC the prolongation of the APTT is linearly related to the amount of PS. More recently another APTT-based assay has been proposed (Wolf et al 1989). When diluted test plasma is mixed with PS-depleted plasma, APTT reagent, activated PC and activated bovine factor V the prolongation of the clotting time is linearly related to the amount of PS.

Despite the fact that a functional PS assay is badly needed, these methods and those derived thereafter have not so far gained widespread acceptance; this is in part due to the need for sophisticated reagents such as monoclonal antibodies and activated PC and also because their reliability has been questioned. A drawback shared by some of the existing methods

(Comp et al 1984, Kamiya et al 1986, Suzuki et al 1988) is the use of undiluted plasma in the test system, which makes the assay susceptible to artefacts when, for instance, activated clotting factors are present in plasma in conditions such as DIC. In addition, plasmas from patients with multiple coagulation defects (liver diseases, oral anticoagulant therapy) are extremely sensitive to the anticoagulant effect of activated PC, leading to the overestimation of PS activity. Besides these two drawbacks, another problem has been associated with the measurement of PS activity. There is evidence that the apparent plasmatic PS activity is dependent on factor II, which in the presence of phospholipid would act as an immediate, dose-dependent inhibitor of activated PC cofactor activity (Mitchel et al 1988). In view of this drawback, the current assessment of PS activity should be done by also measuring factor II levels. The assay is not reliable in individuals with very low or very high factor II levels.

Recently we developed a simple one-stage functional assay for PS which can be performed with standardized reagents using a highly automated centrifugal coagulometer (Preda et al 1990). In this method the PS cofactor activity for activated PC is measured by observing the degree of prolongation of a prothrombin time-based clotting assay in which appropriate amounts of diluted test plasma, PS-depleted plasma previously incubated with Protac to fully activate PC, bovine thromboplastin and calcium ions are mixed together. The method is highly reproducible, the between-assay coefficient of variation being less than 5%; its high sensitivity (approximately 0.5 s clotting time prolongation per 1 U/dl PS activity) allows the assay to be performed on diluted plasma, thus reducing potential artefacts. In addition it avoids the purification and subsequent activation of human PC; the source of PC is the PS-depleted plasma in which PC is activated by the snake venom. Preliminary evaluation of this method by studying a normal population as well as with congenital or acquired deficiency of PS demonstrated that it is both specific for PS and diagnostic.

METHODS

PC functional assay (Francis 1986)

Reagents

Washing buffer (pH 6.0):

0.02 M imidazole hydrochloride
0.3 M sodium chloride.

Elution buffer (pH 6.0):

0.2 M Mes hydrochloride
0.15 M sodium citrate.

Activation buffer (pH 8.0):

0.05 M Trizma base
0.1 M sodium chloride
0.1% bovine serum albumin.

Thrombin–thrombomodulin: Buffer (pH 7.4):

0.1 M Tris
0.02 M sodium chloride

1 M barium chloride
130 mM calcium chloride (for activation)
25 mM calcium chloride (clotting)
~2.5 mg/ml of human thrombin
~0.6 mg/ml of rabbit thrombomodulin
~50 U/ml of antithrombin.

Pooled normal plasma or *international standard* as reference.

Procedure

Adsorption. A 0.5 ml aliquot of the test sample or standard is mixed in a conical plastic tube with 20 µl barium chloride, after which the mixture is stirred for 30 min at 4°C, then centrifuged for 1 min at high speed (12 000 r.p.m.). After discarding the supernatant, the pellet is resuspended (using a wooden stick) in 50 µl of washing buffer, centrifuged again and the supernatant discarded.

Elution. The pellet is resuspended with 100 µl of elution buffer, then centrifuged for 2 min at high speed. The supernatant is harvested and diluted 1:10 in activation buffer. At this stage the eluate can be analysed immediately or stored at –30°C without appreciable lack of activity.

Activation. A 52 µl aliquot of thrombomodulin stock solution is mixed with 5 µl of thrombin stock solution and 943 µl of thrombin–thrombomodulin buffer. The mixture must be prepared just before use and stored at 4°C. The activation is carried out by mixing, in plastic tubes, 100 µl of eluate (previously diluted 1:10 in activation buffer), 5 µl calcium chloride and 25 µl thrombin–thrombomodulin solution. The mixture is then incubated for 1 h at 37°C.

Inhibition of residual thrombin. To each of the tubes 20 µl antithrombin stock solution is added, followed by 15 min incubation at 37°C.

Measurement of activated PC. To a glass tube prewarmed at 37°C the following are added:

60 µl of normal pooled plasma (as substrate)
60 µl of APTT reagent.

A stopwatch is started and the mixture is incubated for the time suggested by the APTT manufacturer. After the required period has elapsed, the following are added:

60 µl of activated eluate (test sample or standard)
60 µl of calcium chloride.

A second stopwatch is started, regularly the tube is tilted back and forth and the clotting time is recorded.

A blank must be run following the same procedure after substitution of the eluate with the same amount of activation buffer.

Standard curve. The eluate of a pooled normal plasma or standard (previously diluted 1:10) is further diluted according to the following scheme:

PC activity (U/dl)	Eluate (diluted 1:10) (µl)	Activation buffer (µl)
100	100	—
75	75	25
50	50	50
25	25	75
10	10	90

Calculation. The actual prolongation of the APTT due to activated PC is obtained by subtracting from each test sample or standard dilution the clotting time of the blank. The prolongations of the standard dilutions are then plotted against the PC activity on linear graph paper and the PC activity of the unknown are derived thereafter.

Note. It is advisable to run the standard curve in duplicate and the test samples at two different dilutions (1:10 and 1:20).

PC electroimmunoassay

Reagents

Migration buffer (pH 8.6):

1.62 g/l of sodium barbitone
7.05 g/l of glycine
5.65 g/l of Trizma base
1.80 g/l of disodium EDTA.

Staining solution. Dissolve 0.5% Coomassie blue in:
4.5 volumes of methyl alcohol
4.5 volumes of distilled water
1 volume of acetic acid.

Incubate the mixture at 56°C for 30 min and filter.

Destaining solution. Mix:

4.5 volumes of methyl alcohol
4.5 volumes of distilled water
1 volume of acetic acid.

Agarose. Dissolve 1% agarose in migration buffer.

Anti-PC antibody. Approximately 1%.

Procedure

Antibody-containing agarose gel plates (18.5 × 9 cm) are prepared according to the standard technique (1 mm gel thickness). After cutting circular wells along the main edge of the gel plate, 15 μl of test sample diluted 1:2 and 1:4 and pooled normal plasma or standard dilutions are pipetted. Electrophoresis (10 mA per gel plate) is carried out overnight at 15°C. After electrophoresis is completed the gel plate is removed from the apparatus, rinsed in saline for 2 h, pressed, dried, stained and destained.

Standard curve. Pooled normal plasma or standard undiluted, 1:2, 1:4 and 1:8 in migration buffer represent 100, 50, 25 and 12.5 U/dl PC antigen concentration.

Calculation. The peak heights of the standard dilutions are plotted against PC antigen concentration on semi-log graph paper and the PC antigen concentration of the unknown derived thereafter.

PS electroimmunoassay

Reagents

Migration buffer.

0.081 M Trizma base
0.024 M Tricine
3 mM disodium EDTA.

Staining solution. As for PC.
Destaining solution. As for PC.
Agarose. Dissolve 1% agarose in migration buffer.
Anti-PS antibody. Approximately 1%.

Procedure

Antibody-containing agarose gel plates (18.5 × 9 cm) are prepared according to the standard technique (1 mm gel thickness). After cutting circular wells along the main edge of the gel plate, 10 μl of test sample diluted 1:2 and 1:4 and pooled normal plasma dilutions are pipetted. Electrophoresis

(25 mA per gel plate) is carried out at 25°C (thermostat) for 4 h. After electrophoresis is completed the gel plate is removed from the apparatus, rinsed in saline for 2 h, pressed, dried, stained and destained.

Standard curve. Pooled normal plasma undiluted, 1:2 1:4 and 1:8 in migration buffer represent 100, 50, 25 and 12.5 U/dl PS antigen concentration.

Calculation. The peak heights of the standard dilutions are plotted against PS antigen concentration on semi-log graph paper and the PS antigen concentration of the unknown derived thereafter.

PS two-dimensional immunoelectrophoresis

Reagents

Migration buffer (pH 8.6). As for PS electroimmunoassay.
Staining and destaining solution. As for PC electroimmunoassay.
Agarose. Dissolve 1% agarose in migration buffer.
Anti-PS antibody. Approximately 1%.

Procedure

Agarose gel plates (9 × 11 cm) are prepared according to the standard technique (1.5 mm gel thickness). After cutting two circular wells (3 cm apart) along the main edge of the gel plate, 10 μl of undiluted test sample and pooled normal plasma as control are pipetted. Test sample and pooled normal plasma can be added with small amounts of bromophenol blue as a tracer to follow the migration. Electrophoresis (12.5 mA per plate) is carried out for 2 h at 10°C (thermostat). After electrophoresis is completed the plate is removed from the apparatus and the gel is cut in two parts. The direction of the cut must be parallel with that of electrophoresis. The part of the agarose layer which contains the protein separated by the first electrophoresis is kept, while the other is removed and substituted with an equivalent amount of antibody-containing agarose gel. The plate is then rotated through 90° and electrophoresis continued overnight at 4 mA per plate at 25°C (thermostat). After electrophoresis is completed the gel plate is removed from the apparatus, rinsed in saline for 2 h, pressed, dried, stained and destained.

REFERENCES

Bertina R M 1987 An international collaborative study on the performance of protein C antigen assay. Thrombosis Haemostasis 57: 112–117

Bertina R M 1988 Prevalence of hereditary thrombophilia and the identification of genetic risk factors. Fibrinolysis 2(suppl 2): 7

Bertina R M, Broekmans A W, Van der Linden I K, Mertens K 1982 Protein C deficiency in Dutch family with thrombotic disease. Thrombosis Haemostasis 48: 1–5

Bertina R M, Broekmans A W, Krommenhoek-van Es C, van Wijngaarden A 1984 The use of functional and immunologic assay for plasma protein C in the study of the heterogeneity of congenital protein C deficiency. Thrombosis Haemostasis 51: 1–5

Bertina R M, Reinalda-Poot J, van Wijngaarden A, Poort S R, Bom V J J 1985 Determination of plasma protein S. The protein cofactor of activated protein C. Thrombosis Haemostasis 53: 268–272

Boyer C, Rothschild C, Wolf M, Amiral J, Meyer D, Larrieu M J 1984 A new method for estimation of protein C by ELISA. Thrombosis Research 36: 579–589

Boyer-Neumann C, Wolf M, Amiral J, Guyader A M, Meyer D, Larrieu M J 1988 Familial type I protein S deficiency associated with severe thrombosis. A study of five cases. Thrombosis Haemostasis 60: 128

Broekmans A W, Veltkamp J J, Bertina R M 1983 Congenital protein C deficiency and venous thromboembolism: a study of three Dutch families. New England Journal of Medicine 309: 340–344.

Broekmans A W, Bertina R M, Reinalda-Poot J, Engesser L, Muller H P, Leeuw J A, Michiels J J, Brommer E J P, Briet E 1985 Hereditary protein S deficiency and venous thrombo-embolism. A study in three Dutch families. Thrombosis Haemostasis 53: 273–277.

Broekmans A W, van der Linden I K, Jansen-Koeter Y, Bertina R M 1986 Prevalence of protein C (PC) and protein S (PS) deficiency in patients with thrombotic disease. Thrombosis Research suppl VI: 135

Clouse H L, Comp P C 1986 The regulation of hemostasis: the protein C system. New England Journal of Medicine 314: 1298–1304

Comp P C, Esmon C T 1979 Activated protein C inhibits platelet prothrombin-converting activity. Blood 54: 1272–1281

Comp P C, Nixon R R, Cooper M R, Esmon C T 1984 Familial protein S deficiency associated with recurrent thrombosis. Journal of Clinical Investigation 74: 2082–2088

Comp P C, Doray D, Patton D, Esmon C T 1986 An abnormal plasma distribution of protein S occurs in functional protein S deficiency. Blood 67: 504–508

Dahlback B 1983 Purification of human C4b-binding protein and formation of its complex with vitamin-K dependent protein S. Biochemical Journal 209: 847–856

Dahlback B, Stenflo J 1981 High molecular weight complex in human plasma between vitamin-K dependent protein S and complement component C4b-binding protein. Proceedings of the National Academy of Science, USA 78: 2512–2516

D'Angelo A, Vigano'-D'Angelo S, Esmon C T, Comp P C 1988 Acquired deficiencies of protein S. Protein S activity during oral anticoagulation, liver disease and disseminated intravascular coagulation. Journal of Clinical Investigation 81: 1445–1454

Epstein D J, Bergum P W, Bajaj S P, Rapaport S I 1984 Radioimmunoassay for protein C and factor X. Plasma antigen levels in abnormal hemostatic states. American Journal of Clinical Pathology 82: 573–581

Esmon C T, Owen W G 1981 Identification of an endothelial cell cofactor for thrombin-catalyzed activation of protein C. Proceedings of the National Academy of Science, USA 78: 2249–2252

Fair D, Revak D 1984 Quantitation of human protein S in the plasma of normal and warfarin treated individuals by radioimmunoassay. Thrombosis Research 36: 527–532

Franchi F, Tripodi A, Valsecchi C, Mannucci P M 1988 Functional assay for protein C: comparison of two snake–venom assays with two thrombin assays. Thrombosis Haemostasis 60: 145–147

Francis R B 1986 A simplified PTT-based protein C activity assay using the thrombin–thrombomodulin complex. Thrombosis Research 37: 337–344

Gladson C L, Scharrer I, Hach V, Beck K H, Griffin J H 1988 The frequency of type I heterozygous protein S and protein C deficiency in 141 unrelated young patients with venous thrombosis. Thrombosis Haemostasis 59: 18–22

Griffin J H, Evatt B, Zimmerman T S, Kleiss A J, Wideman C 1981 Deficiency of protein C in congenital thrombotic disease. Journal of Clinical Investigation 68: 1370–1373

Hubbard A R 1988 Standardization of protein C in plasma: Establishment of an international standard. Thrombosis Haemostasis 59: 464–467

Kamiya T, Sugihara T, Ogata K, Saito H, Suzuki K, Nishioka J, Hashimoto S, Yamagata K 1986 Inherited deficiency of protein S In a Japanese family with recurrent venous thrombosis: a study of three generations. Blood 67: 406–410

Kisiel W, Canfield W M, Ericsson L H, Davie E W 1977 Anticoagulant properties of bovine protein C following activation by thrombin. Biochemistry 16: 5824–5831
Krachmalnicoff A, Valsecchi C, Tombesi S, Albertini A, Mannucci P M 1990 A monoclonal antibody to human protein S used as the capture antibody for measuring total protein S by enzyme immunoassay. Clinical Chemistry 36: 43–47
Loberman H, Kolde H J, Deubel R, Peter R, Tourte E, Becker U 1986 Determination of protein C in plasma. Behring Institut Mitteilungen 79: 112–120
Mahasandana C, Suvatte V, Marlar R, Manco-Johnson M, Jacobson L, Hathaway W E 1989 Neonatal purpura fulminans associated with homozygous protein S deficiency. Thrombosis Haemostasis 62: 301
Malm J, Laurell M, Dahlback B 1988 Changes in the plasma levels of vitamin-K dependent protein C and S and of C4b binding protein during pregnancy and oral contraception. British Journal of Haematology 68: 437–448
Mannucci P M, Tripodi A 1987 Laboratory screening of inherited thrombotic syndromes. Thrombosis Haemostasis 57: 247–251
Mannucci P M, Boyer C, Tripodi A, Vigano'-D'Angelo S, Wolf M, Valsecchi C, D'Angelo A, Meyer D, Larrieu M J 1987 Multicenter comparison of five functional and two immunological assays for protein C. Thrombosis Haemostasis 57: 44–48
Mannucci P M, Valsecchi C, Krachmalnicoff A, Faioni E M, Tripodi A 1989 Familial dysfunction of protein S. Thrombosis Haemostasis 62: 763–766
Martinoli J R, Stocker K 1986 Fast functional protein C assay using Protac, a novel protein C activator. Thrombosis Research 43: 253–264
Mikami S, Tuddenham E G D 1986 Studies on immunological assay of vitamin-K factors. Comparison of four immunoassay methods with functional activity of protein C in human plasma. British Journal of Haematology 62: 183–193
Mitchel C A, Jane S M, Salem H H 1988 Inhibition of the anticoagulant activity of protein S by prothrombin. Journal of Clinical Investigation 82: 2142–2147
Preda L, Tripodi A, Valsecchi C, Lombardi A, Finotto E, Mannucci P M 1990 A new functional assay for protein S. A prothrombin time-based functional assay of protein S. Thrombosis Research 60: 18–32
Sala N, Owen W G, Collen D 1984 Functional assay for protein C in human plasma. Blood 63: 671–675
Sakata Y, Curriden S, Lawrence D, Griffin J H, Loskutoff D J 1985 Activated protein C stimulates the fibrinolytic activity of cultured endothelial cells and decreases antiactivator activity. Proceedings of the National Academy of Science, USA 82: 1121–1125
Schwarz H P, Fisher M, Hopmeier P, Batard M A, Griffin J H 1984 Plasma protein S deficiency in familial thrombotic disease. Blood 64: 1297–1300
Seligsohn U, Berger A, Abend M, Rubin L, Attias D, Zivelin A, Rapaport S I 1984 Homozygous protein C deficiency manifested by massive thrombosis in the newborn. New England Journal of Medicine 310: 559–562
Sharon C, Tirindelli M C, Mannucci P M, Tripodi A, Mariani G 1986 Homozygous protein C deficiency with moderately severe clinical symptoms. Thrombosis Research 41: 483–488
Suzuki K, Nishioka J 1988 Plasma protein S activity measured using Protac, a snake venom derived activator of protein C. Thrombosis Research 49: 241–251
Tripodi A, Valsecchi C, Bottasso M, Sharon C, Mannucci P M 1985 Comparison of a functional assay for protein C with two immunoassays. Thrombosis Research 40: 243–248
Tripodi A, Franchi F, Krachmalnicoff A, Mannucci P M 1990 Asymptomatic protein C deficiency. Acta Haematologica 83: 152–155
van de Waart P, Preissner K T, Bechtold J R, Muller-Berghaus G 1987 A functional test for protein S activity in plasma. Thrombosis Research 48: 427–437
Van Hinsbergh V W M, Bertina R M, Van Wijngaarden A, Van Tilburg N H, Emeis J J, Haverkate F 1985 Activated protein C decreases plasminogen activator inhibitor activity in endothelial cell conditioned medium. Blood 65: 444–451
Vigano'-D'Angelo S, Comp P C, Esmon C T, D'Angelo A 1986 Relationship between protein C antigen and anticoagulant activity during oral anticoagulant and in selected disease states. Journal of Clinical Investigation 77: 416–425
Walker F J 1980 The regulation of activated protein C by a new protein: a possible function for bovine protein S. Journal of Biological Chemistry 255: 5521–5524

Walker F J 1984 Protein S and the regulation of activated protein C. Seminars in Thrombosis and Hemostasis 10: 131–138

Walker F J, Sexton P W, Esmon C T 1979 The inhibition of blood coagulation by activated protein C through the selective inactivation of activated factor V. Biochimica et Biophysica Acta 571: 333–342

Wolf M, Boyer-Neumann C, Martinoli J L, Leroy-Matheron C, Amiral J, Meyer D, Larrieu M J 1989 A new functional assay for human protein S activity using activated factor V as substrate. Thrombosis Haemostasis 62: 1144–1145

3. The serpin inhibitors of blood coagulation: antithrombin and heparin cofactor II

David A. Lane   Michael D. Boisclair

INTRODUCTION

The role of antithrombin as an inhibitor of blood coagulation is now well established (Abildgaard 1968, 1969, Damus et al 1973). Antithrombin is the most important physiological proteinase inhibitor of thrombin. It has a normal plasma concentration of about 125 μg/ml (2.3 μM) (Conard et al 1983). The disappearance of labelled antithrombin from the circulation can be fitted to a curve containing three exponential components, and the plasma half-time of disappearance has been calculated to be about 65 h (Collen et al 1977, Knot et al 1986). Failure to maintain an adequate functional level of this inhibitor in the plasma results in an increased risk of thrombosis and pulmonary embolism. An important functional property of antithrombin is its interaction with heparin. This glycosaminoglycan accelerates its inactivation of thrombin, factor Xa and other proteinases of the blood coagulation system. A second plasma inhibitor of thrombin, whose action is accelerated by heparin, heparin cofactor II (HCII), was suggested by Briginshawe & Shanberge (1974a,b), but conclusively identified and characterized by Tollefsen & Blank (1981) and Tollefsen et al (1982). The plasma concentration of HCII (1.2 μM) is less than that of antithrombin. Its elimination can be fitted to a two-compartment exponential model, and it has a plasma half-time approximately the same as that of antithrombin (Sie et al 1985a). A clear relationship between HCII deficiency and thrombosis has yet to be established. Here, the structure, function and deficiency states of these proteins are summarized. Other reviews concentrating on selected aspects of this subject have been used for the preparation of this chapter (Thaler & Lechner 1981, Travis & Salvesen 1983, Conard et al 1988, Bjork et al 1989, Lane & Caso 1989, Tollefsen 1989).

STRUCTURE AND SEQUENCE HOMOLOGY WITH OTHER PROTEINS, THE SERPINS

Antithrombin and HCII are single-chain glycoproteins of molecular weights 58 200 and 65 600, whose primary structures have been elucidated by protein and cDNA sequencing (Petersen et al 1979, Bock et al 1982,

Chandra et al 1983a, Prochownik et al 1983a, Inhorn and Tollefsen 1986, Ragg 1986, Blinder et al 1988). The molecules are synthesized primarily in the liver with signal peptides of 32 and 19 amino acids, respectively. These peptides are necessary for their intracellular transport through the endoplasmatic reticulum, contain the usual very hydrophobic region and are cleaved at –1Cys– +1His and –1Gly– +1Gly bonds, respectively, prior to secretion. Plasma antithrombin contains 432 amino acids, six of which are cysteines which form three disulphide bonds. There are four glycosylation sites, Asn96, Asn135, Asn155 and Asn192, attached to which are biantennary carbohydrate side-chains. These are presumed to be identical, except for possible variations in sialic acid content. A minor pool of normal antithrombin is not glycosylated at Asn135 (Peterson and Blackburn 1985, Brennan et al 1987). The heterogeneity of the molecule is apparent on isoelectric focusing, which reveals numerous major and minor bands within the pI range of 4.9–5.7. Plasma HCII contains 480 amino acids, three of which are cysteines and which apparently do not form disulphide bonds. There are three potential glycosylation sites, Asn30, Asn169 and Asn368. On isoelectric focusing, HCII migrates as a major band at pI 5.15 and minor bands at pI 4.95 and 5.05 (Tollefsen et al 1982).

A close similarity between primary structures of antithrombin and α_1-antitrypsin (more correctly known as α_1-proteinase inhibitor) was noted by Petersen et al (1979) and Carrell et al (1979). There is a 33% amino acid sequence homology between the two proteins, while comparison of cDNA sequences reveals 46% homology (Bock et al 1982, Chandra et al 1983a,b, Prochownik et al 1983a, Kidd and Woo 1986). Hunt & Dayhoff (1980) identified ovalbumin as another related protein and, subsequently, an increasing number of serine proteinase inhibitors (serpins), including HCII, have been grouped together in what has been termed the serpin superfamily. It is believed that all the family members evolved from a common ancestor approximately 500 million years ago.

The structure of these proteins is usually considered in terms of a model of α_1-antitrypsin derived from the work of Loebermann et al (1984). Their crystallographic studies demonstrated that α_1-antitrypsin is almost completely arranged in well-defined secondary structural elements, with 30% helical (nine helices, denoted A–I) and 40% β sheet (three sheets, denoted A–C) regions (see Fig. 3.1). Recently, X-ray structure determination of bovine antithrombin has validated the interpretation of antithrombin structure in terms of that of α_1-antitrypsin (Samama et al 1989).

When the members of the serpin superfamily are aligned according to this model, consensus sequences are apparent throughout their structures, except at their *N*-terminal regions (corresponding to the antithrombin sequence 1–50 and HCII sequence 1–106) (for a recent analysis see Ye et al 1987). Leaving these regions aside, the structures of all the proteins generally conform to the helical/β sheet model, except in the region of helices C

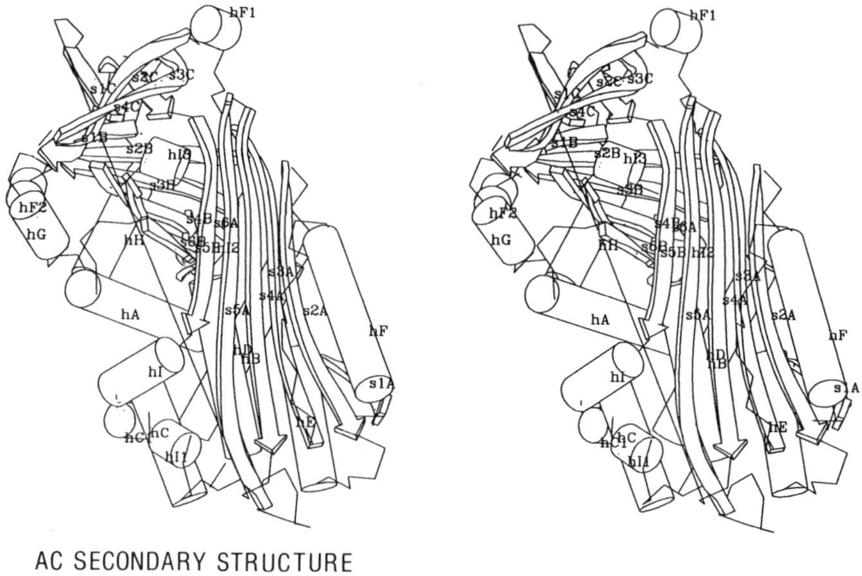

Fig. 3.1 Polypeptide folding structure of α_1-antitrypsin with the secondary structure elements represented by arrows (sheet strands) and cylinders (helices). Key: hX, helix X; sXY, strand X in sheet Y; thXhY, turn between helix X and helix Y; bsXY, bulge in strand X of sheet Y; 1h, left-handed helical conformation. (From Huber and Carrell (1989), kindly supplied by Professor Huber.)

and D. Here there is an extended insertion in placental plasminogen activator inhibitor (PAI) and smaller inserts in chicken ovalbumin, chicken gene Y and angiotensinogen. An exceptionally well-conserved sequence is that of sheet 3A, Val-Leu-Val-Asn-Tyr-Ile-Tyr-Phe-Lys-Gly-Lys. Regions either side of the reactive site, the region that is directly involved in proteinase inhibition, are also very well conserved, particularly the sequences Gly-Thr-Glu-Ala in sheet 4A and Pro-Phe-Leu-Phe in sheet 4B. These sequences are believed to be essential for correct folding of the molecules (the important roles of alanine and proline residues in these sequences are discussed again below in terms of their positions in antithrombin, 382 and 407, respectively). The reactive sites themselves are not highly conserved, as might be expected, as these confer specificity on the inhibitory proteins.

The reactive site of antithrombin is located at the Arg393—Ser394 bond (Bjork et al 1981, 1982) (numbering according to the amino acid sequence derived from the cDNA sequence); see Fig. 3.2. The presence of Arg393 results in the broad specificity of antithrombin, enabling most of the coagulation proteinases to be inhibited. Several other serpins contain arginine at their reactive site and this indicates the importance of the P1' (serine in the case of antithrombin) and surrounding residues in contributing to

	P3	P2	P1	P1′	P2′	P3′
HCII	442 Met	443 Pro	444 Leu	445 Ser	446 Thr	447 Gln
Antithrombin	391 Ala	392 Gly	393 Arg	394 Ser	395 Leu	396 Asn

Fig. 3.2 Amino acid sequences within reactive sites of antithrombin and HCII

specificity. The reactive bonds (P1—P1') of other arginine serpins include Arg—Thr (C1 inhibitor) and Arg—Met (α_2-antiplasmin) (Potempa et al 1988). The reactive site of HCII is Leu444—Ser445 (Griffith et al 1985).

The central role of the P1 residue in determining the specificity of the serpins has been illustrated by the study of natural and recombinant variants of these proteins. An interesting variant of α_1-antitrypsin was described by Owen et al (1983). A young child with a fatal bleeding disorder was found to have an inherited variant (α_1-antitrypsin Pittsburgh). The structural defect was identified as being at the reactive site Met358 to Arg. This substitution altered the specificity of α_1-antitrypsin, such that, rather than being an inhibitor of elastase, its main inhibitory action was redirected towards thrombin and proteinases involved in contact activation of blood coagulation (Schapira et al 1985, Jallat et al 1986, Scott et al 1986). Because α_1-antitrypsin is an acute-phase protein, a rapid increase in the plasma concentration of the mutant inhibitor was stimulated by a bleeding episode. The resulting excess of coagulation proteinase-inhibitory activity in plasma probably exacerbated the bleeding problem and caused the premature death of the patient. Detailed consideration of inherited variants of antithrombin is given below.

A series of recombinant α_1-antitrypsin variants has been studied by Travis et al (1985), Matheson et al (1986) and Jallat et al (1986). They demonstrated that the specificity of the inhibitor is determined by the class of amino acid at the P1 position. Alteration from uncharged to charged residue results in changes of inhibitor specificity and reactivity. Substitution of the P3 residue can additionally modify inhibitor reactivity. Studies with recombinant antithrombin mutants of the P1' position (Ser394) have been described by Stephens et al (1988) (see below). An interesting property of HCII is its restricted specificity: it inhibits chymotrypsin, cathepsin G and thrombin, but none of the other coagulation proteinases. Derechin et al (1990) proposed that this restricted specificity could be caused in part by the leucine residue at the reactive site. As thrombin and other coagulation proteinases usually react with arginine residues in their substrates, Derechin et al prepared recombinant HCII, substituting arginine for Leu444. The rHCII was expressed in yeast and partially purified. In the absence of glycosaminoglycans, rHCII (Leu444 to Arg) inhibited thrombin with a two orders of magnitude increase in second-order rate constant of inhibition over the wild type. Factor Xa, kallikrein and plasmin were also inhibited rapidly by the mutant rHCII, while the inhibition rate of chymotrypsin was reduced.

Hortin et al (1989) have provided an additional explanation for the preference of HCII for thrombin, rather than other coagulation proteinases. They identified a short duplicated amino acid sequence, Glu-Asp-Asp-Asp-Tyr-X-Asp (where X is either Leu or Ile) near the amino terminus of HCII. This region, not homologous with that in any other serpin, is highly polyanionic. Indeed, tyrosine residues in each repeat are sulphated by a post-translational mechanism, and the region is similar to one on hirudin that is implicated in its binding to thrombin. Hortin et al therefore prepared a synthetic peptide, corresponding to HCII (54–75) and studied its interaction with thrombin. HCII (54–75) inhibits cleavage of fibrinogen by thrombin, but does not inhibit the substrate reaction of thrombin. It is proposed that HCII (54–75) binds to the anion-binding exosite of thrombin; this binding may then orient the active site of thrombin to the reactive site of HCII. As pointed out by Blinder et al (1988), the presence of Pro443 at the P2 position may enable HCII to react efficiently with thrombin, as proline is often favoured in this position in effective thrombin substrates.

The second important functional domains of antithrombin and HCII are their heparin-binding sites. Early attempts at the characterization of the interaction between heparin and antithrombin used heparin that was heterogeneous with respect to size and ability to interact with antithrombin. A major advance, therefore, was the finding that only a fraction of commercial heparin binds with high affinity to the protein and that this is responsible for the majority of the anticoagulant activity that is expressed as a consequence of the binding interaction (Hook et al 1976, Lam et al 1976). Furthermore, a series of subsequent studies culminated in the identification of a unique pentasaccharide sequence of heparin that is responsible for high-affinity binding (Lindahl et al 1980, Casu et al 1981, Thunberg et al 1982, Choay et al 1983, Atha et al 1984). High-affinity heparin binds through the pentasaccharide sequence to a single site on antithrombin with a dissociation constant of 2×10^{-8} M (Nordenman et al 1978, Jordan et al 1980a, Olson et al 1981). Binding depends strongly on ionic strength and pH, and it has been suggested that a maximum of five to six charged groups on each molecule is involved (Nordenman & Bjork 1981). Binding alters ultraviolet absorption, circular dichroism and tryptophan fluorescence of antithrombin, suggesting changes in the environment of aromatic amino acids, possibly caused by a conformational change (Einarsson & Andersson 1977, Nordenman et al 1978). The probable involvement of tryptophan residues in a conformational change was indicated by chemical modification studies of Blackburn & Sibley (1980) and Blackburn et al (1984). They identified a role for Trp49 in or near to the heparin-binding site of antithrombin. This amino acid could directly participate in heparin binding or in the resulting conformational change (Karp et al 1984).

Two studies have used V8 protease digestion of antithrombin to locate its heparin-binding domain. Liu & Chang (1987) used limited cleavage with the enzyme with quantitative *N*-terminal sequence analyses to detect changes in structure. They reported that Glu34—Gly35, Glu42—Ala43 and Glu50—Leu51 are preferential cleavage sites for the enzyme. The cleavage of Glu42—Ala43 and Glu50—Leu51, particularly, was drastically inhibited by preincubation of antithrombin with heparin, suggesting that Glu34—Leu51 is involved in the binding region. On the other hand, Smith & Knauer (1987) used extensive digestion of antithrombin and isolated peptides with high-performance liquid chromatography. Incubation with labelled fluorescamine–heparin identified binding peptides that were studied by sequence analysis. They postulated that the region Lys114—Glu156 is a likely heparin-binding domain. This claim was supported by use of charge density and hydropathy plots; Phe123—Val141 has the highest positive charge within the molecule and Leu126—Val140 is exposed on its surface. The sequence is contained on a cyanogen bromide fragment that retains some of the heparin-binding properties of the parent molecule (Rosenfeld & Danishefski 1986).

As mentioned above, part of the normal antithrombin exists without a carbohydrate side-chain at Asn135. This normal variant has increased affinity for heparin, which suggests the close proximity of Asn135 to the heparin-binding domain (Peterson & Blackburn 1985, Brennan et al 1987).

The binding of heparin to antithrombin is known to be mediated primarily through the interaction of specific sulphate groups on the pentasaccharide sequence of heparin with basic amino acids (lysine and arginine residues) of antithrombin. The role of lysine residues of antithrombin was suggested by Rosenberg & Damus (1973) and has been given additional support from experimental work by Peterson et al (1987). They identified Lys125 as an essential amino acid on the basis of chemical modification studies. Chang (1989) used chemical modification of antithrombin with a water-soluble colour reagent specific for lysine residues to show that Lys107, Lys125 and Lys136 are involved in heparin binding. Binding of the glycosaminoglycan diminished modification of these residues, whilst enhancing modification of Lys236. It was concluded that Lys236 is exposed by the conformational change induced by heparin. Indirect support for the involvement of the lysines around the *N*-terminus was obtained from a study of sequential reduction of the three disulphide bonds of antithrombin (Sun & Chang 1989). Reduction of Lys8–Lys128 correlated quantitatively with loss of binding, suggesting the region around Lys128 is important.

Villaneuva (1984) has considered the secondary structure of antithrombin using a predictive scheme based upon amino acid sequencing. Lys290, Lys294 and Lys297 are aligned on one face of an unstable helical region of the molecule. This region is also near to one tryptophan residue, Trp307, which could be perturbed if an interaction of heparin took place with this region of antithrombin. It was predicted that these three lysines could be aligned for maximal interaction with the three sulphate groups of the antithrombin-binding pentasaccharide; the 6-*O*-sulphate at position 2, the 2-*N*-sulphate at position 4 and the 2-*N*-sulphate at position 6. Atha et al (1985) have pointed out that while the critical 3-*O*-sulphate group at position 4 is out of range of these lysines, it may interact simultaneously with a section of the *N*-terminal region of antithrombin.

There is good evidence for a role of arginine residues of antithrombin in heparin binding. Jorgensen et al (1985) conducted a chemical modification study and concluded that up to seven Arg residues are involved; studies of congenital variants of antithrombin that do not bind to heparin have identified one of these as Arg47. Other amino acids identified by this latter route are Pro41 and Ile7 (see below); these may not participate directly in binding but may be important in maintaining secondary structure of the domain.

The tertiary structure model of Loebermann et al (1984) has been used to devise a model of the heparin-binding domain of antithrombin. Borg et al (1988) have proposed that seven basic residues are aligned to form a positive site stretching across the molecule from the A helix (Arg47) to the D helix (Lys125, Arg129, Arg132) and the adjacent Lys133. This interesting model appears to provide a partial explanation for many of the features of the heparin-binding site of antithrombin. It should be appreciated, though, that the model is one of reactive-site cleaved α_1-antitrypsin onto which the amino acids of antithrombin are 'projected'. Furthermore, neither reactive-site cleaved antithrombin nor cleaved α_1-antitrypsin actually binds heparin with high affinity.

The glycosaminoglycan binding domain of HCII does not exhibit the same structural specificity as that of antithrombin. While the latter reacts with high-affinity heparin (and some heparan sulphate fractions containing part of the antithrombin-binding site), HCII action is stimulated by heparin (high and low affinity for antithrombin), dermatan sulphate, fucoidin, and carboxylate- and phosphate-containing polyanions (Tollefsen et al 1983, Scully & Kakkar 1984, Scully et al 1986, Church et al 1989, Pratt et al 1989, Tollefsen 1989).

Chemical modification studies of HCII by Church & Griffith (1984) and Church et al (1986) have indicated that basic amino acids participate in heparin binding. Modification of five arginine residues per molecule with 2,3-butanedione results in loss of heparin binding and inhibitory properties towards thrombin. Modification of 3–4 lysine residues produces a similar effect.

Amino acid sequence alignment of HCII with antithrombin has suggested a potential heparin-binding domain (Blinder et al 1988). Beginning at Arg103 of HCII (or Arg47 of antithrombin), 21 of the following 47 residues are identical (Fig. 3.3). Furthermore, in the region from Ile179 to Arg193 of HCII (corresponding to Ile119–134), eight residues are identical with those of antithrombin, including Lys185 (corresponding to Lys125 in

```
            |<signal peptide >|                            CHO                |degr -->  SO4
HCII   -19  MKHSLNALLIFLIITSAWGGSKGPLDQLEKGGETAQSADPQWEQLNNKNLSMPLLPADFHKENTVTNDWIPEGEEDDDYL
                                          :  :          :                                 :
ATIII                           -32 MYSNVIGTVTSGKRKVYLLSLLLIGFWDCVTCHGSPVDICTAKPRDIPMNPMCIYR
                                    |<-------signal peptide ------>|
                      SO4
HCII    62  DLEKIFSEDDDYIDIVDSLSVSPTDSDVSAGNILQLFHGKSRIQRLNILNAKFAFNLYRVLKDQVNTFDNIFIAPVGIST
              ::   :::                               :   :   :  ::   :  : :  :  ::::  :  :::
ATIII   25  SPEKKATEDDGSEQKIPEATNR-------------------RVWELSKANSRFATTFYQHLADSKNDNDNIFLSPLSIST

                                      CHO
HCII   142  AMGMISLGLKGETHEQVHSILHFKDFVNASSKYEITTIHNLFRKLTHRLFRR-NFGYTLRSVNDLYIQKQFPILLDFKTK
            :  :  ::    :  :      :       :      ::  : ::  :: :  :    :  : : :  :
ATIII   86  AFAMTKLGACNDTLQQLMEVFKFDTISEKTSDQ----IHFFFAKLNCRLYRKANKSSKLVSANRLFGDKSLTFNETYQDI
                     CHO                                        CHO              CHO

HCII   221  VREYYFAEAQIADFSDPAFISKTNNHIMKLTKGLIKDAL----ENIDPATQMMILNCIYFKGSWVNKFPVEMTHNHNFRL
                : :  :  ::   :  :          :           : :   :     : ::::: :  ::  : :    :
ATIII  162  SELVYGAKLQPLDFKENAEQSRAAINKWVSNKTEGRITDVIPSEAINELTVLVLVNTIYFKGLWKSKFSPENTRKELFYK
                                         CHO
                                                                              CHO
HCII   297  NEREVVKVSMMQTKGNFLAANDQELDCDILQLEYVGGISMLIVVPHKMSGMKTLEAQLTPRVVERWQKSMTNRTREVLLP
               :    :::   : :      :             : :    :         :  ::: :   :          :  :
ATIII  242  ADGESCSASMMYQEGKFRYRRVAEGTQVLELPFKGDDITMVLILPKPEKSLAKVEKELTPEVLQEWLDELEEMMLVVHMP

                                                                                   ↓
HCII   377  KFKLEKNYNLVESLKLMGIRMLFDKNGNMAGISDQRIAIDLFK----HQGTITVNEEGTQATTVTTVGFMPLSTQ---VR
             :  :    : : :  ::   ::                ::      :     :::::  :   : :     :     :
ATIII  322  RFRIEDGFSLKEQLQDMGLVDLFSPEKSKLPGIVAEGRDDLYVSDAFHKAFLEVNEEGSEAAASTAVVIAGRSLNPNRVT
                                                                                   ↑
                                                                             reactive site
HCII   450  FTVDRPFLFLIYEHRTSCLLFMGRVANPSRS
            :   ::::  : :       ::::::::
ATIII  402  FKANRPFLVFIREVPLNTIIFMGRVANPCVK
```

Fig. 3.3 Amino acid sequence alignment of antithrombin and HCII.
Asterisks denote residues that have been implicated in heparin binding. From Blinder et al 1988, with kind permission of Dr Tollefsen.

antithrombin). The close correspondence between this region of HCII with a region known to be important in antithrombin implicates its participation in glycosaminoglycan binding. The roles of Arg189 of HCII and Arg129 of antithrombin in glycosaminoglycan binding is discussed below.

LOCATION AND ORGANIZATION OF THE GENE POLYMORPHISMS

Statistical analyses of a number of large families with hereditary thrombosis identified linkage of antithrombin deficiency with chromosome 1q markers (Duffy blood group antigens) Fy and 1qh. Reduced plasma antithrombin levels in carriers of chromosome deletions indicated that the antithrombin gene was in the region of 1q22–25 (Winter et al 1982). The position of the structural gene was conclusively localized to 1q23–25 by in situ hybridization and by quantitative analysis of gene dosage in DNA isolated from carriers of chromosome 1 deletions (Bock et al 1985).

The intron locations of antithrombin have been identified by Jagd et al (1985), Prochownik et al (1985) and Bock et at (1988). The gene appeared initially to contain six exons and five introns distributed over 19 kilobase-pairs (kbp) of DNA. Subsequent reanalysis by Bock et al (1988) identified an additional small (1 kbp) intron in exon 3. The revised structure of the normal antithrombin gene is illustrated in Fig 3.4.

An intragenic sequence polymorphism in the coding region of antithrombin was identified by Prochownik et al (1983a,b). The nucleotide

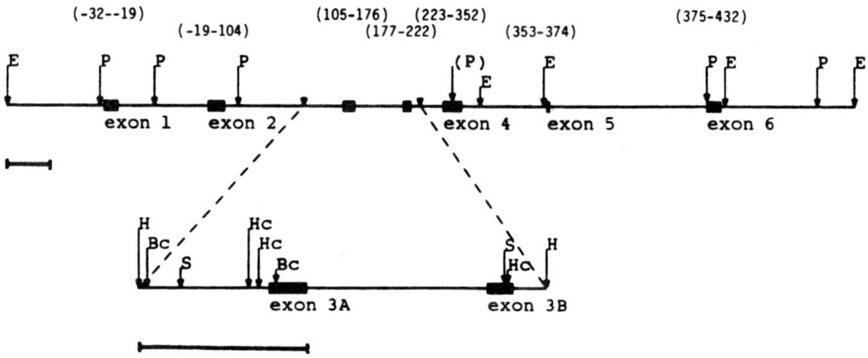

Fig. 3.4 Revised structure of the antithrombin gene. Restriction sites are indicated, (P) is the intragenic polymorphic site (see text). The approximate positions of amino acids coded for by the exons is indicated in parentheses. The scale bar represents 1 kbp. (Adapted from Bock et al (1988).

sequence of Leu304—Gln305 can be either 5'-CTGCAA-3' or 5'-CTGCAG-3', a PstI cleavage site being between the A and the G nucleotides in the latter sequence (a '+' allele). Persons who are homozygous for the presence of the PstI polymorphism (+/+), have four DNA fragments that hybridize with an antithrombin cDNA probe. These fragments are 5.5, 5.0, 2.5 and 1.8 kbp in length. Persons homozygous for the absence of the site (-/-) have fragments of length 10.5, 2.5 and 1.8 kbp. In heterozygotes (-/+), one of the 10.5 kbp bands is cleaved by PstI to fragments 5.5 and 5.0 kbp in length yielding a total of five fragments from both alleles. When 102 individuals (from different ethnic backgrounds) were examined, of the 204 alleles, 103 were (+) and 101 were (–).

Bock and Levitan (1983) conducted a systematic search for DNA polymorphisms using different restriction endonucleases and identified a DNA length polymorphism in the 5' flanking sequence of the antithrombin gene. This length polymorphism is due to the presence of variable DNA fragments of 32 and 108 bp which are non-homologous and are located 345 bp upstream of the initiating ATG codon. The length polymorphism can be detected by various restriction enzymes such as BamHI, AvaII, MspI and SphI. Use of the polymerase chain reaction has greatly simplified the identification of the length polymorphism and the PstI sequence polymorphism; it allows direct visualization of the amplified DNA sequence in ethidium bromide-stained agarose gels. Although the PstI intragenic and the length polymorphisms have been used in the study of the molecular genetics of inherited antithrombin deficiency (see below), the limited number of polymorphic sites linked to the antithrombin gene means that the identification of the abnormal allele in many families has to be accomplished by other methods.

Blinder et al (1988) have studied the chromosome location of the HCII gene and its polymorphisms. Blot hybridization of an HCII probe to DNA isolated from sorted chromosomes localized the HCII gene to chromosome 22. A restriction fragment length polymorphism was identified with BamHI: 2.6 and 3.1 kbp bands visible on Southern blotting probably represent different alleles of the same gene. Their population frequencies have not been determined. Three different nucleotide sequences found by Blinder et al (1988) and Ragg (1986) may also represent polymorphisms. These are at position 1608 in the 3' untranslated region, C–T at position 532 and G–A at position 738 (the latter two being in the coding region).

FUNCTIONS AND PHYSIOLOGICAL ROLES

Inhibition of proteinases by antithrombin and HCII occurs by the formation of an equimolar complex between the reactive site of inhibitor and the active site of proteinase. The mechanism of inhibition of proteinases by antithrombin involves two steps and is similar to that observed with other serpin–proteinase reactions. This was demonstrated when the antithrombin–thrombin reactions were studied at high (>70 μM) concentrations of antithrombin (Olson & Shore 1982). An initial weak complex with a dissociation constant of 1.4×10^{-3} M was formed between antithrombin and proteinase. This was then converted to a stable complex at a rate constant of 10/s. It is thought that the high dissociation constant of the initial complex is mainly responsible for the relatively long half-time (about 40 s) of inhibition of thrombin in plasma (Bjork et al 1989).

The transformation of initial to stable complex involves the formation of a covalent bond between the reactive site (Arg393 of antithrombin and Leu444 of HCII) and the serine residue of the active site of thrombin. The covalent bond forms as a consequence of activation of the inhibitor and trapping of the proteinase. Initially, the reactive bond of the inhibitor acts as a substrate for the enzyme, but once cleavage of the reactive-site bond has taken place, a conformational change occurs that traps the enzyme. The conformational change may not be restricted to the region of the reactive site. Peterson and Blackburn (1987a) used monoclonal antibodies to the *N*-terminal domain of antithrombin to demonstrate a conformational change in response to thrombin binding. This conformational change is thought to be responsible for the reduced binding affinity of the antithrombin–thrombin complex to heparin.

Heparin has an appreciable accelerating effect upon the formation of antithrombin–proteinase complexes. The formation of the antithrombin–thrombin complex is accelerated at least 2000-fold under optimum conditions (rate constant of inhibition of 1.5×10^7 to 3×10^8/M s), and this reduces the half-time of inhibition of thrombin in plasma to about 10 ms (Bjork et al 1989). Similar rate enhancements have been observed for the inactivation of factors Xa and IXa by antithrombin (Jordan et al 1980b) but not for the coagulation proteinases participating in contact activation.

The accelerating effect of heparin occurs when it is present in concentrations very much below those of antithrombin and the proteinases. Each molecule of heparin acts in a catalytic manner, accelerating the formation of many antithrombin–proteinase complexes. Although many polyanions accelerate the thrombin–HCII reaction, heparin and dermatan sulphate are currently of most interest. In the presence of 40–80 μg/ml of heparin and 250–500 μg/ml dermatan sulphate, maximal second-order rate constants for the thrombin–HCII reaction increase ~1000-fold (up to 6.3×10^6 and 1.0×10^7/M s respectively) (Tollefsen et al 1983).

Bjork et al (1989) have reviewed the mechanisms involved in heparin acceleration of antithrombin–proteinase complex formation. Heparin promotes the formation of a ternary complex with antithrombin and proteinase (Pomerantz & Owen 1978, Griffith 1982), in which the active site of the proteinase is brought into close contact with the reactive site of antithrombin. Because of the high affinity of antithrombin to heparin, assembly of the ternary complex proceeds preferentially through formation of a heparin–antithrombin complex. The binding of heparin to antithrombin induces a conformational change in the protein that further enhances heparin binding. Thrombin, and other proteinases that bind with quite high affinity to heparin, bind to the heparin chain adjacent to antithrombin on the relatively non-specific regions of the polysaccharide chain that adjoin the antithrombin-binding pentasaccharide sequence. In this circumstance, a crucial role of heparin seems to be the bringing together of inhibitor and proteinase ('approximation'), rather than just the induction of a conformational change (Peterson & Blackburn 1987b). It should be emphasized that, in the case of thrombin, binding to the heparin chain and approximation are essential for its accelerated inhibition (Lane et al 1984). In contrast, factor Xa and other proteinases which bind only weakly to heparin are inhibited directly by the heparin–antithrombin complex, and approximation of antithrombin and proteinase on the heparin does not need to take place. Rather, the conformational change induced in the inhibitor by heparin appears to enable the inhibition reaction to proceed more rapidly. Once an acyl intermediate has formed between the reactive site of antithrombin and the active site of the proteinase (factor Xa or thrombin), the change in conformation in antithrombin results in a reduced binding affinity of the complex to heparin, enabling its release and participation in additional antithrombin–proteinase reactions.

The prime physiological role of antithrombin is the regulation of coagulation proteinase activity. While the reaction of heparin with antithrombin is of clear clinical importance, it is unlikely to be of physiological importance as heparin is not found within the vasculature under normal circumstances. Nevertheless, evidence has been obtained for the presence of an analogous accelerating mechanism that operates through heparan sulphate proteoglycans, intercalated in the surface membranes of endothelial cells (Marcum & Rosenberg 1984, Marcum et al 1986). The physiological role of HCII is as yet uncertain. There is no firm evidence that it functions as a regulator of thrombin within the circulation. The work of McGuire & Tollefsen (1987) suggests a possible role. They found that human fibroblasts accelerate HCII inhibition of thrombin 2.3–7.5-fold. They were also able to extract proteoglycans from a fibroblast cell line that were rich in dermatan sulphate and which are active against HCII. They suggest that HCII may have a role in inhibiting thrombin in the subendothelial tissues, following injury and disruption of the normal endothelium.

FUNCTIONAL DEFICIENCY: CLINICAL PRESENTATION AND MOLECULAR BASIS

Egeberg (1965) first established an association between antithrombin deficiency and recurrent venous thrombosis in a Norwegian family. Subsequent estimates of the prevalence of antithrombin deficiency in the general population have been 1 per 5000 in a Norwegian study (Abildgaard 1981) and 1 per 2000 in the USA (Rosenberg 1975). The prevalence of hereditary antithrombin deficiency in patients with a history of venous thrombosis or pulmonary embolism has been estimated at 2–3% by Thaler & Lechner (1981) and at about 5% by Engesser (1988) (see also Chapter 1). The pattern of inheritance of antithrombin deficiency is autosomal dominant, males and females being equally affected. Individuals with antithrombin deficiency are usually heterozygous, with antithrombin levels around 40–70% of normal.

Patients with antithrombin deficiency have a high risk of developing venous thrombosis, the risk increasing with increasing age. Thaler & Lechner (1981) reviewed the published reports for the time of onset of the first thrombotic event (80 patients) and the age of affected individuals free of thrombosis at the time of the report (62 persons). They found that thrombosis occurred in only 10% of children below the age of 15 years, but more than 85% of patients older than 50 years had had at least one thrombotic event. In 58% of patients reviewed, the first thrombotic event was probably triggered by a known risk factor, such as surgery, delivery, pregnancy or major trauma. Thrombosis usually occurred in the deep leg veins, but other sites such as mesenteric veins were not uncommon. Pulmonary embolism was frequently suspected. It should be noted that while thrombotic events occur with high frequency in antithrombin deficiency, there is a great variability in frequency between and within families. This variability results in a conservative approach to the treatment of asymptomatic individuals. The prophylaxis and treatment of acute thrombotic events in antithrombin deficiency have been reviewed by Conard et al (1988).

Hereditary deficiency of HCII was originally described in two families (Sie et al 1985b, Tran et al 1985). Deficiency is inherited as an autosomal trait. In one family, thrombotic events were linked with HCII deficiency while, in the other, only the propositus had had thrombosis. A detailed study of the prevalence of HCII deficiency by Bertina et al (1987) identified three additional individuals with HCII deficiency and thrombosis. However, they also found two cases of deficiency not associated with thrombosis in 107 healthy volunteers. They concluded that it is unlikely that heterozygosity for HCII deficiency in itself is a risk factor for thrombosis.

Most patients with antithrombin deficiency have reduced levels of immunologically and functionally determined antithrombin; this is sometimes termed 'classical' deficiency. Diagnosis of classical deficiency is relatively straightforward and is based upon concordance of reduced levels of antithrombin when determined by, for example, heparin cofactor assay and immunodiffusion or immunoelectrophoretic assay. Other individuals with deficiency have normal levels of immunologically determined antithrombin but reduced levels of antithrombin by functional assay. These individuals are heterozygous for a variant (functionally inactive) protein. The first reported case of a variant antithrombin was by Sas et al (1974). They reported a variant with impaired ability to bind to heparin, antithrombin Budapest. Since then, numerous cases of variant proteins have been described (for a recent review, see Hultin et al 1988) and appreciable progress is being made in the characterization of their molecular defects (see below). Variants can be recognized and distinguished by preliminary investigation of patients' plasma, using simple tests (see pp.63–64 for details of methodology). Characteristically, they all have reduced levels (mostly about 50%) when assayed by a heparin cofactor assay. This arises because the heparin cofactor assay depends upon both the functional domains of the molecule. A distinction can be drawn between reactive site and heparin-binding site variants using cross immunoelectrophoresis in the presence of heparin (see Fig. 3.5). The former display normal electrophoretic patterns while the latter have at least two components, one normal and one with reduced mobility caused by impaired reaction with heparin. Confirmation of the nature of the defect relies upon purification from plasma, additional functional studies and, ultimately, elucidation of the molecular defect.

A number of attempts have been made to classify all the cases of antithrombin deficiency (Sas et al 1974, Finazzi et al 1987, Hultin et al 1988). This has been done with regard to their plasma levels and reported functional properties (rather than with regard to their molecular defects, which generally have not been available). Consequently, these classification schemes must remain tentative until the precise nature of more of the abnormalities is known. While a number of cases may well be placed in a wrong subgroup, these schemes have nevertheless been useful in providing a preliminary overview of the relationships between the functional abnormalities and the frequency of thrombosis. For example, Finazzi et al (1987) recently reviewed 404 cases of antithrombin deficiency. They classified deficiency into two types and five subtypes as follows: type I, low functional and immunological antithrombin; subtype Ia, reduced synthesis and/or

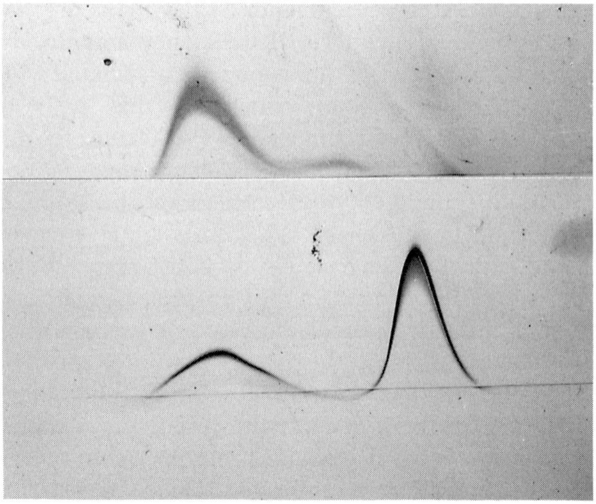

a

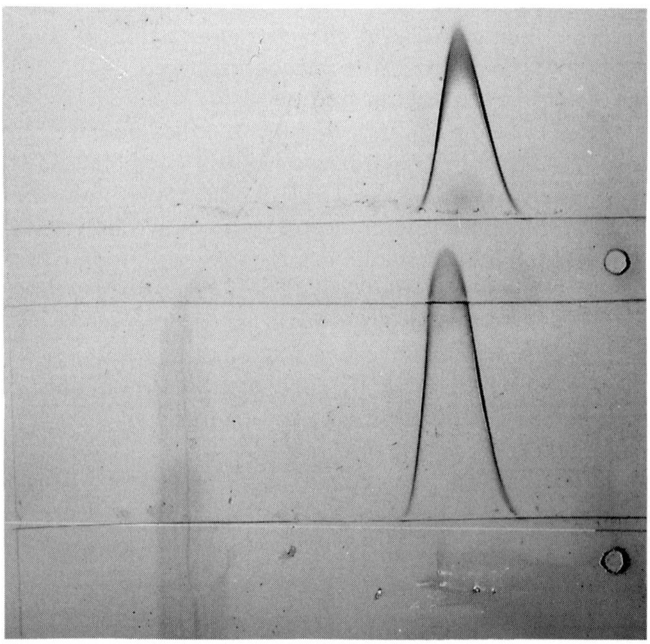

b

Fig. 3.5 Crossed immunoelectrophoresis of antithrombin Padua 2, a type IIc variant with an Arg47 to Cys mutation (Olds et al 1990) in (**a**) the presence and (**b**) absence of heparin. The top trace in each case is a normal control. (Abnormal plasma kindly supplied by Professor A. Girolami).

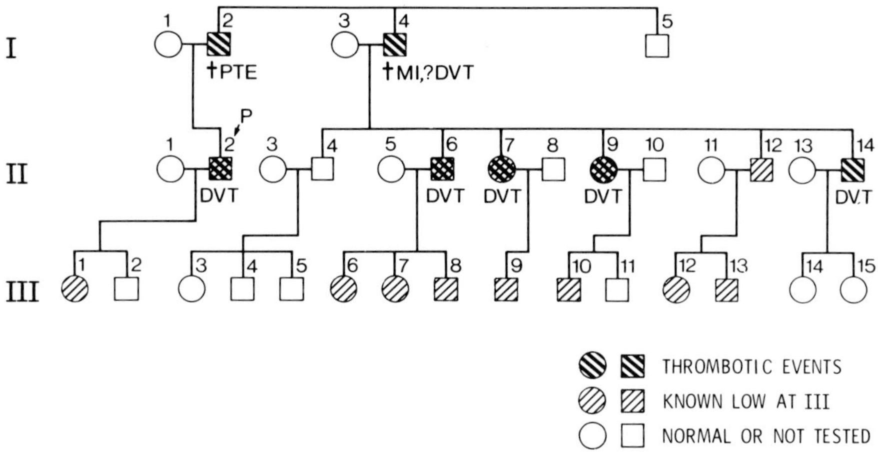

Fig. 3.6 History of thrombosis in a type llb family, antithrombin Glasgow. From Lane et al (1987).

increased turnover of a normal molecule; subtype Ib, reduced synthesis and/or increased turnover of variant antithrombin (note that the original case of deficiency, antithrombin Oslo (Egeberg 1965), has recently been classified as this subtype (Hultin et al 1988)); type II, low functional but normal immunological antithrombin; subtype IIa, functional abnormalities affecting both the reactive site and the heparin-binding site; subtype IIb, functional abnormalities limited to the reactive site; subtype IIc, functional abnormalities limited to the heparin-binding site (see also Chapter 1).

Type I deficiency is associated with an overall incidence of thrombosis of 52–54%. The incidence of thrombosis in subtypes IIa and IIb is possibly even slightly higher (see Fig. 3.6 for a history of thrombosis in a type IIb family). However, patients who are heterozygous for subtype IIc deficiency have a low incidence of thrombosis (6%). It is only in the extremely rare situation where the patients in this subtype are homozygous that the incidence of thrombosis becomes very high (100%) (Finazzi et al 1987). While there will always inevitably be difficulties associated with classification schemes based upon simple functional tests, it is clear that some form of classification scheme is of merit and for the remainder of this chapter the above scheme is adopted.

The molecular genetic basis of type Ia deficiency has been investigated by Prochownik et al (1983b) and Bock & Prochownik (1987). They used the intragenic (PstI) and length polymorphisms described above to study inheritance of abnormal alleles. In a restriction enzyme analysis of 15 type Ia families, only one family was shown to have a deletion of the antithrombin gene. The abnormalities of the antithrombin genes in the other 14 families were not identified but were assumed to involve point mutations, (i.e. minor insertions or deletions, or single base substitutions,

404	406	407	Type Ib: increased turnover of variant
Ala	Arg	Pro	
GCC	AGG	CCT	
↓	↓	↓	
ACC	ATG	CTT	
Thr	Met	Leu	

382	384	384	393	393	393	394	429	Types IIa and IIb: reactive site
Ala	Ala	Ala	Arg	Arg	Arg	Ser	Pro	
GCA	GCA	GCA	CGT	CGT	CGT	TCG	CCT	
↓	↓	↓	↓	↓	↓	↓	↓	
ACA	CCA	TCA	CAT	CCT	TGT	TTG	CTT	
Thr	Pro	Ser	His	Pro	Cys	Leu	Leu	

7	24	41	47	47	47	129	Type IIc: heparin-binding site
Ile	Arg	Pro	Arg	Arg	Arg	Arg	
ATC	CGC	CCG	CGT	CGT	CGT	CGA	
↓	↓	↓	↓	↓	↓	↓	
AAC*	TGC	CTG	TGT	CAT	AGT*	CCA	
Asn	Cys	Leu	Cys	His	Ser	Gln	

Fig. 3.7 Novel amino acid and nucleotide mutations in antithrombin deficiency. CpG dinucleotides are underlined. Asterisks denote assumed nucleotide mutations.

leading to a reduced synthesis of antithrombin). Since linkage to the antithrombin locus was not established, transacting mutations could not be ruled out. Recently, the molecular genetic basis of type Ia deficiency was established in an Italian family. Olds et al (1990a) identified a T deletion in codon 119 that results in a frameshift and introduction of a premature stop codon in codon 126.

More substantial progress has been made in the investigation of type Ib and type II deficiencies, using both protein and genomic sequencing techniques (see references cited below; also Caso et al 1990, Olds et al 1989, 1990b). The novel amino acid substitutions and nucleotide sequence mutations that have been identified are summarized in Fig. 3.7.

Type Ib mutations are an interesting group that appear to present as 'classical' or type Ia defects, in that there is a reduced level of antithrombin by both activity and antigen assays. However, closer analysis of plasma indicates small quantities of variant protein are present. The substitutions in variants of this subtype at positions 404 (antithrombin Oslo), 406 (antithrombin Kyoto (tentative name)) and 407 (antithrombin Utah) all seem to undermine the conformational integrity of the inhibitor (Bock et al 1988, Bock 1989, Nakagawa 1989). This results in inability of the variant to inactivate thrombin and rapid elimination of the variant from the circulation.

Type IIa and/or type IIb variants are unable to inactivate proteinases and have amino acid substitutions in the vicinity of the reactive site. The substitution at Ala382 (antithrombin Hamilton) and Ala384 (antithrombin Charleville) are interesting as they are not immediately adjacent to the reactive site (Devraj-Kizuk et al 1988, Mohlo-Sabatier et al 1989). Comparison of sequence homology between serpins reveals that Ala382 is conserved in all superfamily members that retain inhibitory activity (see also above). It seems that this residue is important for maintaining the conformation of the reactive site. Ala384 may also be important in this regard, as substitution to Pro results in transformation of the inhibitor into a substrate for thrombin (Caso et al 1991). Functional properties have not yet been reported for the variant with the Ala384 to Ser (Perry & Carrell 1991). Substitution of reactive site Arg393 (to Cys, His & Pro) in antithrombins Northwick Park, Glasgow & Pescara prevents any interaction with thrombin (Erdjument et al 1988, Lane et al 1989). The Arg393 to Cys substitution turned out to be particularly interesting, as Cys393 is able to form a disulphide bond with albumin (Erdjument et al 1987). Substitution at the P1' position, Ser394 to Leu (antithrombin Denver), reduces the interaction of antithrombin with thrombin 4000-fold (Stephens et al 1987). Eight mutant proteins have been generated by site-directed mutagenesis (Stephens et al 1988): all of the variants bound heparin but had varying abilities to inactivate thrombin. When Pro or Met were at the P1' position, inhibitory activity was completed abolished. An interesting substitution has been found in the propositus with antithrombin Budapest. He suffers from recurrent thrombosis and has now been found to be homozygous for a substitution Pro429 to Leu (Olds et al 1990c). Although the prospositus is homozygous, two populations of antithrombin can be isolated from the plasma. The first binds strongly to heparin–Sepharose and has reduced ability (30%) to inactivate thrombin. The second binds only weakly to heparin and is devoid of inhibitory activity. It is proposed that the substitution may perturb the conformation of the reactive site in the first population, while a gross alteration in structure may be present in the second. This could be due to an increased sensitivity to proteolysis or possibly to disruption of the disulphide bond between Cys430 and Cys247.

Although abnormalities of type IIc are not associated with a high incidence of thrombosis, the molecular and genetic mutations remain of interest, as they provide an unambiguous means of defining the heparin binding domain of antithrombin. Furthermore, there is an indication that certain amino acid substitutions may be associated with an increased risk of thrombosis (Mohlo-Sabatier et al 1989). A variant, antithrombin Rouen III (Brennan et al 1988), with reduced heparin binding has been shown to have an Ile7 to Asn substitution. This substitution results in generation of a new potential glycosylation site at position 7. It is not clear whether the alteration in heparin binding arises form the amino acid substitution or the incorporation of the sugar side-chain in the antithrombin. A substitution

Arg24 to Cys (antithrombin Rouen IV) has been reported by Perry & Carrell (1989). Its functional properties had not been described at the time of writing. Chang and Tran (1986) identified the mutation Pro41 to Leu in a variant (antithrombin Basel) with a heparin-binding abnormality. Computer analysis predicted an increase in the helical structure and hydrophobicity around residue 41 caused by the substitution. This change in conformation may be responsible for the impaired heparin binding. A recurrent mutation site is at position 47. Both the Arg47 to Cys (antithrombin Toyama) (Koide et al 1984) and Arg47 to His (antithrombin Rouen I) (Owen et al 1987) occur frequently, and one case of Arg47 to Ser (antithrombin Rouen II) has been described (Borg et al 1988). All cases have impaired binding to heparin. Until recently, identified type IIa congenital substitutions were confined to the amino terminal region of antithrombin. However, Gandrille et al (1991) have now shown conclusively that the region near Lys125 is involved in heparin binding. They studied antithrombin Geneva, a variant with impaired binding to heparin, which has a substitution Arg129 to Gln. Church et al (1989) and Gandrille et al (1991) propose that Lys125, Arg129, Arg132, Lys133, Lys136 and Lys139 are all on the same side of a helix and constitute an essential part of the heparin-binding domain. A naturally occurring mutant with a substitution in the corresponding amino acid of HCII, HCII Oslo, has been characterized by Blinder et al (1989). Two asymptomatic individuals have the variant, which interacts normally with heparin, but not dermatan sulphate. A substitution, Arg189 to His, was identified.

It can be seen from Fig. 3.7, that there is a high frequency of mutation of CpG dinucleotides in antithrombin deficiency. This supports the view that the CpG dinucleotide may be a mutation hotspot in the human genome. A mechanism of spontaneous deamination of methyl cytosine to form thymine is a generally accepted mechanism. While this seems to be responsible for many of the recurrent mutations of antithrombin, other mechanisms must also be involved, for example in the recurrent mutation of Ala384

METHODOLOGY FOR THE STUDY OF ANTITHROMBIN AND HCII

Antithrombin

Heparin cofactor assay

This is a particularly good method for screening for cases of functional or absolute deficiency because decreased levels of antithrombin, and any abnormality that affects either the heparin-binding domain or the reactive site, will result in a decreased assay result. The method of Odegard et al (1975), is marketed commercially by KabiVitrum (Heparin Cofactor Coatest), but reagents from other companies are suitable (e.g. Behring,

Berichrom and Diagnostica Stago). The details of the Coatest method are contained on the data sheet supplied by KabiVitrum, but a short account of the principle, which applies to most assays, is given below.

The test plasma is diluted in buffer containing EDTA and an excess of heparin and thrombin is added. This is incubated for 30 s at 37°C and residual thrombin determined. This is achieved by adding chromogenic substrate plus polybrene to neutralize the heparin during the period of substrate hydrolysis. The hydrolysis is monitored on a spectrophotometer at 405 nm, either as an initial rate or as a fixed time (30 s) reaction. The details of the method will vary depending on the substrate used and on the equipment available (autoanalysers are being used with increasing frequency), and all manufacturers of substrates, kits and equipment produce their own detailed procedures.

Antigen concentration

Two common methods of determining antigen concentration are rocket electrophoresis and radial immunodiffusion. Local considerations determine which should be used. Behring NOR-Partigen plates are convenient to use. A disadvantage is the 18 h wait before results are obtained, but this is more than compensated by the simplicity of the method. Reference samples are supplied with preformed plates.

Crossed immunoelectrophoresis

The procedure is usually based on that of Laurell (1965), but may be modified according to Sas et al (1975) to include heparin in the gel. A 0.8% solution of agarose in 0.05 M sodium barbitone buffer, pH 8.4, is prepared containing 16.6 IU/ml of heparin. This is poured onto gel bond, a small sample hole made near one corner for 5 μl plasma, and electrophoresis performed for 2–4 h at ~20 V/(cm gel). The gel is then cut and most of it not containing the sample is discarded. More agarose in buffer, this time containing anti-antithrombin antiserum, is added to the gel bond in the region of the discarded gel. Electrophoresis is performed at right angles to the original direction. This may be carried out at lower voltage, overnight. After electrophoresis, the gel is extensively washed in saline for 2 h, and dried under a filter paper containing paper towels and lead weights above it. The gel is then stained using Coomassie blue.

Isolation of antithrombin from plasma

A method is described by McKay (1981), in which a preliminary precipitation step with dextran sulphate is performed prior to isolation on heparin–Sepharose. Chromatography is simplified by batch elution of the antithrombin. Plasma is applied to the column in 0.1 M Tris HCl, pH 7.4, containing 0.4 M sodium chloride. If the plasma contains a heparin-binding variant, this will pass straight through the column and only the normal component will be retained (assuming that the patient is heterozygous). The normal component is eluted with stepwise addition of 2.0 M sodium chloride in the same buffer. The antithrombin eluted with high salt is ~90% pure and requires an additional purification step only if its kinetic properties are to be studied. (Small amounts of heparin elute from the heparin–Sepharose column and these need to be removed by ion exchange chromatography.) In the case of a reactive-site variant, this will probably bind to the heparin–Sepharose along with the normal component. The normal antithrombin can be separated by passing the antithrombin through a thrombin–Sepharose column (see Lane et al 1989). If a heparin-binding variant is indicated by the presence of antithrombin in the wash through the heparin–Sepharose column (and by crossed immunoelectrophoresis), then the variant must be further purified by chromatography on immobilized antibody to antithrombin (see Caso et al 1990).

This protocol has to be varied according to the precise molecular defect in the variant protein.

Heparin cofactor II

As there has not been as much clinical interest in HCII for the reasons noted above, the reagents for its assay are not widely available commercially. A functional assay can be devised using reagents for the dermatan sulphate assay (Dupouy et al 1988) (see also Chapter 1) obtainable through through Diagnostica Stago. The test plasma is diluted in buffer containing dermatan sulphate and an excess of thrombin is added. This is incubated for 2 min at 37°C and residual thrombin determined by adding chromogenic substrate and monitoring amidolytic activity on a spectrophotometer at 405 nm, either as an initial rate or at a fixed time (90 s). Immunological assays require specific antibodies, which have been raised by individual investigators; see for example Hortin et al (1986) and Bertina et al (1987).

ACKNOWLEDGEMENTS

The work of the authors reported in this article was supported by the British Heart Foundation and Wellcome Trust.

REFERENCES

Abildgaard U 1968 Highly purified antithrombin III with heparin cofactor activity prepared by disc electrophoresis. Scandinavian Journal of Clinical and Laboratory Investigation 21: 89–91

Abildgaard U 1969 Binding of thrombin to antithrombin III. Scandinavian Journal of Clinical and Laboratory Investigation 24: 23–27

Abildgaard U 1981 Antithrombin and related inhibitors of coagulation. In Poller L (ed) Recent advances in blood coagulation. Churchill Livingstone, Edinburgh, vol 3, p 151–173

Atha D H, Stephens A W, Rosenberg R D (1984) Evaluation of critical groups required for binding of heparin to antithrombin. Proceedings of the National Academy of Sciences, USA 81: 1030–1034

Atha D H, Lormeau J-C, Petitou M, Rosenberg R D, Choay J 1985 Contribution of monosaccharide residues in heparin binding to antithrombin III. Biochemistry 24: 6723–6729

Bertina R M, van der Linden I K, Engesser L, Muller H P, Brommer E J P 1987 Hereditary heparin cofactor II deficiency and the risk of development of thrombosis. Thrombosis and Haemostasis 57: 196–200

Bjork I, Danielsson A, Fenton J W, Jornvall H 1981 The site in human antithrombin for functional proteolytic cleavage by human thrombin. Federation of European Biochemical Societies Letters 126: 257–260

Bjork I, Jackson C M, Jornvall H, Lavine K K, Nording K, Salsgiver W J 1982 The active site of antithrombin. Release of the same proteolytically cleaved form of the inhibitor from complexes with Factor IXa, Factor Xa and thrombin. Journal of Biological Chemistry 257: 2406–2411

Bjork I, Olson S T, Shore J D 1989 Molecular mechanisms of the accelerating effect of heparin on the reactions between antithrombin and clotting proteinases. In Lane D A and Lindahl U (eds) Heparin: chemical and biological properties, Clinical applications. Edward Arnold, London, p 229–255

Blackburn M N, Sibley C C 1980 The heparin binding site of antithrombin III. Evidence for a critical tryptophan residue. Journal of Biological Chemistry 255: 824–826

Blackburn M N, Smith R L, Carson J, Sibley C C 1984 The heparin-binding site of antithrombin III. Identification of a critical tryptophan in the amino acid sequence. Journal of Biological Chemistry 259: 939–941

Blinder M A, Marasa J C, Reynolds C H, Deaven L L, Tollefsen D M 1988 Heparin cofactor II: cDNA sequence, chromosome location, restriction fragment length polymorphism, and expression in *Escherichia coli*. Biochemistry 27: 752–759

Blinder M A, Andersson T R, Abildgaard U, Tollefsen D M 1989 Heparin cofactor II Oslo. Mutation of Arg-189 to His decreases the affinity for dermatan sulphate. Journal of Biological Chemistry 264: 5128–5133

Bock S C 1989 Antithrombin III genetics. Thrombosis and Haemostis 62: 468

Bock S C, Levitan D J 1983 Characterization of an unusual DNA length polymorphism 5' to the human antithrombin III gene. Nucleic Acids Research 11: 8569–8582

Bock S C, Prochownik E V 1987 Molecular genetic survey of 16 kindreds with hereditary antithrombin III deficiency. Blood 70: 1273–1278

Bock S C, Wion K L, Vehar G A, Lawn R M 1982 Cloning and expression of the cDNA for human antithrombin III. Nucleic Acids Research 10: 8113–8125

Bock S C, Harris J F, Balazs I, Trent J M 1985 Assignment of the human antithrombin III structural gene to chromosome 1q23–25. Cytogenetics Cell Genetics 39: 67–69

Bock S C, Marrinan J A, Radziejewska E 1988 Antithrombin III Utah: Proline-407 to leucine mutation in a highly conserved region near the inhibitor reactive site. Biochemistry 27: 6171–6178

Borg J Y, Owen M C, Soria C, Soria J, Caen J, Carrell R W 1988 Proposed heparin binding site in antithrombin based on Arginine 47. Journal of Clinical Investigation 81: 1292–1296.

Brennan S O, George P M, Jordan R E 1987 Physiological variant of antithrombin III lacks carbohydrate side chain at Asn135. Federation of European Biochemical Societies Letters 219: 431–436

Brennan S O, Borg J–Y, George P M, Soria C, Soria J, Caen J, Carrell R W 1988 New carbohydrate site in mutant antithrombin (7 Ile-Asn) with decreased heparin affinity. Federation of European Biochemical Societies Letters 237: 118–122

Briginshawe G F, Shanberge J N 1974a Identification of two distinct heparin cofactors in human plasma. Separation and partial purification. Archives of Biochemistry and Biophysics 161: 683–690

Briginshawe G F, Shanberge J N 1974b Identification of two distinct heparin cofactors in plasma. II. Inhibition of thrombin and activated factor X. Thrombosis Research 4: 463–477

Carrell R W, Owen M, Brennan S, Vaughan L 1979 Carboxy terminal fragment of human

α_1–antitrypsin from hydroxylamine cleavage: homology with antithrombin III. Biochemical and Biophysical Research Communications 91: 1032–1037

Caso R, Lane D A, Thompson E A, Zangouras D, Panico M, Morris H R, Olds R J, Thein S L, Girolami A 1990 Antithrombin Padua I: impaired heparin binding caused by an Arg47 to His (CGT to CAT) substitution. Thrombosis Research 58: 185–190

Caso R, Lane D A, Olds R J, Thein S L, Panico M, Morris H, Freysinnet J M, Aiach M, Rodeghiero F, Finazzi G 1991 Antithrombin Vicenza, Ala 384 to Pro (GCA to CCA) mutation, transforming the inhibitor into a substrate. British Journal of Haematology 77: 87–92

Casu B, Oreste P, Torri G, Zoppetti G, Choay J, Lormeau J–C, Petitou M, Sinay P 1981 The structure of heparin oligosaccharide fragments with high anti-(factor Xa) activity containing the minimal antithrombin III binding sequence. Biochemical Journal 197: 599

Chandra T, Stackhouse R, Kidd V J, Woo S L C 1983a Isolation and sequence characterization of a cDNA clone of human antithrombin III. Proceedings of the National Academy of Sciences, USA 80: 1845–1848

Chandra T, Stackhouse R, Kidd V J, Robson J H, Woo S L C 1983b Sequence homology between human α_1–antichymotryspin, α_1–antitrypsin and antithrombin III. Biochemistry 22: 5055–5061

Chang J-Y 1989 Binding of heparin to human antithrombin III activates selective chemical modification at lysine 236. Lys-107, Lys-125 and Lys-136 are situated within the heparin-binding site of antithrombin III. Journal of Biological Chemistry 264: 3111–3115

Chang J-Y, Tran T H 1986 Antithrombin III Basel: Identification of a Pro–Leu substitution in a hereditary abnormal antithrombin with impaired heparin cofactor activity. Journal of Biological Chemistry 261: 1174–1176

Choay J, Petitou M, Lormeau J C, Sinay P, Casu B, Gatti G 1983 Structure–activity relationship in heparin: a synthetic pentasaccharide with high affinity for antithrombin III and eliciting high anti-factor Xa activity. Biochemical and Biophysical Research Communications 116: 492–499

Church F C, Griffith M J 1984 Evidence for essential lysines in heparin cofactor II. Biochemical and Biophysical Research Communications 124: 745–751

Church F C, Villanueva G B, Griffith M J 1986 Structure–function relationships in heparin cofactor II: chemical modification of arginine and tryptophan and demonstration of a two domain structure. Archives of Biochemistry and Biophysics 246: 175–184

Church F C, Meade J B, Treanor R E, Whinna H C 1989 Antithrombin activity of fucoidan. The interaction of fucoidan with heparin cofactor II, antithrombin III, and thrombin. Journal of Biological Chemistry 264: 3618–3623

Collen D, Schetz J, DeCock F, Holmer E, Verstraete M 1977 Metabolism of antithrombin III (heparin cofactor) in man: Effects of venous thrombosis on heparin administration. European Journal of Clinical Investigation 7: 27–35

Conard J, Brosstad F, Larsen M L, Samama M, Abildgaard U 1983 Molar antithrombin concentration in normal human plasma. Haemostasis 13: 363–368

Conard J, Horellou M H, Samama M 1988 Incidence of thromboembolism associated with congenital disorders in coagulation and fibrinolysis. Acta Chirugica Scandanavica suppl 543: 15–25

Damus P S, Hicks, M, Rosenberg R D 1973 Anticoagulant action of heparin. Nature 246: 355–357

Devraj-Kizuk R, Chui D H K, Prochownik E V, Carter C J, Ofosu F A, Blajchman M A 1988 Antithrombin-III-Hamilton: a gene with a point mutation (guanine to adenine) in codon 382 causing impaired serine protease reactivity. Blood 72: 1518–1523

Derechin V M, Blinder M A, Tollefsen M F 1990 Substitution of arginine for Leu444 in the reactive site of heparin cofactor II enhances the rate of thrombin inhibition. Journal of Biological Chemistry 265: 5623–5628

Dupouy D, Sie P, Dol F, Boneu B 1988 A simple method to measure dermatan sulphate at sub-microgram concentrations in plasma. Thrombosis and Haemostasis 60: 236–239

Egeberg O 1965 Inherited antithrombin III deficiency causing thrombophilia. Thrombosis et Diathesis Haemorrhagica 13: 516–530

Einarsson R, Andersson L-O 1977 Binding of heparin to human antithrombin III as studied by measurements of tryptophan fluorescence. Biochimica et Biophysica Acta 490: 104–111

Engesser L 1988 Thrombophilia: disorders of blood coagulation and fibrinolysis. Thesis, University of Leiden

Erdjument H, Lane D A, Ireland H, Panico M, Dimarzo V, Blench I, Morris H R 1987 Formation of a covalent disulfide-linked antithrombin–albumin complex by an antithrombin variant, antithrombin 'Northwick Park'. Journal of Biological Chemistry 262: 13381–13384

Erdjument H, Lane D A, Panico M, DiMarzo V, Morris H R 1988 Single amino acid substitutions in the reactive site of antithrombin leading to thrombosis. Congenital substitution of arginine 393 to cysteine in antithrombin Northwick Park and to histidine in antithrombin Glasgow. Journal of Biological Chemistry 263: 5589–5593

Finazzi G, Caccia R, Barbui T 1987 Different prevalence of thromboembolism in the subtypes of congenital antithrombin III deficiency: review of 404 cases. Thrombosis and Haemostasis 58: 1094

Gandrille S, Aiach M, Lane D A, Vidaud D, Mohlo-Sabatier P, Caso R, de Moerloose P, Fiessinger J-N, Clauser E 1990 Important role of Arg 129 in heparin binding site of antithrombin III: identification of a novel mutation Arg 129 to Gln. Journal of Biological Chemistry 265: 18997–19001

Griffith M J 1982 Kinetics of the heparin-enhanced antithrombin III–thrombin reaction. Evidence for a template mechanism of action of heparin. Journal of Biological Chemistry 257: 7360–7365

Griffith M J, Noyes C M, Tyndall J A, Church F C 1985 Structural evidence for leucine at the reactive site of heparin cofactor II. Biochemistry 24: 6777–6782

Hook M, Bjork I, Hopwood J, Lindahl U 1976 Anticoagulant activity of heparin: separation of high-activity and low-activity heparin species by affinity chromatography on immobilized antithrombin. Federation of European Biochemical Societies Letters 66: 90–93

Hortin G L, Tollefsen D M, Benutto B M 1989 Antithrombin activity of a peptide corresponding to residues 54-75 of heparin cofactor II. Journal of Biological Chemistry 264: 13 979-13 982

Huber R, Carrell R W 1989 Implications of the three dimensional structure of α_1-antitrypsin for structure and function of serpins. Biochemistry 28: 8951–8966

Hultin M B, McKay J, Abildgaard U 1988 Antithrombin Oslo: Type Ib classification of the first reported antithrombin-deficient family with a review of hereditary antithrombin variants. Thrombosis and Haemostasis 59: 468–473

Hunt L T, Dayhoff M O 1980 A surprising new protein superfamily containing ovalbumin, antithrombin III and α_1-proteinase inhibitor. Biochemical and Biophysical Research Communications 95: 864–871

Inhorn R C, Tollefsen D M 1986 Isolation and characterisation of a partial cDNA clone for heparin cofactor II. Biochemical and Biophysical Research Communications 137: 431–436

Jagd S, Vibe-Pedersen K, Magnusson S 1985 Location of two of the introns in the antithrombin III gene. Federation of European Biochemical Societies Letters 193: 213–216

Jallat S, Carvallo D, Tessier L H, Roechklin D, Roitsch C, Ogushi F, Crystal R G, Courtney M 1986 Altered specificities of genetically engineered alpha 1 antitrypsin variants. Protein Engineering 1: 29–35

Jordan R E, Oosta G M, Gardner W T, Rosenberg R D 1980a The binding of low molecular weight heparin to hemostatic enzymes Journal of Biological Chemistry 225: 10 073–10 080

Jordan R E, Oosta G M, Gardner W T, Rosenberg R D 1980b The kinetics of hemostatic enzyme–antithrombin interactions in the presence of low molecular weight heparin. Journal of Biological Chemistry 255: 10 081–10 090

Jorgensen A M, Borders C L, Fish W W 1985 Arginine residues are critical for the heparin-cofactor activity of antithrombin III. Biochemical Journal 231: 59–65

Karp G I, Marcum J A, Rosenberg R D 1984 The role of tryptophan residues in heparin–antithrombin interactions. Archives in Biochemistry Biophysics 233: 712–720

Kidd V J, Woo S L C 1986 Molecular analysis of the serine proteinase inhibitor gene family. In: Barrett A J and Salvesen G (eds) Proteinase inhibitors. Elsevier, Amsterdam, p 421–440

Koide T, Odani S, Takahashi K, Ono T, Sakuragawa N 1984 Antithrombin III Toyama: replacement of arginine 47 by cysteine in hereditary abnormal antithrombin III that lacks heparin-binding ability. Proceedings of the National Academy of Sciences, USA 81: 289–293

Knot E A R, deJong E, ten Cate J W, Iburg A H C, Henny C W P, Bruin T, Stibbe J 1986 Purified radiolabeled antithrombin III metabolism in three families with hereditary ATIII deficiency: Application of a three-compartment model. Blood 67: 93–98

Lam L H, Silbert J E, Rosenberg R D 1976 The separation of active and inactive forms of heparin. Biochemical and Biophysical Research Communications 69: 570–577

Lane D A, Caso R 1989 Antithrombin: Structure, genomic organisation, function and inherited deficiency. Baillières Clinical Haematology 2: 961–998

Lane D A, Denton J, Flynn A M, Thunberg L, Lindahl U 1984 Anticoagulant activities of heparin oligosaccharides and their neutralisation by platelet factor 4. Biochemical Journal 218: 725–732

Lane D A, Lowe G D O, Flynn A, Thompson E, Ireland H, Erdjument H 1987 Antithrombin Glasgow: a variant with increased heparin affinity and reduced ability to inactivate thrombin. British Journal of Haematology 66: 523–527

Lane D A, Erdjument H, Thompson E, Panico M, DiMarzo V, Morris H R, Leone G, De Stefano V, Thein S L 1989. A novel amino acid substitution in the reactive site of a congenital variant antithrombin. Antithrombin Pescara, Arg 393 to Pro, caused by a CGT to CCT mutation. Journal of Biological Chemistry 264, 10 200–10 204

Laurell C B 1985 Antigen–antibody crossed immunoelectrophoresis. Analytical Biochemistry 10: 358–361

Lindahl U, Backstrom G, Thunberg L, Leder I G 1980 Evidence for a 3-*O*-sulfated D-glycosamine residue in the antithrombin-binding sequence of heparin. Proceedings of the National Academy of Sciences of the USA 77: 6551–6555

Liu C-S, Chang J Y 1987 Probing the heparin-binding domain of human antithrombin III with V8 protease. European Journal of Biochemistry 167: 247–252

Loebermann H, Tokuoka R, Deisenhofer J, Huber R 1984 Human alpha$_1$-proteinase inhibitor. Crystal structure analysis of two crystal modifications, molecular model and preliminary analysis of the implications for function. Journal of Molecular Biology 177: 531–556

McGuire E A, Tollefsen D M 1987 Activation of heparin cofactor II by fibroblasts and smooth muscle cells. Journal of Biological Chemistry 262: 169–175

McKay E J 1981 A single two-step procedure for the isolation of antithrombin III from biological fluid. Thrombosis Research 21: 375–382

Marcum J A, Rosenberg R D 1984 Anticoagulantly active heparin-like molecules from vascular tissue. Biochemistry 23: 1730–1737

Marcum J A, Atha D H, Fritze L M S, Nawroth P, Stern D, Rosenberg R D 1986 Cloned bovine aortic endothelial cells synthesize anticoagulantly active heparan sulphate proteoglycans. Journal of Biological Chemistry 261: 7507–7517

Matheson N R, Gibson H L, Hallewell R A, Barr P J, Travis J 1986 Recombinant DNA-derived forms of human α_1-proteinase inhibitor. Journal of Biological Chemistry 261: 10404–10409

Mohlo-Sabatier P, Aiach M, Gaillard I, Fiessinger J N, Fischer A M, Chadeuf G, Clauser E 1989 Molecular characterization of antithrombin III (ATIII) variants using polymerase chain reaction. Identification of the ATIII Charleville as an Ala384 Pro mutation. Journal of Clinical Investigation 84, 1236–1241
Investigation 84: 1236–1241

Nakagawa M 1989 Antithrombin deficiency and its molecular analysis. Proceedings of Kyoto Satellite Symposium 'Recent advances in antithrombin research' of the XII Congress of ISTH.

Nordenman B, Bjork I 1981 Influence of ionic strength and pH on the interaction between high-affinity heparin and antithrombin. Biochimica et Biophysica Acta 672: 227–238

Nordenman B, Danielsson A, Bjork I 1978 The binding of low-affinity and high-affinity heparin to antithrombin. Fluorescence studies. European Journal of Biochemistry 90: 1–6

Odegaard O R, Lie M, Abildgaard U 1975 Heparin cofactor activity measured with an amidolytic method. Thrombosis Research 6: 287–294

Olds R J, Lane D A, Caso R, Tripodi A, Mannucci P M, Thein S L 1989 Antithrombin Milano 2: a single base substitution in the thrombin binding domain detected by PCR and direct genomic sequencing. Nucleic Acids Research 17: 10511

Olds R J, Lane D A, Caso R, Girolami A, Thein S L 1990b Antithrombin III Padua 2: a single base substitution in exon 2 detected with PCR and direct genomic sequencing. Nucleic Acids Research 18: 1926

Olds R J, Lane D A, Caso R, Panico M, Morris H R, Sas G, Thein S L 1990c Antithrombin III Budapest: a single amino acid substitution (429 Pro to Leu) in a region highly conserved in the serpin superfamily. British Journal of Haematology 76: Suppl 1: 2
Olds R J, Lane D A, Finazzi G, Barbui T, Thein S L 1990a A frameshift mutation leading to type I antithrombin deficiency and thrombosis. Blood 76: 2182–2186
Olson S T, Shore J D 1982 Demonstration of a two-step reaction mechanism for inhibition of α-thrombin by antithrombin III and identification of the step affected by heparin. Journal of Biological Chemistry 257: 14 891–14 895
Olson S T, Srinivasan K R, Bjork I, Shore J D 1981 Binding of high-affinity heparin to antithrombin III. Stopped flow kinetic studies of the binding interaction. Journal of Biological Chemistry 256: 11073–11079
Owen M C, Brennan S O, Lewis J H, Carrell R W 1983 Mutation of antitrypsin to antithrombin. α_1-Antitrypsin Pittsburgh (358 Met–Arg), a fatal bleeding disorder. New England Journal of Medicine 309: 694–698
Owen M C, Borg J Y, Soria C, Soria J, Caen J, Carrell R W 1987 Heparin binding defect in new antithrombin III variant: Rouen, 47 Arg to His, Blood 69: 1275–1279
Perry P J, Carrell R W 1989 CpG dinucleotides are 'hotspots' for mutation in the antithrombin III gene. Twelve variants identified using the polymerase chain reaction. Molecular and Biological Medicine 6: 239–243
Perry P J, Carrell R W 1991 To be published.
Petersen T E, Dudek-Wojciechowska G, Sottrup-Jensen L, Magnusson S 1979 Primary structure of antithrombin III (heparin cofactor). Partial homology between α_1-antitrypsin and antithrombin III. In: Collen D, Wiman B, Verstraete M (eds). The physiological inhibitors of blood coagulation and fibrinolysis. Elsevier, Amsterdam, p 43–54
Peterson C B, Blackburn M N 1985 Isolation and characterization of an antithrombin III variant with reduced carbohydrate content and enhanced heparin binding. Journal of Biological Chemistry 260: 610–615
Peterson C B, Blackburn M N 1987a Antithrombin conformation and the catalytic role of heparin. Does cleavage by thrombin induce structural changes in the heparin-binding region of antithrombin? Journal of Biological Chemistry 262: 7552–7558
Peterson C B, Blackburn M N 1987b Antithrombin conformation and the catalytic role of heparin. Is heparin-induced conformational change in antithrombin required for rapid inactivation of thrombin? Journal of Biological Chemistry 262: 7559–7566
Peterson C B, Noyes C M, Pecon J M, Church F C, Blackburn M W 1987 Identification of a lysyl residue in antithrombin which is essential for heparin binding. Journal of Biological Chemistry 262: 8061–8065
Pomerantz M W, Owen W G 1978 A catalytic role for heparin. Evidence for a ternary complex with heparin cofactor, thrombin and heparin. Biochimica et Biophysica Acta 535: 66–77
Potempa J, Shieh B H, Travis J 1988 Alpha$_2$ antiplasmin: a serpin with two separate but overlapping reactive sites. Science 241: 699–700
Pratt C W, Whinna H C, Meade J B, Treanor R E, Church F C 1989 Physicochemical aspects of heparin cofactor II. In: Heparin and related polysaccharides. Structures and activities. Annals of the New York Academy of Sciences 556: 104–115
Prochownik E V, Markham A F, Orkin S H 1983a Isolation of a cDNA clone for human antithrombin III. Journal of Biological Chemistry 258: 8389–8394
Prochownik E V, Antonarakis S, Bauer K A, Rosenberg R D, Fearon E R, Orkin S H 1983b Molecular heterogeneity of inherited antithrombin III deficiency. The New England Journal of Medicine 308: 1549–1552
Prochownik E V, Bock S C, Orkin S H 1985 Intron structure of the human antithrombin III gene differs from that of other members of the serine protease inhibitor superfamily. Journal of Biological Chemistry 260: 9608–9612
Ragg H 1986 A new member of the plasma protease inhibitor gene family. Nucleic Acids Research 14: 1073–1088
Rosenberg R D 1975 Actions and interactions of antithrombin and heparin. New England Journal of Medicine 292: 146–151
Rosenberg R D, Damus P S 1973 The purification and mechanism of action of human antithrombin–heparin cofactor. Journal of Biological Chemistry 248: 6490–6505
Rosenfeld L, Danishefski I 1986 A fragment of antithrombin that binds to both heparin and thrombin. Biochemical Journal 237: 639–646
Samama J P, Delarue M, Monrey L, Choay J, Moras D 1989 Crystallization and preliminary

crystallographic data for bovine antithrombin III. Journal of Molecular Biology 210: 877–879
Sas G, Blasko G, Banhegyi D, Jako J, Palos L A 1974 Abnormal antithrombin III (antithrombin III 'Budapest') as a cause of a familial thrombophilia. Thrombosis et Diathesis Haemorrhagica 32: 105–115
Sas G, Pepper D S, Cash J D 1975 Further investigations on antithrombin III in the plasma of patients with the abnormality antithrombin 'Budapest'. Thrombosis et Diathesis Haemorrhagica 33: 564–572
Schapira M, Ramus M A, Jallat S, Carvallo D, Courtney M 1985 Recombinant alphal-antitrypsin Pittsburgh (Met 358–Arg) is a potent inhibitor of plasma kallikrein and activated factor XII fragment. Journal of Clinical Investigation 76: 635–637
Scott C F, Carrell R W, Glaser C B, Kueppers F, Lewis J H, Colman R W 1986 Alpha-1-antitrypsin-Pittsburgh. A potent inhibitor of human plasma factor XIa, kallikrein and factor XII. Journal of Clinical Investigation 77: 631–634
Scully M F, Kakkar V V 1984 Identification of heparin cofactor II as the principle cofactor of pentosan polysulphate (SP54). Thrombosis Research 36: 187–196
Scully M F, Ellis V, Seno N, Kakkar V V 1986 The anticoagulant properties of mast cell product, chondroitin sulphate E. Biochemical and Biophysical Research Communications 137: 15–22
Sie P, Dupouy D, Pichon J, Boneu B 1985a Turnover study of heparin co-factor II in healthy men. Thrombosis and Haemostasis 54: 635–641
Sie P, Dupouy D, Pichon J, Boneu B 1985b Constitutional heparin cofactor II deficiency associated with recurrent thrombosis. Lancet ii: 414–416
Smith J W, Knauer D J 1987 A heparin binding site in antithrombin III. Journal of Biological Chemistry 262: 11964–11972
Stephens A W, Siddiqui A, Hirs C H W 1987 Antithrombin III Denver, a reaction site variant. Journal of Biological Chemistry 262: 1044–1048
Stephens A W, Siddiqui A, Hirs C H W 1988 Site-directed mutagenesis of the reactive center (serine 394) of antithrombin III. Journal of Biological Chemistry 263: 15849–15852
Sun X J, Chang J-Y 1989 Heparin binding domain of human antithrombin III inferred from the sequential reduction of the three disulphide linkages. An efficient method for structural analysis of partially reduced proteins. Journal of Biological Chemistry 264: 11288–11293
Thaler E, Lechner K 1981 Antithrombin III deficiency and thromboembolism. Clinics in Haematology 10: 369–390
Thunberg L, Backstrom G, Lindahl U 1982 Further characterization of the antithrombin-binding sequence in heparin. Carbohydrate Research 100: 393–410
Tollefsen D M 1989 Heparin cofactor II. In: Lane D A, Lindahl U (eds) Heparin, chemical and biological properties, Clinical applications. Edward Arnold, London, p. 257–273
Tollefsen D M, Blank M K 1981 Detection of a new heparin-dependent inhibitor of thrombin in human plasma. Journal of Clinical Investigation 68: 589–596
Tollefsen D M, Majerus D W, Blank M K 1982 Heparin cofactor II. Purification and properties of a heparin-dependent inhibitor of thrombin in human plasma. Journal of Biological Chemistry 257: 2162–2169
Tollefsen D M, Pestka C, Monafo W J 1983 Activation of heparin cofactor II by dermatan sulfate. Journal of Biological Chemistry 258: 6713–6716
Tran T H, Marbet G A, Duckert F 1985 Association of hereditary heparin cofactor II deficiency with thrombosis. Lancet ii: 413–414
Travis J, Salvesen G S 1983 Human plasma proteinase inhibitors. Annual Review of Biochemistry 52: 655–709
Travis J, Owen M, George P, Carrell R, Rosenberg S, Hallewell R A, Barr P J 1985 Isolation and properties of recombinant DNA produced variants of human $alpha_1$-proteinase inhibitor. Journal of Biological Chemistry 260: 4384–4389
Villaneuva G B 1984 Predictions of the secondary structure of human antithrombin III and the location of the heparin binding site. Journal of Biological Chemistry 259: 2531–2536
Winter J H, Bennett B, Watt J L, Brown T, San Roman C, Schinzel A, King J, Cook P J L 1982 Confirmation of linkage between antithrombin III and Duffy blood group and assignment of ATIII to 1q22–q25. Annals of Human Genetics 46: 29–34
Ye R D, Wun T C, Sadler J E 1987 cDNA cloning and expression in *Escherichia coli* of a plasminogen activator inhibitor from human placenta. Journal of Biological Chemistry 262: 3718–3725

4. The laboratory diagnosis of lupus anticoagulants

Douglas A. Triplett   Linda Barna

INTRODUCTION

The term 'lupus anticoagulant' (LA) is both an unfortunate misnomer and clinically misleading (Triplett & Brandt 1988). The majority of patients with LA *do not* have systematic lupus erythematosus (Shapiro & Thiagarajan 1982). LA are found in a variety of clinical conditions and not infrequently may be detected in an apparently normal individual (Table 4.1). The term 'anticoagulant' suggests to most physicians the possibility of clinical haemorrhage (Margolius et al 1961). However, paradoxically, LA are infrequently associated with bleeding and often linked to thromboembolic

Table 4.1 Clinical conditions associated with LA

I. Autoimmune diseases
- A. Systemic lupus erythematosus
- B. Rheumatoid arthritis
- C. Primary antiphospholipid syndrome
- D. Others, including 'overlap' syndromes

II. Drug exposure
- A. Chlorpromazine
- B. Procainamide
- C. Hydralazine
- D. Quinidine
- E. Antibiotics
- F. Phenytoin

III. Infections
- A. Bacterial
- B. Protozoan (*Pneumocystis carinii*)
- C. Viral

IV. Lymphoproliferative disorders
- A. Hairy cell leukaemia
- B. Malignant lymphoma
- C. Waldenström's macroglobulinemia

V. Miscellaneous disorders
- A. Epithelial malignancies
- B. No underlying disease

Table 4.2 Predisposing causes for bleeding in patients with LA

Specific inhibitors
Factor VIII
Factor II
Thrombocytopaenia
Platelet dysfunction
Uraemia
Concomitant drug administration (e.g. aspirin)

phenomena (Bowie et al 1963, Elias & Eldor 1984, Lechner 1987). Although a variety of alternate names (e.g. phospholipid-dependent anticoagulant, antiphospholipid anticoagulant, non-specific inhibitor of the APTT (activated partial thromboplastin time) and lupus-like anticoagulant) have been proposed, the majority of participants at the 1989 LA Subcommittee of the Scientific and Standardization Committee (SSC) recommended the continued use of the current name.

Two early papers described circulating anticoagulants which in retrospect appear to have been LA (Aggeler et al 1946, Mueller et al 1951). Mueller et al identified a number of characteristics which are now used to diagnose LA. In their study, they found the plasma anticoagulant activity was inversely proportional to the amount of phospholipid present, and the anticoagulant effect could be diminished by addition of 'washed blood cells' which contained platelets. However, the paper by Conley & Hartmann (1952) is generally cited as the first description of LA. Although this report suggested that these anticoagulants were associated with clinical bleeding, it was soon appreciated that LA were only associated with bleeding if there were additional risk factors (Table 4.2) (Shapiro & Thiagarajan 1982, Triplett & Brandt 1988). The term 'lupus anticoagulant' was first proposed by Feinstein and Rapaport (1972).

Patients who are found to have circulating anticoagulants present an important diagnostic challenge to the haemostasis laboratory (Hougie 1985). Anticoagulants which are specific for a single coagulation protein (e.g. factor VIII:C, factor IX) are associated with significant clinical bleeding which on occasion can be life threatening (Hougie 1985). Conversely, LA may be associated with thrombosis (Bowie et al 1963, Lechner 1987). Therefore, the correct identification of an inhibitor is imperative. A classification of circulating anticoagulants is presented in Table 4.3. This chapter will focus on the detection of circulating anticoagulants, and the necessary confirmatory procedures to diagnose LA.

CHARACTERIZATION OF LA

LA may be defined as immunoglobulins either IgG/IgM (or both) which interfere with *in vitro* phospholipid-dependent tests of coagulation (e.g.

Table 4.3 Classification of circulating anticoagulants (Triplett 1985)

1.	Specific
	a. Neutralizing
	Factor VIII
	Factor IX
	Factor XI
	Factor XIII
	Fibrinogen
	von Willebrand factor
	b. Non-neutralizing
	Factor VIII
	von Willebrand factor
	Prothrombin
	Factor X
II.	Non-specific
	LA
	Paraproteins
	Fibrin split products
III.	Global
	Heparin-like activity

prothrombin time (PT), APTT, Russell Viper Venom Time (RVVT) (Triplett & Brandt 1988). These antibodies do not specifically inhibit any of the coagulation proteins, rather, they appear to be directed at phospholipid epitopes. Early case reports of LA emphasized the frequent association with biological false-positive tests for syphilis (BFP–STS), a reaction that depends on the presence of cardiolipin (Laurell & Nilsson 1957, Johansson & Lassus 1974). Also flocculation tests of liver function such as the cephalin flocculation test or thymol turbidity test were often found to be abnormal (Frick 1955). Laurell & Nilsson (1957) were the first to demonstrate the ability of cardiolipin and Kahn antigen to adsorb LA from plasma. However, the first definitive proof of LA phospholipid specificity was provided by Thiagarajan et al (1980). They isolated a monoclonal IgM from a patient plasma which demonstrated LA activity in a variety of in vitro coagulation assays. This antibody reacted with negatively charged phospholipids in agarose gels and also inhibited the binding of radiolabelled prothrombin and factor X to phospholipid micelles. These experiments thus documented the phospholipid specificity of LA and also offered a plausible explanation for the lack of bleeding.

Antiphospholipid antibodies (APA) have stimulated a great deal of interest in a variety of medical specialties including rheumatology, cardiology, neurology, obstetrics, internal medicine and pathology (Hughes 1983, Harris et al 1984a, 1985, Asherson 1988, Harris 1990a). LA represent one member group of this family of antibodies (Table 4.4). The rheuma-

Table 4.4 Family of antiphospholipid antibodies

I.	Reagin (BFP–STS)
II.	Lupus anticoagulants (LA)
III.	Anticardiolipin antibodies (ACA)
IV.	Antibodies to anionic phospholipids (APA)

tologists have recently emphasized the importance of anticardiolipin antibodies (ACA). Initially, Harris et al suggested ACA and LA were very closely related (Harris et al 1983). In their original study, Harris et al (1983) found a strong degree of concordance between ACA detected by a solid phase radioimmunoassay and LA. However, subsequent studies have not confirmed the original observations (Exner et al 1988, Triplett et al 1988, Exner & McRea 1990d). Consequently, it is often necessary for laboratories to test for both LA using coagulation-based assay systems and ACA or APA (e.g. antibodies to all anionic phospholipids) using solid phase assays (radioimmunoassay (RIA), enzyme-linked immunosorbent assay (ELISA)) (Loizou et al 1985).

CLINICAL CONSIDERATIONS

LA may be detected in a wide variety of patients. For years they were regarded as a laboratory nuisance which often initiated an extensive and expensive laboratory evaluation. Not infrequently, the tests were inconclusive and the patient did not bleed despite a surgical challenge. With the increased awareness of the association of LA with several significant clinical complications (Triplett & Brandt 1988), the laboratory is now frequently asked: 'does my patient have a lupus anticoagulant?'. This question is in contrast to the previous situation where the majority of LA were detected by serendipity.

LA have been associated with both venous and arterial thromboembolic events (Lechner 1987). Pulmonary emboli are a frequent complication of venous thrombi while stroke is often seen with cerebral artery thrombosis (Hughes 1983, Sidor et al 1986). A number of obstetrical complications have been linked to LA and ACA (Fig. 4.1) (Triplett 1989a, Triplett & Harris 1990). There is a high incidence of recurrent fetal death or spontaneous abortions in women with these antibodies (Lubbe et al 1984). Initially, there appeared to be an association of placental infarction with the fetal losses (deWolf et al 1982). However, more recent work has emphasized placental insufficiency as the most common placental pathology (Triplett 1989a). Other obstetrical complications include early-onset hypertension, premature delivery, and a peculiar postpartum syndrome characterized by polyserositis.

Patients with LA or ACA may present with a variety of bewildering clini-

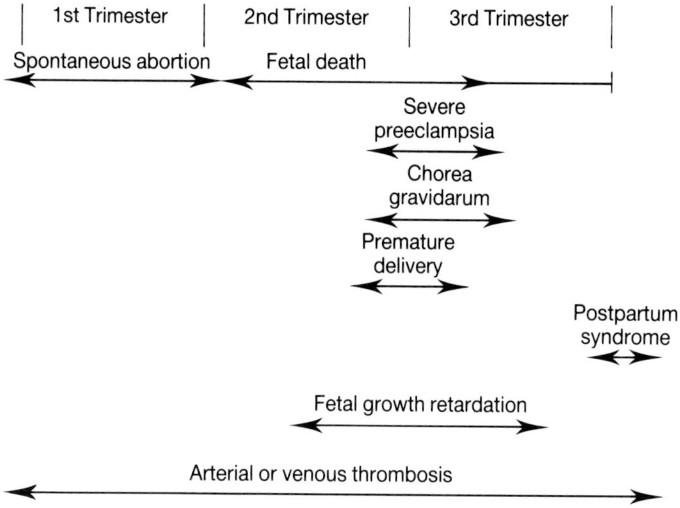

Fig. 4.1 Obstetrical complications and APA.

cal symptoms or physical findings. A number of neurological findings have been linked to LA including Sneddon's syndrome and myelitis (Rebollo et al 1983, Kushner & Simonian 1989). The dermatologic finding of livedo reticularis has been frequently associated with LA (Sontheimer 1987). Thus, awareness of LA is truly of importance to all medical specialities (Harris 1990a).

The pathophysiology of the various clinical complications is still unresolved. Indeed, there remains the question as to whether LA are causative or merely epiphenomena (Triplett & Brandt 1988). Nevertheless, a number of speculative mechanisms have been proposed to explain the thrombotic and obstetrical complications. Carreras et al (1982) were the first to suggest the endothelial cell as a possible target for LA. They demonstrated a decreased production of prostacyclin (PGI_2) by cultured endothelial cells incubated with LA patient samples. Since PGI_2 is a potent vasodilator and an inhibitor of platelet aggregation, these findings offered a very plausible explanation for thrombosis. However, subsequent studies using homologous cultured endothelial cells have been unable to confirm the original study (LeRoux et al 1986, Walker et al 1988, Schorer et al 1989). Other proposed mechanisms have focused on the potential of LA to interfere with the various regulatory systems of haemostasis. Since LA inhibit phospholipid-dependent reactions, the activation of protein C has been an attractive field of study. Several investigators have found LA will inhibit the activation of protein C by the thrombin–thrombomodulin complex on the surface of endothelial cells (Freyssinet et al 1986a, b, Tsakiris et al 1990). A potential second site of inhibition of the protein C system is the assembly and activity of activated protein C and protein S on the surface of endothelial cells or platelets (Marciniak & Romond 1989). Another potential site of LA-induced prothrombotic change is the interaction of heparan sulphate (HS) and antithrombin III (ATIII) (Cosgriff & Martin 1981). The HS–ATIII reaction also occurs on the surface of endothelial cells (Rosenberg & Rosenberg 1984, Nawroth & Stern 1985). Thus, although there is no accepted single explanation for LA-induced thrombosis, there appears to be a growing consensus that the anticoagulant properties on the surface of endothelial cells are the most likely candidates. Based on the laboratory heterogeneity of LA it is logical to assume there will be multiple pathophysiological mechanisms associated with LA (Coots et al 1981, Triplett et al 1985, Horellou et al 1987).

LABORATORY DIAGNOSIS OF LA

Criteria for the diagnosis of LA are not well established. In 1983, the Working Party on Acquired Inhibitors of Coagulation of the International Committee on Thrombosis and Haemostasis (ICTH) proposed the following criteria:

1. Prolongation of the APTT
2. APTT of a 1:1 mixture of patient/normal plasma should be greater than 4 s over the control
3. A decrease in at least two factors (VIII, IX, XI or XII) by one-stage assay, with normal values by two-stage assay
4. A sensitivity to dilution so that the apparent activity of the measured factor increases with dilution (Green et al 1983).

In our experience, these criteria have proved to be too stringent and incompatible with modern laboratory practice. Specifically, mixing studies are very difficult to interpret with mildly prolonged clotting times and factor assays may not show an apparent reduction in activity and non-parallelism of the assay curves (Raman & Saeed 1988). Furthermore, few routine laboratories are capable of performing two-stage factor assays. Based on the working definition of LA, minimal criteria for the diagnosis include:

1. An abnormality of phospholipid-dependent coagulation test(s)
2. Proof that the abnormality is due to an inhibitor
3. Inhibitor activity is directed at phospholipid (not specific coagulation factors) (Triplett & Brandt 1988).

Thus, a logical laboratory approach to the diagnosis of LA is divided into three distinct steps: screening procedures to identify coagulation abnormalities, procedures to identify the inhibitory nature of the abnormality and procedures to identify the phospholipid dependence of the inhibitor.

Prior to discussing these sequential steps, the importance of specimen collection and processing must be emphasized (Triplett and Brandt 1989, Triplett et al 1989b,c). The blood collection should be carefully monitored to ensure a clean venipuncture and expeditious transport to the laboratory. Perhaps the most important preanalytical variable is the preparation of platelet-poor plasma (PPP). The more platelet free the sample, the greater the sensitivity of most test systems to the presence of LA (McGlasson et al 1989). Furthermore, the ability to detect LA when plasma has been frozen is severely compromised by residual platelets in PPP. Ideally the PPP should have a platelet count of less than 10×10^9/litre (LA Working Party 1990). In order to achieve this goal, it is usually necessary to either employ double centrifugation or filtration of the plasma. Filtration of PPP through a 0.22 μm cellulose acetate syringe filter yields an optimal PPP (Exner 1985). If the PPP is going to be frozen, the use of filtration is strongly recommended (Exner 1985). Normal control plasma should also be prepared in a similar fashion. If a commercial source of normal plasma is utilized, it is important to obtain information from the manufacturer regarding residual platelets or platelet fragments.

Prolonged APTT

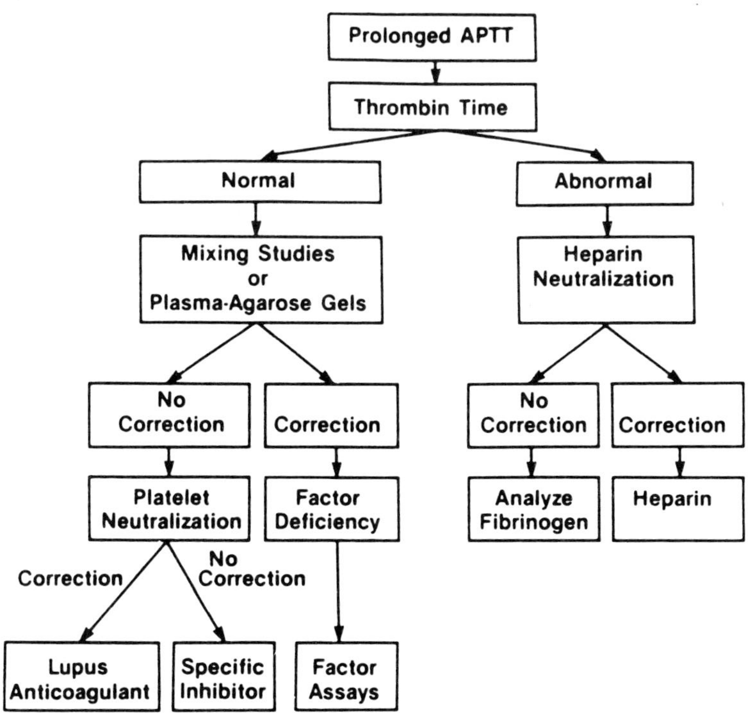

Fig. 4.2 Laboratory approach to an unexplained prolonged HPTT.

A variety of tests have been utilized to screen for the presence of LA. Each of these tests has its advocates, and there is often discussion as to the most 'sensitive' test (Lesperance et al 1988). Presently, there is no agreement regarding the most sensitive test. However, it is apparent that no *single* test will detect all LA (Triplett 1989b). This is no doubt due to the marked heterogeneity of LA. Therefore, laboratories should offer more than one screening test. This is of particular importance when a clinician refers a patient with a highly suggestive clinical history for LA. If the routinely performed screening procedure is normal, the laboratory should then employ a second screening test.

Activated Partial Thromboplastin Time

Commonly used screening tests are summarized in Table 4.5. The APTT is the most commonly used procedure (Kitchen 1988). The popularity of the APTT is due to its ease of performance, ready availability in virtually every laboratory, ease of automation, and the high quality of commercial reagents (Triplett 1989b). The sensitivity of the APTT to LA varies depending on the test system (i.e. reagent–instrument combination). Until recently, reagent manufacturers did not consider LA sensitivity of their reagents important. With the increasing interest in LA, many manufacturers are now designing reagents which are sensitive to LA. Nevertheless, there is well-document variability among APTT reagents (Mannucci et al 1979, Brandt et al 1987). Consequently, laboratories should carefully evaluate reagents and select a product which is sensitive to LA (Triplett 1989b). Several different approaches have been used to evaluate APTT reagent sensitivity to LA. These include individual institutional evaluations, interlaboratory evaluations and national/international proficiency testing programmes (Machin et al 1990, Exner et al, 1991). A major problem with any such study is the choice of the 'reference reagent' which was used to identify the LA. As a result, each study has an inherent bias. The availability of LA standards or a reference system which simulates a LA effect in coagulation testing is highly desirable. Perhaps the use of the antibiotic polymyxin B will provide a useful means of evaluating reagent sensitivity to LA (Uchman & Triplett 1989). An extract of Brown Recluse Spider Venom also offers promise as a potential artificial reference system (McGlasson et al 1988).

The sensitivity of any APTT is dependent on the quality of PPP. The effect of residual platelets will be most evident on APTT performed on freeze–thawed plasma. Other variables include the choice of reagent and instrumentation. In most cases, instruments and reagents made by the same company perform the best.

APTT reagents contain an activator and phospholipid (Proctor & Rapaport 1961). The phospholipid may be of animal or vegetable origin. APTT reagents which utilize the same source of phospholipid often differ

Table 4.5 Screening tests for LA

	Test system				
Test	Phospholipid	Other features	Advantages	Disadvantages	Sensitivity ranking
APTT	Varying animal or vegetable sources Varying PL composition and concentration	Variable activators: ellagic acid (soluble); kaolin, micronized silica (particulate)	Readily available, easily automated, can be used in PL confirmatory step	Reagents vary widely in sensitivity to LA	2
Kaolin clotting time (KCT)	No added PL, few residual platelets	Add kaolin; use mixtures of normal and patient plasma	May be used if patient is on oral anticoagulants	Very sensitive to residual platelets. Not readily automated; cannot be used for PL confirmation	4
Dilute, Russell's viper venom time (dRVVT)	Dilute PL	Variable source of RVV	Easy to perform, readily available	Manual technique; affected by heparin or oral anticoagulants	3
Plasma clot time (PCT)	No added PL, use PRP	Addition of platelets to patient PRP may shorten prolonged value due to LA	Requires no reagents or equipment	Must be performed on freshly drawn blood, manual technique	1

This table summarizes characteristics of the various screening tests used to evaluate patient samples for the presence of LA. Each of these tests has been evaluated in non-pregnant populations. Consequently, the sensitivity ranking is based on a population of males and non-pregnant females. Pregnancy presumably has the most effect on the ability of the APTT to detect LA. The other tests are not significantly altered by the changes in blood coagulation associated with pregnancy.

PL, phospholipid; RVV, Russell viper venom; PRP, platelet-rich plasma.

in their sensitivity to LA. Thus, other properties of the phospholipid apparently determine sensitivity to LA. The composition (e.g. relative amounts of individual phospholipids: phosphatidylserine (PS), phosphatidic acid (PA), phosphatidylinositol (PI)) and concentration of phospholipid may significantly affect reagent sensitivity. Kelsey et al (1984) found an inverse relationship between concentration of PS and LA sensitivity. In addition, the physical state of the phospholipid may be of great importance (Stevenson et al 1986). Rauch et al (1986) have reported that monoclonal LA recognize phospholipids in a hexagonal configuration but not in the physiological lamellar state. Unfortunately, reagent manufacturers do not provide extensive information regarding the phospholipid properties of their reagents.

A number of performance characteristics are useful in evaluating APTT reagents. These include: sensitivity (ability to differentiate normal from abnormal); responsiveness (time to clot formation); range of responsiveness (range of values over which the response remains predictable and can be measured by the technique used); precision (coefficient of variation); stability (inter- and intra-lot performance) (Brandt et al 1987). Generally, sensitive reagents are also responsive. However, this is not always the case. Responsiveness is an important criterion for reagent selection since a responsive reagent will yield fewer borderline prolonged APTT results which often lead to confusing and frustrating mixing studies. Another important variable in reagent evaluation is the *heterogeneity* of individual patient samples (Triplett et al 1985). Thus, it is not uncommon to encounter a patient whose LA is readily demonstrable with an 'insensitive' reagent and only minimally prolonged with a 'sensitive' reagent.

A number of comparative studies on APTT LA sensitivity have been reported (Table 4.6). However, it is difficult to identify the most sensitive reagent since the study results vary widely even with the same reagent. These differences may be due to study design, patient population, techniques, preparation of PPP, and lot-to-lot variability of reagents. Consequently, each laboratory should carefully select a reagent which has been thoroughly evaluated with respect to LA sensitivity and responsiveness. In addition, each laboratory must carefully determine their own normal range. Minimally prolonged APTT should not be ignored (Fig. 4.2)!

Kaolin clotting time

The Kaolin clotting time (KCT) is simply an APTT without added platelet substitute (Margolis 1958). The KCT has proved to be a sensitive screening test for identification of LA (Exner et al 1978). In order to optimize the KCT, meticulous attention must be used in preparing PPP. The presence of residual platelets will significantly impair sensitivity (Exner 1985). The KCT is more sensitive to residual platelets than either the prothrombin time (PT) or APTT.

Table 4.6 Comparative evaluations of APTT reagent sensitivity to LA

Mannucci et al (1979)	Green et al (1983)	Stevenson et al (1986)	Triplett et al (1985)	Johns et al (1989)	Lupus Anticoagulant Working Party (1990)
Bio–Merieux 10/10	GD (Platelin-Plus) 23/23	Manchester APTT 7/7	GD (Automated APTT) 50/50	Dade (Actin FSL) 33/45	Manchester
Manchester 9/10	Dade (Actin) 23/23	Dade (Actin) 6/7	Diatech (Diacelin) 49/49	Bio–Merieux (Cephalite) 18/45	Diagen BA
Immuno 9/10	Behring PTT 23/23	GD (Automated APTT 6/7	Dade (Actin) 49/49	GD (Automated APTT) 10/45	Diagen KP
Behringwerke 8/10		Ortho (Activated Thrombofax) 6/7	Ortho (Activated Thrombofax) 47/47		Boehringer BCL
Hyland 8/10		Dade (Actin FS) 5/7	Helena (APTT) 45/50		
Nygaard 8/10			Pacific Hemostasis (Thromboscreen) 44/50		
Boehringer 7/10			Dade (Actin FS) 40/49		
Dade (Actin) 6/10					
Ortho 6/10					
GD (Automated APTT) 5/10					

Several studies have evaluated the sensitivity of APTT reagents to LA. The ratios following each reagent represent in the denominator the number of patients studied and in the numerator the number of patients identified with an abnormal APTT. Reagents are listed in order of decreasing sensitivity to LA.

Margolis (1958) suggested a platelet count of less than 15 000 × 10^9/litre was necessary for optimal sensitivity and precision. More recently, the LA Working Party of the BCSH Haemostasis and Thrombosis Task Force of the British Society for Haematology recommended less than 10 000 × 10^9/litre (1990). Perhaps the best screen of an adequate KCT test is to evaluate normal individuals. If normal subjects give a KCT of less than 60 s then there is a high probability of significant residual platelets in the PPP.

Two variations of the KCT have been utilized. Exner et al (1978) have emphasized the use of mixtures of patient and normal plasmas with multiple determinations of the KCT on the mixtures. This approach has yielded four patterns of graphical results. The presence of a LA is characterized by convexity of the curve near the origin. Since the KCT is a manual procedure, this method is extremely time consuming and it also requires significant volumes of patient plasma. The second approach uses a KCT determined on the patient plasma only (Gibson et al 1988). For laboratories with a large volume of patient samples, the simple KCT is recommended. Although comparative studies evaluating screening procedures for LA suggest the KCT is not as sensitive as the APTT (Table 4.7), Lubbe and Liggins (1988) suggested that the KCT is the most sensitive test system for identifying LA in the setting of pregnancy. A distinct disadvantage of the KCT is an inability to use this test in the confirmatory step of LA diagnosis (e.g. phospholipid correction).

A slightly different approach which utilizes the KCT has been suggested by Rosner et al (1987). Their format expresses the result of the KCT as the KCT index. The KCT index is derived from the following formula: $\frac{(c-b)/}{/a} \times 100$ where *a* is the KCT of patient plasma, *b* is the KCT of normal plasma and *c* is the KCT of the mixture of patient and normal plasma. The most sensitive mixture is 4:1 (normal:patient) (Gibson et al 1988). The normal KCT index is <15%,

Dilute Russell viper venom time

The dilute Russell viper venom time (dRVVT) has been used both as a screening test and a confirmatory test in the diagnosis of LA (Thiagarajan et al 1986) (Fig. 4.3). The dRVVT suffers from many of the same problems encountered with the APTT. The source of phospholipid used in the assay will significantly alter the results. Brandt and Triplett (1989) evaluated three different phospholipids in the dRVVT system. There was a marked variability among the three dRVVT and the sensitivity was significantly less than the APTT. This lack of sensitivity may be due to the fact the dRVVT evaluates two phospholipid coagulation steps whereas the APTT evaluates three. Exner et al (1990a) have observed patients with abnormal APTT results and normal dRVVT. In their experience these LA are most often IgM isotypes.

Table 4.7 Comparative studies of screening procedures

Study	KCT		APTT		dRVVT		PCT	
	Ratio	Percentage	Ratio	Percentage	Ratio	Percentage	Ratio	Percentage
Gastineau et al (1985)	—	—	96/111	86	—	—	196/202	97
Thiagarajan et al (1986)	—	—	24/29	83	29/29	100	—	—
Raman & Saeed (1988)	59/84	70	84/84	100	47/84	56	—	—
Lo et al (1989)	18/18	100	16/18	89	17/18	94	15/18	83
Liu et al (1989)	14/14	100	9/14	64	14/14	100	—	—
Lazarchick & Kizer (1989)	—	—	19/21	90	13/14	93	—	—
Brandt et al (1989)	56/62	90	52/62	85	37/62	60	—	—
Forastiero et al (1989)	33/52	63	50/52	96	48/52	92	—	—
Johns et al (1989)	20/45	44	33/45	73	35/45	78	—	—
Summary	200/275	73	384/415	93	261/318	82	211/220	96

The ratios listed under each procedure heading are the number of patients studied in the denominator and the number of abnormal results in the numerator (Triplett 1989b)

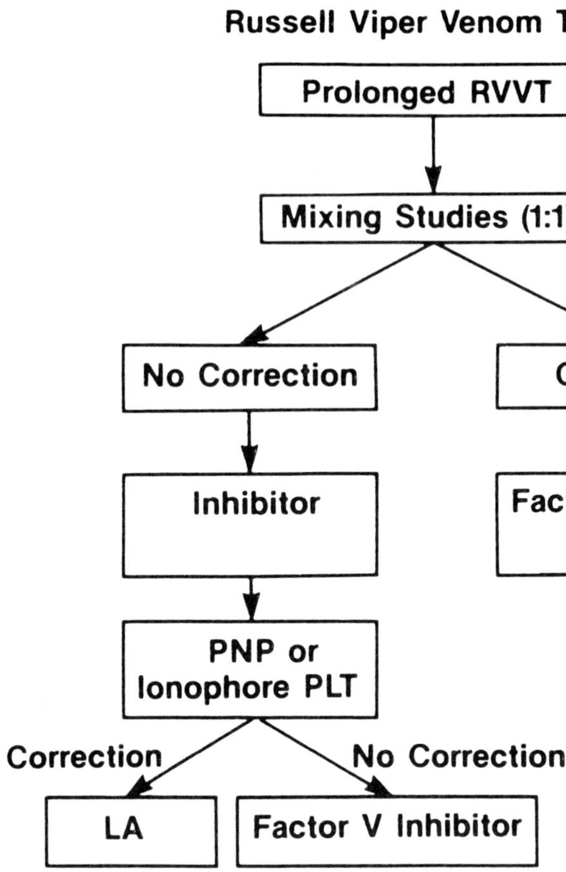

Fig. 4.3 Suggested laboratory approach for detection of LA utilising the dRVVT. PNP: platelet neutralization procedure; ionophore treated platelets.

Another disadvantage of the dRVVT is the need to perform the test manually. However, this will be addressed by the availability of a combined reagent (Russell viper venom and phospholipid) (Exner et al 1990a). With this reagent, the dRVVT can be automated utilizing the PT mode on available coagulation analysers. However, with the combined reagent, it will no longer be possible to utilize the dRVVT as a confirmatory test.

Plasma clot time

The plasma clot time (PCT) has been used by several investigators as a screening procedure to identify LA (Gastineau et al 1985). An obvious paradox in this test system is the use of platelet-rich plasma (PRP). Gastineau et al (1985) found the PCT to be more sensitive than the APTT in identifying LA. A potential explanation for the sensitivity of the PCT despite the presence of platelets is the possible inhibitor effect of LA on platelet function in the PCT. Perhaps the platelets are 'coated' with LA, thus preventing the assembly of the prothrombinase complex in vitro. Supporting this concept is the corrective effect (shortened PCT) of heterologous platelets when added to the patients' PRP.

A major disadvantage of the PCT is the absolute requirement for a fresh sample. The sample *cannot* be frozen to be evaluated at a later time or referred to another laboratory .

Summary of screening tests for LA

Table 4.7 summarizes a comprehensive review of the literature evaluating comparative studies of screening tests (Triplett 1989b). The PCT appears to be slightly more sensitive than the APTT; however, for most laboratory settings, the PCT is not practical. In addition, the PCT can only be performed on fresh plasma. Consequently, the APTT appears to be the best test to screen for LA. However, there is no single test which will identify all patients with LA. Therefore, it is appropriate for a laboratory to use *two* screening tests when evaluating difficult patients.

Demonstration of an inhibitor

Mixing studies

Once an abnormality of a screening procedure has been identified, it is necessary to document the presence of an inhibitor. In a hospital setting, the presence of heparin must be excluded before proceeding with this step in establishing the diagnosis of LA. Usually a thrombin time will successfully identify heparin. Once heparin has been excluded, mixing studies are performed. A variety of approaches has been described; however, the use of a ratio of patient to normal plasma of 4:1 will detect the majority of inhibitors including those with a minimally prolonged APTT (Biggs and Bidwell 1959, Ewing & Kaspar 1982, Raman & Saeed 1988).

Appropriate attention to the source of 'normal' plasma is required (Kaczor et al 1991). The presence of residual platelets in a pooled 'normal' plasma may result in correction of a prolonged screening test thus suggesting that the patient's abnormality is a factor deficiency. Unless a well-characterized commercial plasma is available, it is suggested that the laboratory utilize a filtered pooled 'normal' plasma for mixing studies.

Although most textbooks stress the 'immediate' effect of LA in mixing studies, recent studies have found this not to be the case (Clyne & White 1988). Consequently, it is important to incubate mixtures of patient and normal plasmas for at least 60 min and preferably 120 min. If this is not a part of the laboratory testing, approximately 15–20% of LA may be missed.

Plasma–agarose gels

The plasma–agarose gel is an alternate approach which is particularly useful in situations where the APTT is minimally prolonged (Bird 1975, Bird & Rizza 1975). These gels are easy to prepare, require no special equipment, and remove the ambiguity of interpreting 'borderline' mixing studies. Various modifications of the plasma–agarose gel have been described. The original technique utilized PPP mixed with 2% low-melting point agarose (Bird 1975). However, the modification reported by Cassidy and colleagues (1985) included a source of phospholipid added to the plasma–agarose mixture. Presumably, residual platelets in the PPP supplied the source of phospholipid in the original procedure.

Originally, the plasma–agarose gels were utilized to demonstrate factor VIII:C inhibitors (Bird et al 1975, Coots et al 1985). In the presence of inhibitors, the typical opacity which forms following the addition of calcium chloride solution to the plate will not occur in concentric areas surrounding patient application wells. In many respects, this finding is analogous to the zone of inhibition seen with the Kirby–Bauer antibiotic sensitivity plates utilized in microbiology. Unfortunately, these gels will not differentiate between the various inhibitors encountered in patient plasmas.

Attempts to incubate either freeze–thawed platelets or phospholipid with patient plasmas prior to gel application have no effect on the zone of inhibition seen with LA samples (Exner et al 1990b). Correspondingly, no effect was seen when the phospholipid or platelets were included in the gels. Thus, this test system is not sensitive to the 'bypass' or 'neutralizing' effect of phospholipid on LA. The plasma–agarose gels may be very useful in detecting LA in plasmas which have been frozen with significant residual platelets.

Austen and Rhymes test

This procedure detects immunoglobulin inhibitors and is not specific for LA (Austen & Rhymes 1975). The patient plasma is first adsorbed by aluminium hydroxide for 3 min followed by centrifugation for 15 min. The supernatant is then pipetted into a second test tube and incubated at 56°C for 30 min. To demonstrate an inhibitor, the treated plasma is mixed with an equal volume of normal plasma and an APTT is performed. In addition to a lack of specificity, this test is not particularly sensitive. In a recent UK National External Quality Assessment Scheme (NEQAS) survey, this test performed very poorly when compared to the KCT, dilute tissue thromboplastin inhibition test (TTI) and dRVVT (Machin et al 1990).

ESTABLISHING PHOSPHOLIPID DEPENDENCE OF THE INHIBITOR

Following the identification of an inhibitor as the cause of a prolonged screening test, it must be further characterized. LA must be clearly distinguished from specific factor inhibitors (e.g. factor VIII:C) because the latter are associated with a significant risk of bleeding while the former are not. Therefore, it is imperative to correctly characterize any inhibitor.

Two basic approaches have been utilized in the design of test systems to document phospholipid dependence (Table 4.8). Both approaches rely on the inverse relationship between the phospholipid content of the test system and the degree of prolongation of the coagulation test. In some tests (KCT, TTI, dilute phospholipid APTT or dRVVT), the amount of phospholipid is reduced to accentuate the prolonged coagulation times in the presence of LA (Alving et al 1985). The second approach is designed to 'neutralize' or 'bypass' the inhibitor by increasing the amount of phospholipid in the test system (platelet neutralization procedure (PNP) or rabbit brain neutralization procedure (RBNP)).

Only the most commonly used confirmatory procedures will be discussed. Both the dRVVT and APTT were mentioned earlier in the section dealing with screening procedures; however, these tests may be modified for confirmatory testing. Due to its exquisite sensitivity to platelets, the KCT cannot be used as a confirmatory procedure.

Table 4.8 Confirmatory procedures to identify LA

I.	Test systems with decreased phospholipid
	Tissue thromboplastin inhibition
	Dilute Russell viper venom time
	Kaolin clotting time
	Dilute phospholipid APTT
II.	Test systems with increased phospholipid
	Platelet neutralization procedure
	High-phospholipid APTT
	Rabbit brain neutralization
	Phosphatidylserine–liposome APTT
	Hexagonal phospholipid neutralization
	Platelet-derived vesicles

Confirmatory procedures: reduced phospholipid

Tissue thromboplastin inhibition test. The TTI was previously the most commonly used test to confirm the diagnosis of LA (Schleider et al 1976, Liu et al 1989). Unfortunately, TTI is not specific for LA; consequently, reliance on the test as a diagnostic procedure is unfounded (Triplett et al 1983, Rosove et al 1986). False-positive results may be seen with specific factor inhibitors (e.g. factor VIII:C inhibitors), factor deficiencies (e.g. factor VIII:C, factor IX) and with anticoagulant therapy (Triplett et al 1983). One study suggested 40% of normal individuals will have an abnormal TTI (Rosove et al 1986)!

Too low a dilution of thromboplastin impairs sensitivity while higher dilution will affect specificity (Machin et al 1990). Although not as yet well studied, the origin of thromboplastin appears to significantly alter test results. Also, laboratories must utilize a well-characterized source of PPP for the 'normal' in this test system. IgM LA may yield normal TTI values (Shapiro et al 1982).

Dilute Russell viper venom time. The dRVVT is also used as a confirmatory procedure for LA. In some patients who are receiving immunosuppressive therapy, the APTT will return to normal, but the dRVVT will remain prolonged (Thiagarajan et al 1986).

Freeze–thawed platelets or ionophore-treated platelets may be substituted for phospholipid in the dRVVT test system (Thiagarajan et al 1986). Typically, addition of either will cause significant shortening of a prolonged dRVVT due to LA. False positives may be seen with heparin or factor V inhibitors. Presumably, the presence of platelet factor 4 in the freeze–thawed platelet preparation neutralizes heparin. Similarly, platelets are a source of factor V which potentially could neutralize a weak factor V inhibitor (Brandt et al 1986).

Confirmatory procedures: increased or altered phospholipid

Platelet neutralization procedure. The PNP is based on the ability of platelets to 'neutralize' or 'bypass' the in vitro effect of LA (Triplett et al 1983, Howard & Firkin 1983). Whether the platelet fragments 'neutralize' the LA immunoglobulin in a true antigen–antibody reaction or merely provide an 'excess' of phospholipid surface to bypass the LA is unknown. Given the marked heterogeneity of LA, both mechanisms may be important, although their relative contribution may vary from patient to patient. In early studies, platelets activated by ADP, collagen or ionophore A23187 were utilized (Howard & Firkin 1983, Thiagarajan et al 1986). Subse-

Table 4.9 Comparative sensitivity of TTI and PNP

Study	TTI		PNP	
	Ratio	Percentage	Ratio	Percentage
Lazarchick & Kizer (1989)	20/21	95	15/18	83
Kornberg et al (1989)	38/48	79	47/48	98
Triplett et al (1985)	8/10	80	10/10	100
Brandt et al (1987)	46/50	92	40/50	90
Brandt et al (1989)	65/93	70	86/93	92
Forastiero et al (1989)	24/52	46	46/50	92
Summary	201/274	73	249/269	93

Ratios represent the number of patients studied in the denominator and patients with abnormal results in the numerator (Triplett 1989b).

quently, the use of washed freeze–thawed platelets proved to be effective in significantly correcting the inhibitory effect of LA (Triplett et al 1983).

Because of its simplicity and relative sensitivity and specificity, the PNP has recently become the most commonly used confirmatory procedure for LA (Taberner et al 1987, Machin et al 1990). The PNP may be used with either the APTT or dRVVT (Dayton et al 1990). Recently, the LA Working Party on behalf of the BCSH Haemostasis and Thrombosis Task Force of the British Society for Haematology (1990) recommended the PNP with the dRVVT as the appropriate confirmatory test system. In the USA, the PNP is most frequently employed in the APTT test.

The TTI and PNP are the two most frequently used confirmatory tests. Several studies have compared these tests (Table 4.9) (Forastiero et al 1989, Johns et al 1989, Lo et al 1989). Based on the cumulative literature, the PNP is clearly the most sensitive and specific test.

False-positive PNP results may be seen with heparinized plasma or weak factor V inhibitors (Triplett et al 1983, Brandt et al 1986). Theoretically, factor XI inhibitors may also result in a false-positive result. Platelet membranes contain a factor XI-like material which appears to differ from plasma XI (Walsh 1974). Perhaps, in some cases, the factor XI antibody may be neutralized by the platelet XI. To date, this property of the PNP has not been systematically evaluated. One case of a factor XI inhibitor with an appropriately negative PNP has been reported (Musclow et al 1988).

Other tests with increased or altered phospholipid. A variety of additional tests have been described including the high-phospholipid APTT of Clyne et al (1980), the rabbit brain neutralization of Rosove et al (1980) and the phosphatidylserine liposome APTT of Kelsey et al (1984). Perhaps the most interesting recently described test is the hexagonal phospholipid neutralization procedure of Rauch et al (Rauch et al 1989).

Rauch and Janoff (1990) recently demonstrated the immunogenicity of hexagonal II phase phosphatidyl ethanolamine in an animal model. Previously, lipids were thought to be non-immunogenic. The antibodies to the hexagonal II phase phospholipid were found to react with cardiolipin and in addition they demonstrated LA activity. Perhaps in vivo membrane damage with hexagonal phase rearrangement of the physiological bilayer phase phospholipid may explain the appearance of APA in human subjects (Janoff & Rauch 1986).

Prior to demonstrating the immunogenicity of hexagonal II phase phosphatidylethanolamine, Rauch and coworkers (1986) had shown monoclonal hybridoma lupus anticoagulants could be inhibited by hexagonal II phase phosphatidylethanolamine. In a recent publication this group evaluated the ability of hexagonal II phase phosphatidylethanolamine to differentiate LA, factor deficiencies, specific factor inhibitors and heparin (Rauch et al 1989). Their test system utilized a dilute APTT in which patient plasma was preincubated with hexagonal II phase phosphatidylethanolamine. The hexagonal II phase phosphatidylethanolamine corrected the LA-containing plasmas by 81.2–99.5%. In contrast, plasmas with antibodies to factor VIII:C, factor deficiencies (e.g. XII, XI, VIII, V) and heparin were not affected by hexagonal II phase phosphatidylethanolamine. Thus, this system may be the most specific test for LA. Unfortunately, no commercial preparation of this phospholipid is currently available.

Another recently described test utilizes platelet vesicles which are generated by treating platelets with an ionophore. These vesicles were able to 'bypass' or 'neutralize' LA in a highly selective fashion (Arnout et al 1990).

Confirmatory procedures: factor assays

Occasionally, it is necessary to perform factor assays in order to establish the diagnosis of LA. When one-stage factor assays are performed on LA plasma the factors of the proximal intrinsic pathway are most commonly affected (Green et al 1983). Typically factors XII and XI are more affected than factors VIII and IX. With dilution of the patient's plasma, the apparent factor activity will increase. This lack of parallelism of the factor assay curves is typical of plasma containing an inhibitor.

When two-stage factor assays are performed, there is no apparent LA effect on the factor activity. Also, factor assays performed using synthetic substrates are usually not affected by the presence of LA.

Solid phase immunological assays for APA

Various tests for reagin have been used since the introduction of the Wassermann test in 1906. However, these tests are relatively insensitive. Consequently, Harris et al (1983) developed a solid phase radioimmunoassay for ACA. Since its introduction, ACA immunological assays have been modified in a number of laboratories. Currently, the preferred assay is an ELISA using cardiolipin, phosphatidylserine, or mixtures of phospholipids as the antigen coating the microtitre plates. Three international workshops have been conducted in an attempt to standardize the ELISA assay for ACA (Harris et al 1984b, 1985, Harris & Hughes 1988). As a result of these workshops, various sources of error have been identified. Harris et al (1985) have also provided a source of reference sera for IgG and IgM ACA.

Interpretation of ACA test results have been a source of frustration for many laboratories. Ideally, only strongly positive results should be used in decisions involving patient management. As a further precaution, the positive test should be reconfirmed after an appropriate time interval (e.g. 6 – 8 weeks). The incorporation of a reference sera with each run of patient tests will allow individual laboratories to express their results in G or M units as proposed by Harris et al (1985). The presence of a high-titre IgG ACA is of greater significance in identifying women at risk for abortion or thrombosis than IgM ACA. False-positive ACA tests are seen in patient samples with hypergammaglobulinaemia or rheumatoid factor. The incidence of ACA in a normal obstetrical population has varied from 22% reported by Laskin & Solonika (1988) to 1.2% identified by Harmon et al (1986). With the exception of Laskin's data these values are similar to those observed in normal blood donors or volunteers. Fields et al (1987) evaluated 706 blood donors and found an incidence of 5% ACA positivity. Manoussakis et al (1987) found an incidence of 2.3% in 261 blood donors. The positive results seen in normal pregnancies or blood donors are almost always of low titre. Therefore, each laboratory should establish a threshold value to identify a high-titre positive result (e.g. > 5 SD above the mean of the normal range).

An exciting recent observation was the description of a cofactor necessary for the expression of ACA activity in the ELISA test system (Galli et al 1990, McNeil et al 1990, Matsuura et al 1990). This plasma protein had been previously described as β_2-glycoprotein I or apolipoprotein H. This protein binds to anionic phospholipids and also functions as an inhibitor of the intrinsic pathway of coagulation. In the absence of this protein, known ACA-positive plasma will yield negative results in an ELISA assay (Galli et al 1990, McNeil et al 1990). Perhaps ACA recognize the antigenic configuration of cardiolipin and β_2-glycoprotein I when they are complexed. Appropriate experiments to study the effect of β_2-glycoprotein I in coagulation assays have not as yet been performed.

Summary

The laboratory diagnosis of LA is a common problem. Every laboratory should establish a systematic approach based on the three specific steps as outlined in this chapter. Since APTT reagents vary widely in their sensitivity to LA, a sensitive reagent should be used to screen patients for LA. Appropriate attention to the preparation of PPP is imperative for each of the three sequential diagnostic steps. The PNP test is the most specific of the various confirmatory procedures; however, on occasion, factor assays may be necessary.

Due to the marked individual variability of LA from patient to patient, more than one screening procedure may be indicated when there is a high index of clinical suspicion.

SCREENING PROCEDURES

Activated partial thromboplastin time

Principle

The APTT test consists of recalcifying plasma in the presence of a platelet-like phospholipid and an activator of the contact system (Proctor, & Rapaport 1961). Formation of a fibrin clot is measured manually or by mechanical or photo-optical instrumentation. This test is commonly employed in the clinical laboratory to monitor patients on heparin therapy (Brandt & Triplett 1981). It is a screening test for factor deficiencies in the intrinsic pathway, namely Fletcher factor (prekallikrein), Fitzgerald factor (high-molecular-weight kininogen), factors XII, XI, VIII, IX, V, X and II, and fibrinogen. The APTT test will not detect qualitative or quantitative platelet disorders nor factor VII and XIII deficiencies. The test is sensitive to the presence of specific and non-specific coagulation inhibitors including LA.

Specimen collection and preparation

Collect blood into 0.129 or 0.109 M sodium citrate in a ratio of blood to anticoagulant of 9:1. Place on ice immediately. Centrifuge at 1500 g for 10 min at 4°C. Draw off plasma, staying 0. 5–1 ml above the platelet layer and transfer to a stoppered plastic test tube. Keep plasma in an ice bath to prevent loss of labile coagulation factors. If testing is delayed, store plasma at –20°C or below. Further details of specimen handling are described by Triplett (1980).

Reagents

APTT reagents. Many commercial APTT reagents are available. They vary in phospholipid content and concentration and types of activator used. Follow the manufacturer's instructions for reagent preparation and handling.

Calcium chloride. Either 0.025 or 0.020 M calcium chloride is used depending on the manufacturer's recommendations for their APTT reagent. Calcium chloride solution is available commercially. Alternatively it may be prepared by weighing out anhydrous calcium chloride (0.025 M, 2.77 g; 0.020 M, 2.22 g) and using distilled water to make up a 1 litre solution. Once prepared, the solution should be stored at between 2 and 8°C.

Quality control

Lyophilized control plasmas for normal and abnormal ranges are commercially available through manufacturers of APTT reagents. Controls are run with each new vial of APTT reagent opened and reconstituted according to the manufacturer's directions. Control ranges for each new lot number of reagents and controls are determined.

Ideally the normal range for the APTT is established by collecting blood from at least 40 individuals representing the institutional population. Calculate the mean and standard deviation. In most laboratories the normal range is defined as ±2 SD from the mean.

Procedure

A. Photo-optical instrument.

1. Prepare the instrument for a run according to the manufacturer's directions.
2. Reconstitute reagents and controls.
3. Pipette 100 µl (0.1 ml) of test plasma into each cuvette or well.
4. Prime reagents lines.
5. Initiate test run.
6. After the run is complete, deprime reagents.

B. Fibrometer.

1. Place a test-tube with calcium chloride solution in the heat block to prewarm.
2. Add 100 µl of test sample and 100 µl of APTT reagent to a Fibrometer cup and incubate for the required time interval.
3. At the end of incubation add 100 µl of prewarmed calcium chloride solution and start timer.
4. The Fibrometer probe will stop when a fibrin clot is detected. Run samples in duplicate and average results .

C. *A manual method* (*tilt tube*) may also be used.

Normal values

Normal values are established by each laboratory.

Interpretation

Values significantly prolonged above the upper limit of normal suggest the following possibilities:

1. Heparin contamination from line draws

2. Patient taking oral anticoagulants or receiving heparin therapy
3. Factor deficiencies in the intrinsic pathway
4. Circulating anticoagulants:
   Specific
   Non-specific, e.g. LA
5. Vitamin K deficiency due to malabsorption or prolonged antibiotic therapy
6. Liver disease
7. Obstructive jaundice
8. Disseminated intravascular coagulation (DIC)
9. Fibrinolysis.

Shortened values occur in the presence of activated clotting factors in the plasma. Check the tube for evidence of clots or fibrin strands. Activated clotting factors in DIC patients may significantly shorten the APTT. Thus the APTT in DIC patients is variable. Haemolysed specimens shorten results due to the release of procoagulant substances, ADP and phospholipid, from the red cell membrane.

Heparin therapy and heparin contamination from line draws are the most common reasons for prolonged APTT in the clinical laboratory (Triplett 1982). LA, once viewed as 'laboratory nuisances' are an important cause of a prolonged APTT. LA are associated with thrombotic problems in several clinical situations. The most frequent congenital factor deficiencies are factor VIII (haemophilia A), factor IX (haemophilia B), and Von Willebrand's disease. Investigation of an abnormal APTT result must be pursued.

Technical notes

1. Severe lipaemia interferes with most photo-optical instruments.
2. Redraw specimens with evidence of clot formation, severe haemolysis or lipaemia.
3. Duplicate results should agree within 10% of each other. If they do not, repeat the test.

Kaolin clotting time

Principle

The KCT is an APTT without the addition of platelet phospholipid substitute and with kaolin added as the activator. This test is particularly sensitive to LA (Exner et al 1978). Depleting the test system of phospholipids accentuates the inhibitory effect of this antibody. Presumably platelet microparticles not removed by centrifugation or filtration provide a level of phospholipid adequate to support the clotting event. The KCT has not been successfully automated due to the particulate properties of kaolin.

Specimen collection and preparation (see p. 92)

Stability of frozen plasma is increased by filtration or double centrifugation.

Instrumentation

Fibrometer or a manual technique.

Reagents

2 % Kaolin

Kaolin (Sigma K-7375).

Weigh out 2 g of kaolin and make up to 100 ml with distilled water. For more practical usage, weigh out 500 mg of kaolin and make up to 25 ml with distilled water.

0.025 M calcium chloride. See p. 92.

Procedure

Fibrometer.

1. Pipette 0.2 ml of test plasma into a Fibrometer cup.
2. Add 0.1 ml of the 2% kaolin suspension and incubate for 3 min at 37°C.
3. Pipette 0.2 ml of prewarmed 0.025 M calcium chloride into the Fibrometer cup while simultaneously starting the Fibrometer.
4. Record the clotting time.

Manual method (tilt tube).

1. Preincubate 0.2 ml test plasma with 0.1 ml of 2% kaolin suspension for 3 min.
2. Add 0.2 ml prewarmed 0.025 M calcium chloride and start timing.
3. The endpoint is reached when the appearance of irreversible kaolin/fibrin aggregates is observed.

Normal values

Unfiltered platelet-poor plasma	70–120 s
Filtered platelet-free plasma	100–150 s

Interpretation

Prolonged values may be due to:

1. Heparin contamination from line draws
2. Patient taking oral anticoagulants or receiving heparin therapy

3. Factor deficiencies in the intrinsic pathway
4. Circulating anticoagulants
   Specific
   Non-specific, e.g. LA
5. Vitamin K deficiency due to malabsorption or prolonged antibiotic therapy
6. Liver disease
7. Obstructive jaundice
8. DIC
9. Fibrinolysis.

Technical notes

1. Residual platelets significantly shorten test results.
2. Freezing plasma may break platelets into microparticles not removed by centrifugation. Double centrifuge or filter plasma before freezing.
3. One of the disadvantages of the KCT is its inability to serve as a confirmatory test. Because it is extremely sensitive to residual platelets or other phospholipids, 'bypass' or 'neutralization' studies cannot be used.

Dilute Russell viper venom time

Principle

Russell viper venom directly activates factor X to Xa. The addition of viper venom to citrated plasma is therefore a useful test for measuring the formation of the prothrombinase complex: factors Xa, V, and II in the presence of phospholipid and calcium ions. Diluting the phospholipid in the RVVT increases test sensitivity to LA (Thiagarajan et al 1986). An advantage of the dRVVT is that it is not affected by contact factor abnormalities, factor IX deficiency, or the more common occurrences of congenital factor VIII deficiency and acquired factor VIII inhibitor (Triplett & Brandt 1988).

Specimen collection and preparation (See p. 92)

Note. The sensitivity of the dRVVT to LA is increased by ensuring the complete removal of platelets from plasma. This may be accomplished by double centrifugation or filtration. Use 0.22 μm syringe filters.

Instrumentation

Fibrometer.

Reagents

1. *Russell viper venom* (*Burroughs-Wellcome HA21*). Reconstitute according to the manufacturer's directions. Dilute the reconstituted venom 1:200 with Tris-buffered saline pH 7.4.
2. *Tris-buffered saline (0.15 M sodium chloride, 0.02 M Tris, pH 7.4).*
   Trizma base (Sigma T-1503)
   Sodium chloride (Sigma S-9625).
   To make a 1 litre solution use 8.77 g of sodium chloride and 2.42 g of Tris.
3. *0.03 M calcium chloride.* Weigh out 3.33 g of anhydrous calcium chloride and make up a 1 litre solution with distilled water.
4. *Phospholipid* (*e.g. Platelin* (*Organon Teknika*)). Reconstitute according to the manufacturer's directions. Dilute 1:8 with Tris-buffered saline.

Quality control

Pooled normal plasma may be used for a negative control and a known LA plasma for the positive control.

Procedure

1. Prewarm the calcium chloride solution to 37°C.
2. Into a Fibrometer cup pipette the following:
   0.1 ml of test plasma
   0.1 ml of diluted Russell viper venom
   0.1 ml of diluted phospholipid.
3. Incubate this mixture for 30 s.
4. At the end of 30 s, pipette 0.1 ml of calcium chloride into the Fibrometer cup while simultaneously starting the Fibrometer.
5. Record the clotting time.

Note. This test may also be performed manually.

Normal values

Normal plasma gives a dRVVT value of <35 s. See technical note 2.

Interpretation

The dRVVT is prolonged in:

1. The presence of LA
2. The presence of a factor V inhibitor
3. The plasma of patients with deficiencies of factors V and X, and fibrinogen. Addition of normal plasma will correct the dRVVT

4. Patients taking oral anticoagulants
5. The presence of heparin.

Technical notes

1. Several phospholipid reagents are commercially available. The sensitivity of the dRVVT to LA is affected by the phospholipid source (Brandt & Triplett 1989).
2. It is necessary that each laboratory establish its own normal range.

DEMONSTRATION OF AN INHIBITOR

Mixing studies

Principle

Performance of mixing studies is the first step in evaluating a prolonged APTT once heparin contamination has been ruled out. Mixing an equal volume of normal plasma with test plasma provides a quick screen to assist in differentiating between a factor deficiency and an inhibitor to coagulation. Normal plasma added to factor-deficient plasma will generally correct the APTT to within 5 s of the normal plasma value. If the prolonged APTT is due to an inhibitor, normal plasma will not correct the value (Feinstein & Rapaport 1972). Some shortening may be observed but there will still be a significant difference between the normal plasma value and that of the 1:1 mixture.

In the case of a factor deficiency, normal plasma returns a sufficient factor concentration level to the mixture for coagulation to proceed. If an inhibitor to a specific factor is present it will also inhibit the factor in the normal plasma, subsequently prolonging the APTT. With the lupus inhibitor, activity against the phospholipid in the test system will still be evident by a prolonged APTT. Addition of normal plasma will not correct this effect.

Mixing studies can be used with several test systems including the APTT, PT, KCT and the dRVVT.

Specimen collection and preparation (See p. 92)

Reagents

The test system used will depend on which screening test was prolonged. The most commonly performed test is the APTT but the PT may also be indicated.

APTT reagents. Many commercial APTT reagents are available. Follow the manufacturer's instructions for reagent preparation and handling.

Thromboplastin for the PT. Many thromboplastin reagents are available commercially. Follow the manufacturer's instructions for reagent preparation and handling.

Calcium chloride. Either 0.025 or 0.020 M calcium chloride is used, depending on the manufacturer's recommendations for their APTT reagent (See p. 92).

Normal plasma. Several sources are commonly used and include fresh pooled plasma, frozen pooled plasma and lyophilized commercial normal controls. The best results are gained with platelet-free pooled normal plasma. Citrated plasma is obtained from at least 20 healthy donors and double centrifuged or filtered to ensure platelet removal. The plasma is then pooled, divided into aliquots in plastic test tubes and stored at –20°C or below. Thaw at 37°C and use as needed.

The concentration of coagulation factors is often not known in normal lyophilized plasma. Once diluted in mixing studies a factor may be below its haemostatic level thus causing misinterpretation of test results. In addition, residual platelets or platelet membrane fragments in lyophilized plasma may yield a false-negative mixing study in a patient with LA.

Quality control

Incubate the patient plasma and pooled normal plasma separately at 37°C. Mix just prior to performing the APTT or other selected tests. This control will correct for non-specific time- and temperature-dependent loss of clotting activity in both the normal and patient plasmas.

Procedure

1. Prepare reagents according to the test to be performed.
2. Prepare test mixtures:

Tube	1	2	3	4	5
Patient plasma (ml)	—	0.2	0.5	0.8	1.0
Normal plasma (ml)	1.0	0.8	0.5	0.2	—

3. Immediately perform an APTT or PT on all tubes.
4. Incubate all plasmas at 37°C for 1 h and repeat step 3 above.
5. Repeat testing again after incubation for 2 h.
6. In addition, at the end of 2 h, mix equal volumes of incubated patient plasma and normal plasma. Perform an APTT and/or PT. (See section on quality control).

Interpretation

1. Immediate correction of a 1:1 mixture generally indicates a factor deficiency. However, factor VIII antibodies and occasionally LA are

time dependent and may not be detected by the immediate test. Testing at 1 and 2 h is recommended.
2. LA usually act immediately and are relatively infrequently time dependent. Most frequently, the 1:1 mixture does not correct the abnormal test.
3. A factor IX inhibitor is immediate acting. The 1:1 mixture does not correct.
4. The 4:1 patient plasma:normal plasma mixture (tube 4) is more sensitive to the presence of weak inhibitors (Triplett 1989).
5. Failure to correct in the 1:4 patient plasma:normal plasma mixture (tube 2) indicates a strong inhibitor.
6. Occasionally a mixing study APTT will yield a result more prolonged than the baseline APTT. This is known as the 'lupus cofactor effect'. The cause of this is unknown. Several plasma proteins in the normal plasma have been indicated. The 'cofactor effect' is most often demonstrated in the 4:1 patient plasma:normal plasma mixture.

Plasma–agarose gel for detection of coagulation inhibitors

Principle

Agarose containing fresh normal plasma and a source of phospholipid is poured onto a plate. The fresh normal plasma provides a haemostatic level of factors required for coagulation to proceed when calcium chloride solution is added. Patient and control plasmas are placed in wells cut into the agar and allowed to diffuse into the gel. After incubation for 1 h at 37°C, the plate is flooded with prewarmed calcium chloride solution. The agarose will turn cloudy or opaque as fibrin is formed in the agarose. If a patient has an inhibitor, a clear area, or zone of inhibition, will be seen surrounding the well containing that plasma (Bird 1975, Bird & Rizza 1975, Rainsford & Hall 1976).

Specimen collection and preparation (see p. 92)

Equipment and supplies

Gel bond (plate size, cut 8.3 × 10.3 cm) obtainable from FMC (1-800-341-1574) thickness 0.2 mm, size 100 × 150 mm
Levelling table
Well cutter (3.0 mm)
Water bath (54°C)
Pipettes (5.0 ml, 0.2 ml, 5 µl)
Plastic tubes
Parafilm.

Reagents

1. *Imidazole-buffered saline (IBS).*
   a. 5.85 g of sodium chloride
      3.4 g of imidazole
      186 ml of 0.01 N hydrochloric acid

      Place in 1 litre
      volumetric
      flask and add distilled water,
      to nearly 1 litre.
   b. Adjust pH to 7.3 ± 0.1 with hydrochloric acid or sodium hydroxide.
   c. Adjust final volume to 1 litre and mix well.
   d. Store at 4°C.
2. *(2%) agarose.*
   a. 1 g of ME agarose
      (SeaKem ME Agarose. FMC Co).
      50 ml of IBS
      Place in 125 ml Erlenmeyer flask and gently heat with continuous stirring until the agarose is completely dissolved.

   b. Place in water bath at 54°C and maintain at this temperature until needed. (A beaker may be placed over the top of the flask to prevent evaporation.)
3 *Pooled normal plasma.* Ideally collect citrated plasma from at least 20 normal donors. Remove residual platelets by double centrifugation or filtration to increase test sensitivity to LA. Use fresh or store at –20°C or below.
4. *APTT reagent.*
5. *Calcium chloride.* Either 0.025 or 0.020 M calcium chloride is used depending on the manufacturer's recommendations for their APTT reagent (See p. 92).
6. *4% formaldehyde.* Add distilled water to 40% formaldehyde and make up to 1 litre.

Quality control

1. Negative control. Pooled normal plasma.
2. Positive control. Use a known plasma that has an inhibitor.

Procedure

A. Preparation of plates

1. Prewarm 5.0 ml of pooled normal plasma in a water bath at 54°C for 3 min. (*Note*: Do not exceed 3 min as over-incubation will result in loss of factor activity.)

2. Add 0.2 ml of APTT reagent.
3. Immediately add 5.0 ml of the melted (54°C) 2% agarose.
4. Cover with parafilm and invert 4–5 times.
5. Pour plasma/agarose/phospholipid mixture onto a 8.3 × 10.3 cm gel bond plate.
6. Allow to solidify.
7. Cut 20 wells of 3.0 mm diameter using the pattern below.

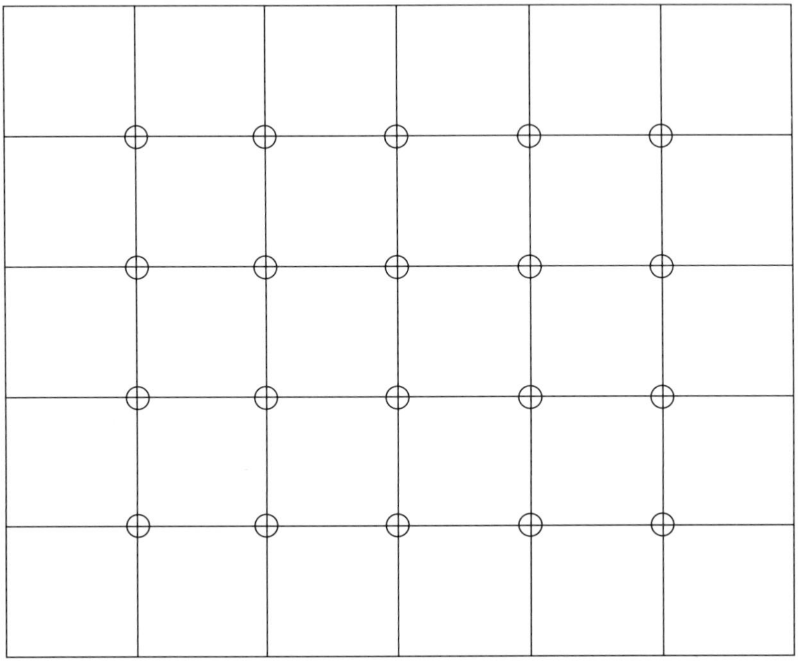

8. Plates should be prepared daily; however, they may be stored in a sealed humidified chamber at 4°C until application of test samples.

B. *Application of samples*

1. Innoculate each appropriately labelled well with 5 µl of undiluted corresponding test sample or control.
2. Duplicate plates are recommended.

C. *Processing*

1. Place plates in a sealed humidified chamber. (A sealed humidified chamber may be made by placing wet paper towels in the bottom of a plastic box and sealing with tape.)
2. Incubate plates at 37°C for 1 h.
3. After the incubation period, immerse the plates in *prewarmed* calcium chloride solution.

4. Maintain at 37°C in calcium chloride solution for 3 min.
5. Remove from calcium chloride solution and immediately immerse in cold (4°C) 4% formaldehyde for 5 min.
6. Rinse plates with distilled water.

Reading results

Place plates on a black background and record the presence or absence of ring formation:

1. Positive: zone of inhibition
2. Negative: no zone of inhibition.

There will be a cloudy or opaque ring of fibrin formation surrounding the well.

Normal values

A normal value would be a negative result.

Interpretation

A zone of inhibition around a well indicates the presence of an inhibitor to coagulation. For example, if an inhibitor to factor VIII is present in a patient's plasma it will diffuse into the agar and inhibit factor VIII. When calcium chloride solution is poured over the plate, fibrin will not form around this well because of the inactivation of factor VIII:C.

This principle also applies to other types of inhibitors (e.g. LA, factor IX inhibitors, heparin). Therefore, this test is only a screening method for the detection of an inhibitor. Further testing is required for the identification of the specific inhibitor type.

Inhibitors to factor VIII occur in less than 20% of patients with classic haemophilia, in post-partum females, in older patients with no underlying diseases and occasionally in patients with immunological disorders such as rheumatoid arthritis.

Inhibitors to factor IX occur in less than 10% of patients with classic haemophilia B and may be seen rarely in other clinical settings similar to those in which factor VIII inhibitors arise.

LA are inhibitors directed against phospholipids. They are spontaneously occurring inhibitors and appear in the plasma of patients with autoimmune diseases, including systemic lupus erythematosus, and drug reactions. These patients are not subject to bleeding episodes as in the case of other inhibitors.

Heparin is an anticoagulant administered primarily in the treatment of deep vein thrombosis, pulmonary embolism and in patients undergoing major abdominothoracic surgery. Heparin acts as a global anticoagulant preventing the formation of fibrin.

Technical notes

1. Smaller plates may be made according to the following reagent adjustments:

   Half plate.

   2.5 ml of pooled normal plasma
   2.5 ml of agarose
   100 µl of APTT reagent.

   Quarter plate.

   1.25 ml of pooled normal plasma
   1.25 ml of agarose
   50 µl of APTT reagent.

DEMONSTRATION OF PHOSPHOLIPID DEPENDENCE OF THE INHIBITOR

Platelet neutralization procedure

Principle

The PNP is a confirmatory test for LA based on the ability of platelets to neutralize or bypass the antibody's effect on in vitro coagulation (Exner et al 1978). This test is a modified APTT in which washed, freeze–thawed platelets are added in equal volume to patient plasma prior to 37°C incubation. Freeze–thawing 'activates' platelets by altering their membrane structure. Intact platelets do not neutralize the LA effect (Triplett et al 1983).

Specimen collection and preparation (See p. 92)

To enhance the sensitivity of the PNP to LA, double centrifuge or filter the plasma with 0.22 µm syringe filters (Nalgene) to remove any residual platelets. If testing is delayed, store plasma at –20°C or below. The stability of frozen plasma is increased by filtration or double centrifugation.

Reagents

APTT reagent or *platelet extract (e.g. Bio/Data).*

Calcium chloride. Either 0.025 or 0.020 M calcium chloride is used depending on the manufacturer's recommendations for their APTT reagent (See p. 92).

Tris-buffered saline.

0.15 M sodium chloride (8.766 g/l).

0.05 M Trizma (6.055 g/l).
900 ml of distilled water.

Adjust pH to 7.4 then make up to 1 litre with distilled water.

Washed platelets. Obtain a newly expired unit of platelet concentrate. Place 20 ml aliquots of the concentrate into large plastic centrifuge tubes and add an equal volume of cold Tris-buffered saline. Centrifuge at 197 g for 10 min to remove red cell contamination. Transfer the platelet-rich supernatant to a plastic centrifuge tube and centrifuge at 2000 g for 10 min. Repeat the washing procedure an additional two times. Following the third wash, resuspend the platelets in Tris-buffered saline and adjust the platelet count to 200 000–300 000/mm^3. Add aliquot to plastic test tubes and store in a freezer at –70°C until use. Experience has shown that frozen platelets remain stable for approximately 3 months.

Quality control

A control for dilutional effect is run on each patient. The reaction mixtures is:

0.1 ml of Tris-buffered saline
0.1 ml of patient plasma
0.1 ml of APTT reagent.

In addition, run pooled normal plasma for the negative control and a known LA plasma for the positive control.

Procedure

1. Thaw frozen platelets at room temperature.
2. Prepare the photo-optical instrument for the APTT run according to the manufacturer's directions if a coagulometer is used.
3. For each patient:
   a. Pipette 0.1 ml of test plasma and 0.1 ml of platelet suspension into a test-tube or cuvette. This is the 'PNP APTT'
   b. Pipette 0.1 ml of patient plasma and 0.1 ml of Tris-buffered saline into a second test-tube or cuvette. This is the buffer control.
4. Ensure that the APTT reagent and calcium chloride solution are in their correct positions on the instrument and that the tubing is primed if a coagulometer is used.
5. Start the test.

Results and interpretation

A positive result is when the patient's baseline APTT is shortened by the addition of platelets. The degree of shortening depends on the titre of inhibitor present. Platelets generally shorten the baseline APTT by 4 s or more. Addition of an equal volume of platelets to the patient plasma will result in dilution of an inhibitor with subsequent shortening of the APTT. Therefore, to rule out the 'dilution effect', compare the buffer control to the PNP APTT. The time obtained on the patient plasma + thawed platelets should be *shorter* than that obtained on the patient plasma + buffer mixture.

Reporting results

The patient report should include the following results:

Baseline APTT
Patient plasma + platelets.
Patient plasma + buffer.

(See technical note 3.)

Technical notes

1. Low titre inhibitors may only minimally prolong the initial APTT making interpretation of test results less obvious. To optimize test results, run the PNP on fresh plasma that has been filtered or centrifuged twice to remove any residual platelets from the patient plasma. Specimen preparation is especially important if the sample is to be frozen for later testing. The presence of residual platelets in a thawed specimen will shorten the APTT and mask a low-titre LA.
2. If the specimen is frozen, repeat the baseline APTT. The results may vary slightly from fresh plasma due to the changes that occur during freezing and thawing.
3. The higher the antibody titre, the greater the effect noted with addition of buffer and platelets to the patient sample. The addition of an equal volume of buffer to the patient plasma will dilute out the effect of the lupus inhibitor and shorten the baseline APTT. However, the addition of freeze–thawed platelets will shorten the APTT to a greater extent, i.e. 4 s or more.

Tissue thromboplastin inhibition test

Principle

The tissue thromboplastin inhibition test (TTI) is commonly used to confirm the presence of LA. Decreased phospholipid concentration in the test system accentuates sensitivity to LA. Plasma is incubated with two different dilutions of thromboplastin, 1:50 and 1:500. A fibrin endpoint is determined after recalcification of the reaction mixture. Test results are interpreted from the ratio of patient seconds to normal control seconds. The TTI is sensitive but non-specific for LA.

Specimen collection and preparation (See p. 92)

To enhance the sensitivity of the TTI to LA, double centrifuge or filter the plasma with 0.22 μm syringe filters to remove any residual platelets. If testing is delayed, store the plasma at –20°C or below. Stability of frozen plasma is increased by filtration or double centrifugation.

Reagents

1. *Tissue thromboplastin.* This is available commercially.
2. *0.02 M calcium chloride.* See p. 92
3. *0.9% sodium chloride.* Obtain normal saline from blood bank or pharmacy.

Quality control

Normal control: pooled normal plasma or commercial normal lyophilized plasma
Positive control: known LA plasma.

Run controls the same as patient plasma for both the 1:50 and 1:500 thromboplastin dilutions.

Procedure

Thromboplastin dilutions. Prepare 1:50 and 1:500 dilutions of thromboplastin in 0.9% sodium chloride solution as follows:

Tube 1 (1:50):

4.9 ml of saline
0.1 ml of thromboplastin.

Tube 2 (1:500):

0.9 ml of saline
0.1 ml of mixture from tube 1
(Modify volume for automated testing: 0.5 ml of mixture from tube 1 and 4.5 ml of saline.)

A. Photo-optical instrumentation.

1. Prepare instrument for run according to the manufacturer's directions.

2. Place 1:50 thromboplastin dilution into the APTT reagent position.
   Place calcium chloride solution into the correction position.
3. Pipette 0.1 ml of test or control plasma into the instrument cuvettes.
4. Initiate test run for the APTT.
5. Repeat procedure for the 1:500 thromboplastin dilution.

B. *Fibrometer.*

1. Mix 0.1 ml of the 1:50 dilution of thromboplastin with 0.1 ml of patient plasma (this will make a final thromboplastin dilution of 1:100). Incubate at 37°C for 3 min.
2. Add 0.1 ml of prewarmed calcium chloride solution and start timer.
3. Record time. Run in duplicate.
4. Repeat above procedure using the 1:500 dilution of thromboplastin (final dilution of thromboplastin is 1:1000).

C. *A manual method (tilt tube)* may also be used.

Results

Calculate the ratio of patient plasma:normal control for both the 1:100 and 1:1000 dilutions of thromboplastin.
Example

	1:100 Dilution	*1:1000 Dilution*
Control	35.1 s	64.6 s
Patient	63.4 s	147.3 s
Ratio	1.8	2.3.

Interpretation.

Patient: Control Ratio	<1.1	Normal
	1.2–1.3	Borderline
	>1.3	Abnormal.

Reported false positives

1. 30% normal subjects
2. Specific factor inhibitors for factors V, VIII and IX (Triplett, ASCP check sample TH 85–5)
3. Hereditary coagulation deficiencies of factors VIII, IX, V, VII and X (Triplett et al 1983)
4. Patients on warfarin or heparin.

Reported false negatives: 10% of LA plasmas.

REFERENCES

Aggeler P M, Lindsay S, Lucia S P 1946 Studies on the coagulation defect in a case of thrombocytopenia purpura complicated by thrombosis. American Journal of Pathology 22: 1181–1203

Alving B M, Baldwin P E, Richard R L, Jackson B J 1985 The dilute phospholipid APTT: a sensitive assay for verification of lupus anticoagulants. Thrombosis and Haemostasis 54: 709–712

Arnout J, Huybrechts E, Vermylen J 1990 A new lupus anticoagulant neutralization test based on platelet derived vesicles. Clinical and Experimental Rheumatology 8: 202 (abstract 3A)

Asherson R A 1988 A "primary" antiphospholipid syndrome? Journal of Rheumatology 15: 1742–1746 (editorial)

Austen D E, Rhymes I L 1975 Laboratory manual of blood coagulation. Blackwell Scientific Publications, Oxford

Biggs R, Bidwell E 1959 A method for the study of antihaemophilic globulin inhibitors with reference to six cases. British Journal of Haematology 5: 379–395

Bird P 1975 Coagulation in an agarose gel and its application to the detection and measurement of factor VIII antibodies. British Journal of Haematology 29: 329–340

Bird P, Rizza C R 1975 A method for detecting factor VIII clotting activity associated with factor VIII related antigen in agarose gels. British Journal of Haematology 31: 5–12

Bowie E J W, Thompson J H, Pascuzzi C A, Owen C A 1963 Thrombosis in systemic lupus erythematosus despite circulating anticoagulants. Journal of Laboratory and Clinical Medicine 62: 416–430

Brandt J T, Triplett D A 1981 Laboratory monitoring of heparin: effects of reagents and instruments on the activated partial thromboplastin time. American Journal of Clinical Pathology 76 (suppl): 530–537

Brandt J T, Triplett D A 1989 The effect of phospholipid on the detection of lupus anticoagulants by the dilute Russell viper venom time. Archives of Pathology and Laboratory Medicine 113: 1376–1378

Brandt J T, Britton A, Kraut E 1986 A spontaneous factor V inhibitor with unexpected laboratory features. Archives of Pathology and Laboratory Medicine 110: 224–227

Brandt J T, Triplett D A, Musgrave K, Orr C 1987 The sensitivity of different coagulation reagents to the presence of lupus anticoagulants. Archives of Pathology and Laboratory Medicine 111: 120–124

Brandt J T, Wurst A, Iams J 1989 Comparative sensitivity of the APTT, kaolin clotting time (KCT), dilute Russell viper venom time (dRVVT) and antiphospholipid antibodies in detecting patients with recurrent pregnancy loss. Thrombosis and Haemostasis 62: 297 (abstract 955)

Carreras L O, Vermylen J G 1982 "Lupus" anticoagulant and thrombosis — possible role of inhibition of prostacyclin formation. Thrombosis and Haemostasis 48: 38–40

Cassidy P G, Triplett D A, LaDuca F M 1985 Use of the agarose gel method to identity and quantitate factor VIII:C inhibitors. American Journal of Clinical Pathology 83: 697–706

Clyne L P, White P F 1988 Time dependency of lupus like anticoagulants. Archives of Internal Medicine 148: 1060–1063

Clyne L P, Dainiak N, Hoffman R, Hardin J 1980 In vitro correction of anticoagulant activity and specific clotting factor assays in SLE. Thrombosis Research 18: 643–655

Conley C L, Hartmann R C 1952 A hemorrhagic disorder caused by circulating anticoagulant in patients with disseminated lupus erythematosus. Journal of Clinical Investigation 31: 621–622

Coots M C, Miller M A, Glueck H I 1981 The lupus inhibitor: a study of its heterogeneity. Thrombosis and Haemostasis 46: 734–739

Coots M C, Glueck H I, Miller M A 1985 Agarose gel method: its usefulness in assaying factor VIII inhibitors, evaluating treatment and suggesting a mechanism of action for factor IX concentrates. British Journal of Haematology 60: 735–750

Cosgriff T M, Martin B A 1981 Low functional and high antigenic antithrombin III level in a patient with the lupus anticoagulant and recurrent thrombosis. Arthritis and Rheumatology 24: 94–96

Dayton V D, Olson S, Peterson L C 1990 Laboratory diagnosis of lupus anticoagulant: comparison of these methods of antibody neutralization. Laboratory Medicine 21: 30–32

deWolf F, Carreras L O, Moerman P, Vermylen J, VanAssche A, Renaer M 1982 Decidual

vasculopathy and extensive placental infarction in a patient with repeated thromboembolic accidents, recurrent fetal loss, and lupus anticoagulant. American Journal of Obstetrics and Gynecology 142: 829–834
Elias M, Eldor A 1984 Thromboembolism in patients with the 'lupus'-like circulating anticoagulant. Archives of Internal Medicine 144: 510–515
Ewing N P, Kasper C K 1982 In vitro detection of mild inhibitors to factor VIII in hemophilia. American Journal of Clinical Pathology 77: 749–752
Exner T 1985 Comparison of two simple tests for the lupus anticoagulant. American Journal of Clinical Pathology 83: 215–218
Exner T, McRea J 1990 Studies on the relatonship between 'antiphospholipid' antibodies and the lupus anticoagulant. Blood Coagulation and Fibrinolysis 1: 17–21
Exner T, Rickard K A, Kronenberg H 1978 A sensitive test demonstrating lupus anticoagulant and its behavioural patterns. British Journal of Haematology 40: 143–151
Exner T, Sahman N, Trudinger B 1988 Separation of anticardiolipin antibodies from lupus anticoagulant on a phospholipid-coated polystyrene column. Biochemical and Biophysical Research Communications 155: 1001–1007
Exner T, Smyth R, Papadopoulos G 1990a Use of a simplified dilute Russell's viper venom time (DRVVT) confirms heterogeneity among lupus anticoagulants. Clinical and Experimental Rheumatology 8: 203 (abstract 7A)
Exner T, Papadopoulos G, Koutts J 1990b Lack of interaction of lupus anticoagulants with phospholipids studied with the agarose gel technique. Clinical and Experimental Rheumatology 8: 202 (abstract 6A)
Exner T, Triplett D A, Taberner D A, Howard M A, Harris E N 1991 Comparison of test methods for the lupus anticoagulant: international survey on lupus anticoagulants-I (ISLA-1). Thrombosis and Haemostasis 64: 478–484
Feinstein D I, Rapaport S I 1972 Acquired inhibitors of blood coagulation in progress. In: Spaet T (ed) Progress in hemostasis and thrombosis. Grune and Stratton, New York, vol 1, p 75–95
Fields R, Toubbeh H, Dixon M, Hurst D 1987 Prevalence of anticardiolipin antibodies in normal blood donors. Arthritis Rheumatism 30: 553 (abstract A92)
Forastiero R R, Cerrato G S, Falcon C R, Carreras L O 1989 A comparison between coagulation tests used for detection of lupus anticoagulants. Thrombosis and Haemostasis 62: 379 (abstract 1191)
Freyssinet J M, Gauchy J, Cazenave J P 1986a The effect of phospholipids on the activation of protein C by the human thrombin–thrombomodulin complex. Biochemical Journal 238: 151–157
Freyssinet J M, Wiesel M L, Gauchy J, Boneu B, Cazenave J P 1986b An IgM lupus anticoagulant that neutralizes the enhancing effect of phospholipid on purified endothelial thrombomodulin activity — a mechanism for thrombosis. Thrombosis and Haemostasis 55: 309–313
Frick P G 1955 Acquired circulating anticoagulants in systemic collagen disease. Blood 10: 691–706
Galli M, Comfurius P, Maassen C, Hemker H C, DeBaets M H, vanBreda-Vriesman P J C, Barbui T, Zwaal R F A, Bevers E M 1990 Anticardiolipin antibodies (ACA) directed not to cardiolipin but to a plasma protein cofactor. Lancet 335: 1544–1547
Gastineau D A, Kazmier F J, Nichols W L, Bowie E J W 1985 Lupus anticoagulant: an analysis of the clinical and laboratory features of 219 cases. American Journal of Hematology 19: 265–275
Gibson J, Starling E, Date C, Rickhard K A, Kronenberg H 1988 Simplified screening procedure for detecting lupus inhibitor. Journal of Clinical Pathology 41: 226–228
Green D, Hougie C, Kazmier F J, Lechner K, Mannucci P M, Rizza C R, Sultan Y 1983 Report of the working party on acquired inhibitors of coagulation: studies of the 'lupus' anticoagulant. Thrombosis and Haemostasis 49: 144–146
Harmon C E, Lee L A, Provost T T 1986 Anticardiolipin antibodies in normal and lupus pregnancies. Arthritis and Rheumatism 29: S96 Abstract E23
Harris E N 1990a A reassessment of the antiphospholipid syndrome. Journal of Rheumatology 17: 733–735 (editorial)
Harris E N 1990b Antiphospholipid antibodies. British Journal of Haematology 74: 1–9 (annotation)
Harris E N, Hughes G R V 1988 Conference report: third international antiphospholipid

conference barbeques, rum, punches, and KAPS. Annals of Rheumatic Disease 47: 612
Harris E N, Gharavi A E, Boey M L, Patel B M, Macworth-Young C G, Loizou S, Hughes G R V 1983 Anticardiolipin antibodies: detection by radioimmunoassay and association with thrombosis in systemic lupus erythematosus. Lancet ii: 1211–1214
Harris E N, Gharavi A E, Asherson R A, Hughes G R V 1984a Antiphospholipid antibodies: a review. European Journal of Rheumatology and Inflammation 7: 5–8
Harris E N, Gharavi A E, Hughes G R V 1984b Proceeding of first world symposium on antiphospholipid antibodies. European Journal of Rheumatology and Inflammation 7: 1–24
Harris E N, Gharavi A E, Hughes G R V 1985 Antiphospholipid antibodies. Clinics in Rheumatic Diseases 11: 591–609
Horellou M H, Aurousseau M H, Boffa M C, Conrad J, Wiesel M L, Samama M 1987 Biological and clinical heterogeneity of lupus and lupus-like anticoagulant in fifty-seven patients. Journal of Medicine 18: 199–217
Hougie C 1985 Circulating anticoagulants. Recent Advances in Blood Coagulation 4: 63–90
Howard M A, Firkin B G 1983 Investigations of the lupus-like inhibitor by-passing activity of platelets. Thrombosis and Haemostasis 50: 775–779
Hughes G R V 1983 Thrombosis, abortion, cerebral disease and the lupus anticoagulant. British Medical Journal 287: 1088–1089
Janoff A S, Rauch J 1986 The structural specificity of antiphospholipid antibodies and autoimmune disease. Chemistry and Physics of Lipids 40: 315–332
Johansson E, Lassus A 1974 The occurrence of circulating anticoagulants in patients with syphilitic and biologically false positive antilipoidol antibodies. Annals of Clinical Research 6: 105–108
Johns A S, Ockelford P A, Chamley L, Pattison N S, McKay E J, Corkill M, Hart H 1989 Comparison of tests for the lupus anticoagulant and phospholipid antibodies in systemic lupus erythematosus. Thrombosis and Haemostasis 62: 380 (abstract 1192)
Kaczor D A, Bickford N M, Triplett D A 1991 Evaluation of different mixing study reagents and dilution effect in lupus anticoagulant testing. American Journal of Clinical Pathology (in press)
Kelsey P R, Stevenson K J, Poller L 1984 The diagnosis of lupus anticoagulants by the activated partial thromboplastin time — the central role of phosphatidyl serine. Thrombosis and Haemostasis 52: 172–175
Kitchens C S 1988 Prolonged activated partial thromboplastin time of unknown etiology. American Journal of Hematology 27: 39–45
Kornberg A Silber L, Yona R, Kaufman S 1989 Clinical manifestations and laboratory findings in patients with lupus anticoagulants. European Journal of Haematology 42: 90–95
Kushner M, Simonian N 1989 Lupus anticoagulants, anticardiolipin antibodies and cerebral ischemia. Stroke 20: 225–229
Laskin C A, Solonika C A 1988 Anticardiolipin antibodies: smoking gun or smoke screen? Journal of Rheumatology 15: 7–9
Laurell A B, Nilsson I M 1957 Hypergammaglobulinemia, circulating anticoagulant and biologically false positive Wasserman reaction. Journal of Laboratory and Clinical Medicine 49: 694–707
LA Working Party of the BCSH Haemostasis and Thrombosis Task Force of the British Society for Haematology 1990 Guidelines on testing for the lupus anticoagulant
Lazarchick J, Kizer J 1989 The laboratory diagnosis of lupus anticoagulants. Archives of Pathology and Laboratory Medicine 113: 177–180
Lechner K, 1987 Lupus anticoagulants and thrombosis. In: Verstraete M, Vermylen J, Lijnen R, Arnout J (eds) Thrombosis and Haemostasis. Leuven University Press, Leuven, p 525–547
LeRoux G, Wautier M P, Guillevin L, Wautier J L 1986 IgG binding to endothelial cells in systemic lupus erythematosus. Thrombosis and Haemostasis 56: 144–146
Lesperance B, David M, Rauch J, Infante-Rivard C, Rivard G E 1988 Relative sensitivity of different tests in the detection of low titre lupus anticoagulants. Thrombosis and Haemostasis 60: 217–219
Liu H W, Wong K L, Lin C K, Wong W S, Tse P W T, Chan G T C 1989 The reappraisal of dilute tissue thromboplastin inhibition test in the diagnosis of lupus anticoagulant. British Journal of Haematology 72: 229–234
Lo S C L, Oldmeadow M J, Howard M A, Firkin B G 1989 Comparison of laboratory tests

used for identification of the lupus anticoagulant. American Journal of Hematology 30: 213–220
Loizou S, McCrea J D, Rudge A C, Reynolds R, Boyle C C, Harris E N 1985 Measurement of anticardiolipin antibodies by an enzyme linked immunosorbent assay (ELISA): standardization and quantitation of results. Clinical and Experimental Immunology 62: 738–745
Lubbe W F, Liggins G C 1988 Role of lupus anticoagulant and autoimmunity in recurrent pregnancy loss. Seminars in Reproductive Endocrinology 6: 181–190
Lubbe W F, Butler W S, Palmer S J, Liggins G C 1984 Lupus anticoagulant in pregnancy. British Journal of Obstetrics and Gynaecology 91: 357–363
McGlasson D L, Brey R L, Strickland D M, Patterson W R 1989 Differences in kaolin-clotting times and platelet counts resulting from variations in specimen processing. Clinical Laboratory Science 2: 109–110
McGlasson D, Brown G, Babcock J, Triplett D A 1988 Evaluation of the lupus like anticoagulant effect of brown recluse spider venom. Blood 72(Supp 1): 303a (abstract 1121)
Machin S J, Giddings J, Greaves M, Hutton, Mackie I J, Malia R G, Taberner D A 1990 Detection of lupus like anticoagulant: current laboratory practices in the United Kingdom. Journal of Clinical pathology 43: 73–75
McNeil H P, Simpson R J, Chesterman C H, Krilis S A 1990 Antiphospholipid antibodies are directed against a complex antigen that includes a lipid-binding inhibitor of coagulation: β_2-Glycoprotein I (apolipoprotein H). Proceedings of the National Academy of Sciences, USA 87: 4120–4124
Mannucci P M, Canciani M T, Mari D, Muecci P 1979 The varied sensitivity of partial thromboplastin and prothrombin time reagents in the demonstration of the lupus-like anticoagulant. Scandinavian Journal of Haematology 22: 423–433
Manoussakis M N, Tzioufas G, Silis M P, Pange P J E, Goudevenos J, Moutsopoulos H M 1987 High prevalence of anticardiolipin and other autoantibodies in a healthy elderly population. Clinical and Experimental Immunology 69: 557–565
Marciniak E, Romond E H 1989 Impaired catalytic function of activated protein C: a new in vitro manifestation of lupus anticoagulant. Blood 74: 2426–2437
Margolis J 1958 The kaolin clotting time. A rapid one stage method for diagnosis of coagulation defects. Journal of Clinical Pathology 11: 406–409
Margolius A, Jackson D P, Ratnoff O D 1961 Circulating anticoagulants: a study of 40 cases and a review of the literature. Medicine 40: 145–202
Matsuura E, Igarashi Y, Fujimoto M, Ichikawa K, Koike T 1990 Anticardiolipin cofactor(s) and differential diagnosis of autoimmune disease. Lancet 336: 177–178 (letter to editor)
Mueller J F, Ratnoff O D, Heinke R V 1951 Observations on the characteristics of an unusual circulating anticoagulant. Journal of Laboratory and Clinical Medicine 38: 254–261
Musclow C E, Amato D, Ofosu F, Armstrong A L, Abbott D 1988 Transfusion induced specific anti-factor XI inhibitor in a patient with previously unrecognized factor XI deficiency. American Journal of Clinical Pathology 89: 418–422
Nawroth P P, Stern D M 1985 A pathway of coagulation on endothelial cells. Journal of Cellular Biochemistry 28: 253–264
Proctor R R, Rapaport S I 1961 The partial thromboplastin time with kaolin: a simple screening test for first stage clotting factor deficiencies. American Journal of Clinical Pathology 36: 212–219
Rainsford S G, Hall A 1976 Detection and measurement of factor VIII antibodies in an agarose gel: a modified method. British Journal of Haematology 33: 309 (letter)
Raman S B K, Saeed S M 1988 Lupus anticoagulant: evaluation of sensitivity of various laboratory tests at different levels of APTT. American Journal of Clinical Pathology 90: 508 (abstract)
Rauch J, Janoff A S 1990 Phospholipid in the hexagonal II phase is immunogenic: evidence for immuno recognition of nonbilayer lipid phases in vivo. Proceedings of the National Academy of Sciences, USA 87: 4112–4114
Rauch J, Tannenbaum M, Tannenbaum H, Ramelson H, Cullis P R, Tilcock C P S, Hope M J, Janoff A S 1986 Human hybridoma lupus anticoagulants distinguish between lamellar and hexagonal phase lipid systems. Journal of Biological Chemistry 261: 9627–9677
Rauch J, Tannenbaum M, Janoff A S 1989 Distinguishing plasma lupus anticoagulants from

anti-factor antibodies using hexagonal (II) phase phospholipids. Thrombosis and Haemostasis 62: 892–896

Rebollo M, Val J F, Garijo F, Quintana F, Berciano J 1983 Livedo reticularis and cerebrovascular lesions (Sneddons's syndrome). Brain 106: 965–979

Rosenberg R D, Rosenberg J S 1984 Natural anticoagulant mechanisms. Journal of Clinical Investigation 74: 1–6

Rosner E, Pauzner R, Lusky A, Modan M, Many A 1987 Detection and quantitative evaluation of lupus circulating anticoagulant activity. Thrombosis and Haemostasis 57: 144–147

Rosove M H, Ismail M, Koizol B J, Runge A, Kasper C K 1986 Lupus anticoagulants: improved diagnosis with a kaolin clotting time using rabbit brain phospholipid in standard and high concentrations. Blood 68: 472–478

Schleider M A, Nachman R L, Jaffe E A, Coleman M 1976 A clinical study of the lupus anticoagulant. Blood 48: 499–509

Schorer A E, Wickham N W R, Watson K V 1989 Lupus anticoagulant induces a selective defect in thrombin-mediated endothelial prostacyclin release and platelet aggregation. British Journal of Haematology 71: 399–407

Shapiro S S, Thiagarajan P 1982 Lupus anticoagulants. Progress in Hemostasis and Thrombosis 6: 263–285

Sidor C F, Martin S E, Abel R, Blatt P M 1986 Lupus anticoagulants. Delaware Medical Journal 58: 239–245

Sontheimer R D 1987 The anticardiolipin syndrome. Archives of Dermatology 123: 590–595

Stevenson K J, Easton A C, Curry A, Thomson J M, Poller L 1986 The reliability of activated partial thromboplastin time methods and the relationship to lipin composition and ultrastructure. Thrombosis and Haemostasis 55: 250–258

Taberner D, Machin S, Mackie I, Giddings J, Malia R, Greaves M 1987 Quality control of the lupus anticoagulant test in the UK. Postgraduate Medical Journal 65: 698–699

Thiagarajan P, Shapiro S S, DeMarco L 1980 Monoclonal immunoglobulin M coagulation inhibitor with phospholipid specificity. Mechanism of a lupus anticoagulant. Journal of Clinical Investigation 66: 397–405

Thiagarajan P, Pengo V, Shapiro S S 1986 The use of the dilute Russell viper venom time for the diagnosis of lupus anticoagulants. Blood 68: 869–874

Triplett D A (ed) 1980 Standardization of coagulation assays: an overview. College of American Pathologists Press, Skokie, Illinois, p 4

Triplett D A (ed) 1982 Laboratory evaluation of coagulation. American Society of Clinical Pathologist Press, Chicago, Illinois

Triplett D A 1985 The clinical importance of lupus anticoagulants; ASCP Check Sample. Thrombosis and Hemostasis TH85–5 (TH–41); vol 7

Triplett D A 1989a Antiphospholipid antibodies and recurrent pregnancy loss. American Journal of Reproductive Immunology 20: 52–67

Triplett D A 1989b Screening for the lupus anticoagulant. Research in Clinic and Laboratory 19: 379–389

Triplett D A, Brandt J T 1988 Lupus anticoagulants: misnomer, paradox, riddle, epiphenomenon. Hematologic Pathology 2: 121–143 (review)

Triplett D A, Brandt J T 1989 Laboratory identification of the lupus anticoagulant. British Journal of Haematology 73: 139–142 (annotation)

Triplett D A, Harris E N 1990 Antiphospholipid Antibodies and Reproduction. American Journal of Reproductive Immunology 21: 123–131

Triplett D A, Brandt J T, Kaczor D, Schaeffer J 1983 Laboratory diagnosis of lupus inhibitors: a comparison of the tissue thromboplastin inhibition procedure with a new platelet neutralization procedure. American Journal of Clinical Pathology 79: 678–682

Triplett D A, Brandt J T, Maas R L 1985 The laboratory heterogeneity of lupus anticoagulants. Archives of Pathology and Laboratory Medicine 109: 946–951

Triplett D A, Brandt J T, Musgrave K A, Orr C A 1988a The relationship between lupus anticoagulants and antibodies to phospholipid. Journal of the American Medical Association 259: 550–554

Tsakiris D A, Settas L, Makris P E, Marbet G A 1990 Lupus anticoagulant antiphospholipid antibodies and thrombophilia. Relationship to protein C – protein S thrombomodulin. Journal of Rheumatology 17: 785–789

Uchman B, Triplett D A 1989 Inhibitory effect of polymyxin B on X-ase and prothrombinase complex formation. Thrombosis and Haemostasis 62: 375 (abstract 1174)

Walker T S, Triplett D A, Javed N, Musgrave K 1988 Evaluation of lupus anticoagulants: antiphospholipid antibodies, endothelium associated immunoglobulin, endothelial prostacyclin secretion, and antigenic protein S levels. Thrombosis Research 51: 267–281

Walsh P N 1974 Platelet coagulation activities and hemostasis: a hypothesis. Blood 43: 597–605

5. The laboratory investigation of the fibrinolytic system

Nuala A. Booth

Fibrinolysis is the physiological process by which fibrin is dissolved in vivo; such fibrin occurs in thrombi and in injured tissues. The balance between the dissolution of fibrin and its formation, as a result of coagulation, is crucial to haemostasis. As in coagulation, there is within the fibrinolytic system a balance between the active and inhibitory elements. This internal balance is disrupted in some situations, leading on the one hand to bleeding and on the other to a thrombotic tendency.

This chapter considers the components of the fibrinolytic system and their physiological regulation. It concentrates on methods available for studying the system. Some situations where fibrinolysis is disordered are used to exemplify the use of the various methods. A comprehensive discussion of such disorders is outside the scope of the chapter and the reader is referred to previous editions of this book and to relevant reviews.

PRINCIPAL COMPONENTS OF THE FIBRINOLYTIC SYSTEM

The main components of the system are shown schematically in Figure 5.1. The central reaction is the activation of plasminogen to form plasmin, the protease that effects fibrin lysis; indeed, plasmin was known originally as fibrinolysin.

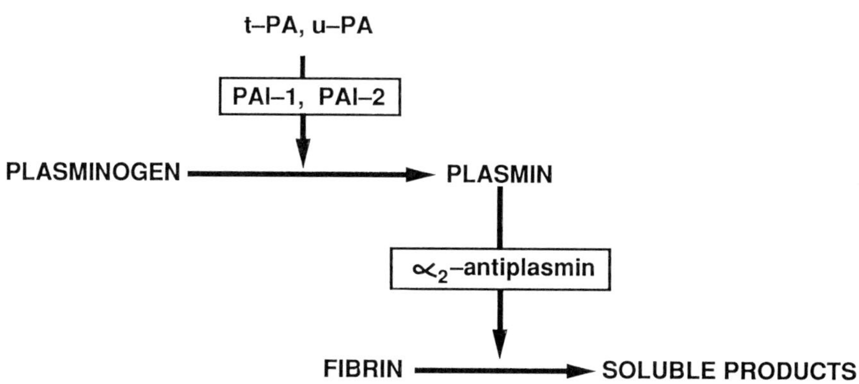

Fig. 5.1 An outline of the fibrinolytic system.

Plasminogen is activated to plasmin by the plasminogen activators. There are two human enzymes that carry out this reaction, t-PA (tissue plasminogen activator) and u-PA (urokinase). The active proteases are inhibited by specific inhibitors. The main plasminogen activator inhibitors are PAI-1 and PAI-2. Plasmin is inhibited principally by α_2-antiplasmin.

These proteins are now considered in more detail.

Proteases of the fibrinolytic system

The enzymes involved in fibrinolysis are all serine proteases; their mechanism of action involves an active-site serine residue. Histidine and aspartate residues complete the catalytic triad. The active sites of this class of enzymes can be blocked by treatment with diisopropylfluorophosphate (DFP) and similar reagents (Kraut 1977). This family of proteases includes trypsin, chymotrypsin, thrombin, elastase, plasmin and the plasminogen activators t-PA and u-PA.

The other common feature of the serine proteases is that the precursor or zymogen is an inactive single-chain molecule and the two-chain product of activation is an active enzyme, the two chains being held together by disulphide bonds. The A (heavy) chain corresponds to the *N*-terminal part of the zymogen; the B (light) chain comes from the *C*-terminal part. The active site of all the serine proteases is located in the B (light) chain, while the A (heavy) chain contains structural domains that have important binding properties. These domains are each encoded by distinct exons and the significance of this for the evolution of this family of proteins has been reviewed by Patthy (1985).

The general features of plasmin, t-PA and u-PA, the three principal enzymes of fibrinolysis, are summarized in Table 5.1.

Plasminogen and plasmin

Plasminogen (reviewed by Castellino 1984) is a single-chain glycoprotein of

Table 5.1 Serine proteases of the fibrinolytic system

Zymogen	Protease	Activation bond	A-Chain domains	B-Chain catalytic triad		
				His	Asp	Ser
plasminogen	plasmin	Arg560—Val561	5 kringles	602	645	740
scu-PA	tcu-PA	Lys158—Ile159	Growth factor 1 kringle	204	255	356
sct-PA[a]	tct-PA	Arg275—Ile276	Finger Growth factor 2 kringles	322	371	478

[a] The single-chain form of t-PA has significant activity.

scu-PA, single-chain urokinase; tcu-PA, two-chain urokinase; sct-PA, single-chain tissue plasminogen activator; tct-PA, two-chain tissue plasminogen activator.

92 kDa. It circulates at a relatively high concentration (0.2 mg/ml, 2 μM) and it has a plasma half-life of about 2 days. Plasminogen has no proteolytic activity. It is activated by cleavage of a specific peptide bond, Arg560—Val561, by t-PA and u-PA to form a two-chain molecule. The active site of plasmin, involving His602, Asp645 and Ser740, is located in the B chain.

The A chain contains five homologous regions, known as kringles. These domains contain lysine-binding sites, which interact with lysine and its analogues, including 6-aminocaproic acid and tranexamic acid. Kringle 1 (the one closest to the *N*-terminus) contains the lysine-binding site that has the highest affinity for lysine (K_d 9 μM). Kringles 2–5 contain low-affinity lysine-binding sites (K_d 5 mM). This property underlines the use of lysine–agarose in affinity purification of plasminogen (Deutsch & Mertz 1970).

These lysine-binding sites are responsible for the binding of plasminogen (and plasmin) to fibrin, a property that is of particular significance for the regulation of fibrinolysis. Interactions between plasmin and its principal inhibitor, α_2-antiplasmin, are also dependent on these sites (Wiman & Collen 1978).

Plasminogen is susceptible to proteolysis, causing removal of small *N*-terminal peptides. The native Glu-plasminogen can thus be converted to Lys-plasminogen. Proteolysis can be prevented by inclusion of an inhibitor such as aprotinin during purification of plasminogen. It is uncertain whether this proteolytic conversion of plasminogen occurs in vivo. Laboratory studies on the two forms of plasminogen show quite significant differences in their activation by t-PA and indicate that Lys-plasminogen mimics fibrin-bound plasminogen in its properties (Hoylaerts et al 1982).

A number of forms of plasminogen can be distinguished by isoelectric focusing in blood from a single individual. This microheterogeneity is due to differences in carbohydrate composition (Collen & De Maeyer 1975).

In plasma, a significant proportion of plasminogen is normally bound to histidine-rich glycoprotein, which reduces the concentration of plasminogen available for potential activation to about half (1 μM). The lysine-binding sites of plasminogen are involved in this interaction.

Tissue plasminogen activator

t-PA was purified originally from uterine and other tissues (Rijken et al 1979); hence its name. It circulates in plasma at a low concentration (about 5 ng/ml) but the concentration rises markedly in response to various stresses, including exercise and venous occlusion. In this context t-PA was previously described as extrinsic plasminogen activator (Collen 1980) but this nomenclature is no longer widely used.

t-PA is a glycoprotein of about 65 kDa. It is unusual among the serine proteases in that it has considerable activity in its single-chain form (Ranby et al 1982, Rijken et al 1982). Cleavage of the Arg275—Ile276 bond gives rise to the two-chain form. The active-site region is homologous to the other serine proteases and the catalytic residues are His322, Asp371 and Ser478.

The A chain of t-PA is composed of discrete domains, comprising a finger region homologous to that in fibronectin, a growth factor domain homologous to epidermal growth factor and two kringles homologous to those of plasminogen. The binding of t-PA to fibrin depends principally on the finger region and on the second kringle (van Zonneveld et al 1986).

The affinity of t-PA for fibrin is one of its most important characteristics. In addition, the activity of t-PA is fibrin specific. The activation of plasminogen by t-PA is relatively inefficient in the absence of fibrin but greatly enhanced in its presence. This is due to an increased affinity of t-PA for plasminogen when fibrin is present (a K_m of 0.15 μM contrasted with a K_m of 65 μM in the absence of fibrin) (Hoylaerts et al 1982). These two properties of t-PA, fibrin affinity and fibrin specificity, are of crucial importance in the regulation of fibrinolysis. They also underlie its use as a therapeutic thrombolytic agent.

Urokinase

This plasminogen activator was purified originally from urine, from which its name is derived. It cleaves the same bond in plasminogen as does t-PA. There are, however, important differences between these two activators, the most striking being that u-PA cleaves plasminogen efficiently in the absence of fibrin (Wallen 1977).

Urokinase exists in a number of forms. The two most important are single-chain (scu-PA or ProUK) and two-chain (tcu-PA, u-PA or UK), both 54 kDa proteins. The single-chain form is a zymogen, expressing less than 1% of the activity of the corresponding two-chain form. Activation of scu-PA to tcu-PA can be achieved by plasmin or by kallikrein. This activation, analogous with the activation of plasminogen to plasmin, depends on cleavage of the Lys158—Ile159 bond.

The active site of u-PA is located in the B chain and the catalytic triad residues are His204, Asp255 and Ser356. The A chain contains two domains that are similar to those in t-PA. These are a growth factor domain and a kringle. The absence of a finger domain and of the second kringle explains why u-PA (either single-chain or two-chain) does not bind fibrin. Despite this, scu-PA does achieve plasminogen activation localized to fibrin, as explained below, and is therefore of great interest as a therapeutic thrombolytic agent (Collen 1987).

The A chain of u-PA contains the site by which u-PA binds to its receptor. This receptor occurs on the surface of several cell types (reviewed by Blasi et al 1987).

In addition to the two 54 kDa forms, degradation products of urokinase occur. The principal one is a 31 kDa molecule, which results from proteolytic cleavage of Lys134—Lys135, and releases a 23 kDa peptide from the *N*-terminus of native u-PA. The loss of its amino terminal fragment means that this form of u-PA does not bind to the u-PA receptor. The cleaved form is found in urine and occurs in many commercial preparations of urokinase that have been purified from urine. It is frequently referred to as low molecular weight UK, high molecular weight UK being the 54 kDa form.

For many years it was believed that t-PA was the only important activator in the circulation and that u-PA had no role in haemostasis. Over the last several years it has become clear that u-PA occurs in the circulation, primarily in its single-chain form. The plasma concentration is normally about 2 ng/ml. The role of plasma u-PA in normal physiology and in disease is not as well defined as other components of the system and it merits further study.

Inhibitors of fibrinolysis

Like the serine proteases, these inhibitors are closely related. They are members of the SERPIN (*ser*ine *p*rotease *in*hibitor) family of inhibitors (reviewed by Carrell et al 1987). These inhibitors contain a region (the reactive centre) that mimics the protease's natural substrate. Unlike the situaton where the enzyme cleaves its substrate and is then available to cleave other substrate molecules, the enzyme forms an inactive 1:1 complex with its inhibitor. This complex is covalent and does not dissociate in sodium dodecyl sulphate (SDS). A fragment is released from the *C*-terminal end of the inhibitor on complex formation.

The reactive centre of the inhibitor is important in defining its protease specificity. The inhibitors of plasmin and of the plasminogen activators all have an arginine residue in their reactive centre, consistent with the fact that these proteases cleave Arg—X bonds in their substrates.

α_2-Antiplasmin

This is the major inhibitor of plasmin. It is a glycoprotein of 70 kDa and circulates at a concentration of about 1 μM. It reacts very rapidly with

Table 5.2 Inhibitors of fibrinolysis and rate constants (/M s)

	α_2-Antiplasmin	PAI-1	PAI-2	PAI-3
sct-PA		10^7	9×10^2	$<10^3$
tct-PA		$>10^7$	2×10^5	$<10^3$
tcu-PA		$>10^7$	10^6	8×10^3
Plasmin	3×10^7			10^2
Plasma concentration	70 μg/ml (1 μM)	20 ng/ml (0.4 nM)	0[a]	2 μg/ml (40 nM)

[a] Late pregnancy plasma concentration is 250 ng/ml (4 nM).

plasmin; the rate constant for their reaction together is about 2×10^7/M s, which is one of the fastest known protein–protein interactions (Table 5.2). This fast reaction, coupled with the relatively high plasma concentration of α_2-antiplasmin means that the half-life of free plasmin in the circulation would be only 100 ms (Wiman & Collen 1978). This inhibitor is therefore an important element in the regulation of fibrinolysis.

Plasminogen activator inhibitors

Plasminogen activator inhibitor 1. For many years the existence of these inhibitors was disputed. This was due to the methodological difficulties in distinguishing between inhibitors of plasmin and of the activators. Most assays for plasminogen activators depend on plasmin generation, which explains the difficulty in distinguishing between inhibition at the level of plasmin and at the level of plasminogen activators. The development of better functional assays for t-PA led to the discovery of a 'fast-acting anti-activator' in blood (Chmielewska et al 1983, Kruitof et al 1983, Verheijen et al 1984). Parallel studies in cultured endothelial cells defined the same inhibitor (Loskutoff et al 1983), which we now know as PAI-1 (Collen 1986).

PAI-1 is a 48 kDa glycoprotein that occurs in normal plasma and platelets and in a number of cultured cells, notably endothelial cells, fibroblasts and hepatocytes. It is widely distributed in tissues, as shown by immunohistochemical techniques (Simpson et al 1989).

PAI-1 is a very potent inhibitor of t-PA and u-PA, with a rate constant in the order of 10^7/M s, comparable to that for α_2-antiplasmin–plasmin (Table 5.2). In contrast to α_2-antiplasmin, however, its plasma concentration is low, about 20 ng/ml (Booth et al 1988, Declerck et al 1988a, Kruithof et al 1988).

Platelets are an important source of PAI-1 and account for more than 90% of the total blood PAI-1. The independence of these two pools of PAI-1 has been shown unequivocally; plasma PAI-1 does not arise simply by leakage from platelets (Booth et al 1988). Both endothelium and the liver have been suggested to be the source of plasma PAI-1 and there is no conclusive evidence on this point (Sprengers & Kluft 1987).

Plasma and platelet PAI-1 differ, not only in their concentrations in their respective pools, but also in activity. It is now known that PAI-1 may occur in an inactive (latent) form that can be activated under denaturing conditions (Hekman & Loskutoff 1985). While plasma PAI-1 is almost all active, platelet PAI-1 is only 3–5% active (Booth et al 1988, Declerck et al 1988a) but can be reactivated following denaturation (Booth et al 1990). Whether there are physiological conditions under which such activation occurs is not yet understood. It should be noted that platelets still account for about half the circulating PAI-1 activity, the relatively poor activity of this PAI-1 being compensated for by its high concentration.

Plasminogen activator inhibitor 2. A distinct but related inhibitor, PAI-2, has been purified form the histiocytic lymphoma cell line U 937 (Kruithof et al 1986). PAI-2 is identical to the inhibitor previously known as placental urokinase inhibitor (Kawano et al 1970). This inhibitor is also found in maternal plasma during pregnancy and is thought to be primarily a placental protein that functions in securing haemostasis at the placento-uterine interface (Astedt et al 1987). It occurs in peripheral blood monocytes (Golder & Stephens 1983), which suggests that PAI-2 may have a more general role in non-pregnant individuals.

PAI-2 is immunologically distinct from PAI-1 but has similar specificity. It has a lower affinity than PAI-1 for both t-PA and u-PA (Table 5.2). It is notable that it is a very poor inhibitor of sct-PA, which is exploited in the design of assays with increased specificity for PAI-1.

Plasminogen activator inhibitor 3. A third plasminogen activator inhibitor, PAI-3, was discovered in urine, and it occurs also in plasma (Stump et al 1986). It is now known to be primarily an inhibitor of activated protein C (Heeb et al 1987). At its normal plasma concentration of about 2 μg/ml, it is unlikely to contribute to physiological inhibition of t-PA and u-PA (Table 5.2).

Other inhibitors of fibrinolysis

A number of plasma protease inhibitors are capable of inhibiting plasmin, t-PA and u-Pa under extreme conditions (Rijken et al 1983, Booth et al 1987b). These inhibitors include α_1-antitrypsin and C1 inhibitor, both of which are SERPINs, and α_2-macroglobulin.

Streptokinase

This is not a component of the human fibrinolytic system but has been included since it is widely used as a therapeutic agent for thrombolysis. It is a product of some streptococcal strains. Streptokinase has no enzymatic activity but it forms a 1:1 complex with plasminogen that has fibrinolytic activity (Brogden et al 1973).

Intrinsic fibrinolytic system

It is uncertain whether all the fibrinolytic activity in the circulation is accounted for by t-PA and scu-PA. Some 20 years ago the fibrinolytic activity in the circulation was considered as being intrinsic or extrinsic, by analogy with the coagulation system. The extrinsic activity is now known to be due to t-PA. The intrinsic activity was that generated from normal plasma by treatment with kaolin, ellagic acid or dextran. It was dependent on the presence of factor XII, prekallikrein and high-molecular-weight kininogen (Saito et al 1975). It is not yet clear whether these phenomena are explained fully by activation of scu-PA to u-PA, which can certainly be effected by kallikrein (Ichinose et al 1986, Hauert et al 1989), or whether another mechanism also operates (Kluft et al 1987).

REGULATION OF THE FIBRINOLYTIC SYSTEM

A number of related mechanisms regulate fibrinolytic activity. As in all serine protease cascades, the activation of zymogens to active enzymes and the specific inhibition of the active enzymes are two important mechanisms. Regulation of the circulating concentrations of these proteins is also vital. Over and above these general mechanisms, fibrin plays a pivotal role in controlling the interactions of the proteins of the system.

Fibrin, the substrate for the fibrinolytic system, has a central and important role in its regulation. Plasminogen binds to fibrin by its lysine-binding sites, which are located in the kringles (Castellino 1984). Its activator, t-PA, also binds strongly to fibrin (Collen 1980). Therefore plasminogen activation can occur on a fibrin surface, so that plasmin can be produced at its site of action.

Even more importantly, activation occurs very much more efficiently on the fibrin surface than in the absence of fibrin. In free solution, t-PA is a relatively poor activator of plasminogen but its affinity for plasminogen is greatly enhanced in the presence of fibrin; the K_m for plasminogen falls from 65 to 0.15 μM (Hoylaerts et al 1982). These effects provide for well-regulated plasminogen activation. Plasminogen in the circulation is not normally activated to form plasmin, activation occurring preferentially on the fibrin surface.

The regulatory mechanism is further enhanced by the effects of the major plasmin inhibitor, α_2-antiplasmin. This is avid in sequestering any plasmin formed in the circulation, which can be calculated to have a half-life of only about 100 ms (Wiman & Collen 1978). When plasmin is formed on the fibrin surface, as a result of the action of fibrin-bound t-PA on fibrin-bound plasminogen, it is relatively protected from the action of its inhibitor. Not only is plasmin's active site occupied by its substrate, fibrin, its lysine-binding sites are also occupied by fibrin. Thus its capacity to interact with α_2-antiplasmin is greatly diminished.

The model for the regulation of plasminogen by t-PA (Collen 1980) also explains the fibrin specificity of u-PA. Even though u-PA does not bind to fibrin, its single-chain form does promote fibrin-specific lysis (reviewed by Collen 1987). This can be explained in terms of plasmin activation of scu-PA to form tcu-PA. Since it is only on a fibrin surface that plasmin can act effectively, protected from inhibition, it follows that the activation of scu-PA will occur preferentially on the fibrin surface.

These interactions limit fibrinolytic activity to the fibrin surface, so that generation of plasmin in the circulation is prevented. Another important consideration is the normal availability of the components of the system and their balance. The plasma concentration of plasminogen (Table 5.3) is relatively high and is therefore unlikely to be a limiting factor in the generation of plasmin. The concentration of α_2-antiplasmin is similarly high. Both of these proteins have plasma half-lives of the order of days and so they normally represent a rather stable part of the system.

Table 5.3 Constituents of the fibrinolytic system in plasma

	Plasma concentration	Half-life in plasma
t-PA	80 pM	5 min
scu-PA	40 pM	8 min
PAI-1	400 pM	7 min
Plasminogen	2 μM[a]	2.2 d
α_2-Antiplasmin	1 μM	3.3 d

[a] Effective concentration reduced to 1 μM by binding to histidine-rich glycoprotein.

The plasminogen activators t-PA and u-PA, and their major inhibitor PAI-1, represent a more dynamic part of the pathway. Their plasma concentrations are low, 2000- to 10 000-fold lower than those of plasminogen and α_2-antiplasmin. They are cleared rapidly from the plasma, with half-lives of the order of minutes rather than days (Table 5.3). Continuous release of these proteins into the circulation must occur to maintain their concentrations in plasma. Their synthesis and release must be finely controlled to maintain the proper balance between these components.

The normal circulating concentration of t-PA is low, only 3–5 ng/ml (80 pM). Plasma PAI-1 is normally present at about 20 ng/ml (400 pM). Given the high affinity of the inhibitor for t-PA, it is likely that complex formation between t-PA and PAI-1 occurs to a significant extent in the circulation, despite the low plasma concentration of these proteins. In plasma samples virtually all the t-PA appears to be in the form of t-PA–PAI-1 complex (Thorsen & Philips 1984). In vivo, rapid clearance of these proteins from the circulation is also occurring, balanced presumably by synthesis and release into the blood. In this situation there may well be a higher proportion of free t-PA present than occurs in the collected blood sample (Wun & Capuano 1987).

In response to physiological stress, such as exercise or venous occlusion, t-PA is released from the vascular endothelium into the bloodstream. Such release also occurs after administration of vasopressin or its analogue desmopressin (DDAVP) (Cash 1978). In plasma taken after these treatments, t-PA activity can be readily detected, indicating that the released t-PA overwhelms the low plasma PAI-1 concentration. It is noteworthy that this important change in balance only requires a relatively small increase in plasma t-PA, from about 3–5 ng/ml to about 10–15 ng/ml (MacGregor et al 1988). These responses form the basis of tests of fibrinolytic potential, where the effects of these treatments on the patient's fibrinolytic activity is measured.

Some individuals, whose tendency to thrombosis had previously been explained as being due to defective t-PA release, were re-examined and shown to have high PAI-1 activity in their plasma (Nilsson et al 1985). PAI-1 would neutralize t-PA on release and would therefore account for the earlier findings. A series of 120 patients with idiopathic deep-vein thrombosis were examined and one-third were found to have a poor fibrinolytic response. Of these almost three-quarters had high baseline PAI-1, while about one-quarter had defective t-PA release. Interestingly, the latter group had a higher incidence of further thrombosis (Juhan-Vague et al 1987).

The plasma concentration of PAI-1 is raised in a number of pathological conditions (Juhan-Vague et al 1984, Wiman & Chmielewska 1985) and it behaves as an acute-phase reactant (Juhan-Vague et al 1985, Kluft et al 1985). There have been a number of studies suggesting an association between high plasma PAI-1 activity and thrombotic disease. Plasma PAI-1 activity was found to be high in young survivors of myocardial infarction (Hamsten et al 1985) and the extent of the elevation was reported to be a risk factor for recurrence (Hamsten et al 1987). In contrast to plasma PAI-1, the platelet pool of PAI-1 varies little in several diseases, the only exceptions observed being chronic renal failure and type II diabetes (Simpson et al 1991). The local role of platelet PAI-1 in the protection of platelet-rich thrombi from dissolution is not yet clear. It is tempting to speculate that PAI-1, which can bind to fibrin (Wagner et al 1989), may have some effect on the t-PA/fibrin interaction but this area requires further investigation.

Abnormalities in t-PA and PAI-1 have also been associated with bleeding. Excess circulating t-PA caused a life-long bleeding tendency in one patient (Booth et al 1983). More recent studies indicate that this was not due to a deficiency of PAI-1. Another similar case has been reported (Aznar et al 1984). Bleeding associated with PAI-1 deficiency has been reported by Schleef et al (1989). These findings all indicate the importance of the balance of plasma t-PA and PAI-1 in haemostasis.

The normal role of u-PA in the circulation is less clear. Plasma u-PA appears to be exclusively in the single-chain form (Wun et al 1982), which has very little activity and which does not react with PAI-1 (reviewed by Blasi et al 1987). Whether u-PA activity is normally generated in the circulation, perhaps on cell surfaces with scu-PA bound to its receptor, is not yet completely understood. A small number of patients with acute promyelocytic leukaemia had high fibrinolytic activity that was due to u-PA, and u-PA activity was associated with their isolated promyelocytes (Bennett et al 1989).

PAI-2 is not normally detectable in the plasma of non-pregnant individuals but it has been observed in patients with advanced liver disease and in those with pancreatitis (Leiper et al 1990). The role of PAI-2 and its origin in non-pregnant subjects merits further study.

A number of deficiencies in α_2-antiplasmin have been described (reviewed by Aoki 1984). In all cases bleeding was observed. It is noteworthy that this bleeding occurred only after minor surgery or other trauma. This is consistent with our understanding of the regulation of the fibrinolytic system. Since plasmin is not normally produced to any extent in the circulation, a lack in its inhibitor would not give rise to obvious problems. Trauma, with its associated release of t-PA, represents a challenge to the haemostatic mechanism and a deficiency in α_2-antiplasmin would become apparent.

α_2-Antiplasmin is present at a reduced level in a number of diseases. This may be due to defective synthesis, for example in liver disease, or consumption, as occurs in DIC.

Thrombolytic therapy

Therapies exploiting the body's fibrinolytic system have been available for two decades, depending originally on a bacterial plasminogen activator, streptokinase, and on urokinase purified from human urine in a two-chain form. Both agents had the disadvantage that they were not well absorbed onto fibrin so that their activity was expressed throughout the circulation, sometimes resulting in haemorrhagic problems.

The regulatory mechanisms of fibrinolysis provide for localized activity on the fibrin surface, avoiding systemic plasminogen activation and consequent bleeding. In recent years these mechanisms have been harnessed for therapeutic use and the growing interest in t-PA and scu-PA as thrombolytic agents illustrates the power of this physiological system.

There has also been a resurgence of interest in streptokinase and recent studies have shown that treatment of myocardial infarction with this agent improves the prognosis of patients (ISIS-2 Collaborative Group 1988). This topic is addressed separately in Chapter 7.

LABORATORY INVESTIGATION OF THE FIBRINOLYTIC SYSTEM

The fibrinolytic system can be examined in a number of ways. Firstly, assays can be carried out to assess the overall activity of the system. These include lysis times of clots formed from whole blood, plasma or euglobulin fraction and lysis of preformed fibrin by euglobulin or plasma. Secondly, individual components can each be measured by specific assays, either functional or immunological. These two general approaches are complementary; results of the simple assays provide useful background for the selection and interpretation of the more specific methods. Thirdly, evidence of fibrinolytic activity can be gained by examining products of the activity, i.e. plasmin–α_2-antiplasmin complex and fibrin degradation products. This last aspect is addressed in Chapter 6.

The above methods, arranged as follows, are now discussed in some detail; technical details follow in the Appendix.

Sample collection	
Overall assays of fibrinolysis	Clot lysis times Fibrin plates; zymography
Specific functional assays	t-PA

	Plasminogen u-PA α_2-Antiplasmin PAI
Immunological assays	Rocket immunoelectrophoresis Enzyme-linked immunosorbent assay (ELISA)

Sample collection

It is generally accepted that assessment of fibrinolysis should ideally be done on samples collected from subjects who are at rest, since t-PA is released into the circulation after exercise. There is a considerable diurnal variation in t-PA and PAI-1 and so a fixed time of sampling is important. Food intake, in particular alcohol and caffeine, may affect components of the system. Ideally, therefore, subjects should be resting and fasted overnight and samples taken at a standardized time, e.g. about 9.00 a.m. This is generally achieved fairly easily in hospital in-patients and in control subjects. Patients attending out-patient clinics and those being assessed in relation to some acute event or to treatment cannot be standardized so easily. In such cases the time of sampling and other relevant details should be noted.

For most purposes it is wise to limit strict criteria to critical variables; exercise and diurnal variations are the principal ones. A short period of rest (e.g. 10 min) is usually sufficient. More rigid criteria are inconvenient and may, indeed, introduce bias in selecting individuals who are not truly representative of a normal population. Significant changes in the system will be detectable against the normal varied background. Control populations should match patients in age and sex (Hashimoto et al 1987).

Citrate is the most usual anticoagulant for these studies. Blood should be collected with minimal stasis but unfortunately this cannot be truly standardized because of variations among subjects.

The anticoagulated blood should be cooled immediately and spun as soon as possible. Platelet contamination of the plasma should be avoided since platelets are a rich source of PAI-1 antigen and are therefore a potential problem in assays of fibrinolytic activity. For most situations anticoagulants designed to avoid platelet release are not necessary (Booth et al 1988) but they are helpful when platelet counts are very high or when samples cannot be spun quickly after collection (Kluft & Verheijen 1990).

Clot lysis times

This type of assay gives an overall view of the balance of the components of fibrinolysis. They measure the time taken to lyse a clot and so give some estimate of plasmin formation and activity.

In blood from normal individuals and in the vast majority of patients, the balance of proteases and inhibitors is such that fibrinolytic activity cannot be measured easily. Therefore, various means are adopted to reduce or remove the effects of the inhibitors and so allow activity to be detected. The usual methods are either to dilute blood or plasma or to make a euglobulin precipitate. A clot is then prepared from this material.

Clots prepared from blood or plasma from most individuals lyse so slowly that precise measurement of these clot lysis times is impractical. Only in samples from patients with hyperfibrinolysis can lysis be achieved in a reasonable time and in such cases these methods do provide useful data. For instance, we have reported a patient with bleeding due to excess t-PA activity, whose whole blood clot lysed spontaneously in less than 6 h (Booth et al 1983).

A more usual approach is either to dilute plasma or to prepare a euglobulin precipitate; this is the fraction of plasma precipitated on dilution and acidification. It contains virtually all the t-PA and plasminogen present in the original plasma. Most of the plasma inhibitors, such as α_2-antiplasmin and α_2-macroglobulin, remain in the discarded supernatant, known as the pseudoglobulin fraction. It is often assumed that PAI-1 is similarly removed from the euglobulin but, as shown in Figure 5.2, this is not the case. Virtually all of the PAI-1 that is in complex with t-PA precipitates in the euglobulin. More importantly, when free PAI-1 is examined, it is clear that this partitions between the precipitate and the supernatant in a ratio of about 3:5. These distributions of PAI-1 need to be borne in mind when interpreting the results of euglobulin clot lysis times. Similarly, much of the plasma C1 inhibitor may precipitate (Kluft & Brakman 1975).

Euglobulin from normal individuals lyses in a few hours at 37°C. Each laboratory should define its own normal range. Lysis of euglobulins from individuals with enhanced fibrinolysis is very much faster; post-exercise

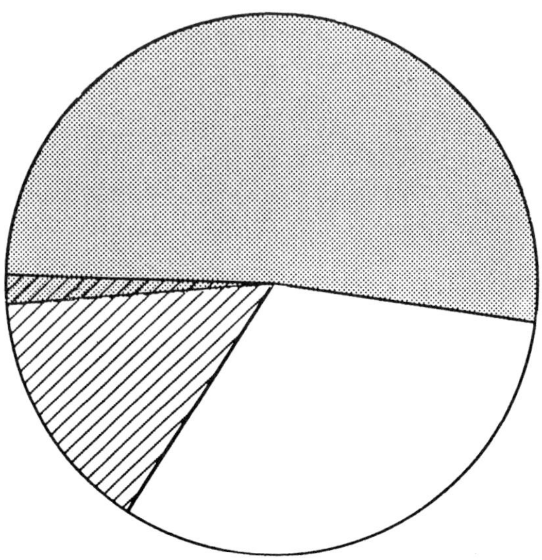

Fig. 5.2 The distribution of the plasma PAI-1 in euglobulin and pseudoglobulin fractions: □ euglobulin; ▩ pseudoglobulin; ▨ PAI-1 in complex with t-PA.

samples may lyse in as little as 15 min (Booth et al 1987b). Similarly, fast lysis is seen in samples from patients with enhanced fibrinolysis and associated bleeding (Booth & Bennett 1984). For most studies, where the emphasis is on thrombosis rather than bleeding, clot lysis assays are much less useful. The variation in lysis times between normal individuals is sufficiently large to make it difficult to find a significant lengthening of the lysis times in affected patients. It is well suited, however, to studying the 'fibrinolytic potential' in patients, where release of t-PA in response to venous occlusion or DDAVP is assessed.

Fibrin plates

Plasma or its euglobulin fraction may be applied to preformed fibrin and the extent of lysis measured. Fibrin plates have the advantage over clots made from patients' samples that the fibrin concentration is standardized. In other respects the limitations of clot lysis assays apply equally here. Untreated normal plasma applied to a fibrin plate results in no measurable lysis. Plasma obtained from normal individuals after exercise or venous occlusion produces a zone of lysis (Booth et al 1987b). This is also seen in plasma from patients with liver disease and other disorders (Booth et al 1984, Bennett et al 1990).

It is more usual to study lysis caused by the euglobulin fraction, since normal euglobulin produces an easily detected zone of lysis. It is therefore possible to observe overall hypofibrinolysis by this method, although, of course, overactivity is still much more easily detected (Fig. 5.3).

Two methods for fibrin plates are given in the Appendix. One is for a tra-

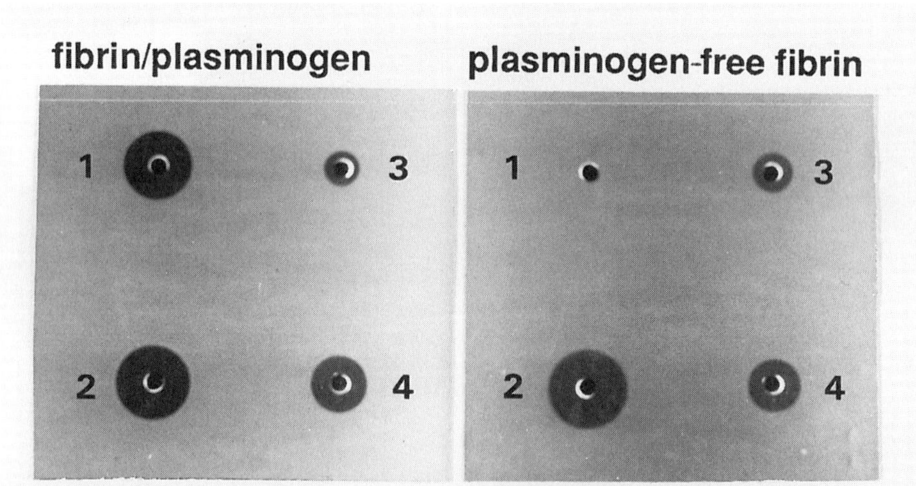

Fig. 5.3 Fibrin plates ± plasminogen. Samples were: **1,** u-PA; **2,** plasmin; **3,** normal plasma euglobulin; **4,** disseminated intravascular coagulation (DIC) plasma euglobulin.

ditional fibrin plate made in a Petri dish. Zones of lysis in these plates will only be regular if care is taken in loading samples, since the sample stays in place by surface tension.

An alternative method is to incorporate agarose in the fibrin plate. This allows wells to be cut in the plate and the samples are then loaded into the wells. It has the advantage that the zones of lysis are quite regular. Another benefit is that any size of plate can be prepared. Glass plates may be used but a flexible support of agarose-coated polyester, e.g. GelBond, is recommended for this application and also for immunoelectrophoresis, where it has the advantage over glass that the gels can be washed without danger of sliding off.

Normally, fibrin plates are made with commercial preparations of fibrinogen, which are contaminated with plasminogen. The contaminating plasminogen is activated by plasminogen activators in the applied sample. Such plates are sensitive to both plasminogen activators and plasmin. In order to discriminate between plasmin and plasminogen activators, plasminogen-free fibrinogen can be used. Plates made from this material are sensitive only to plasmin, as shown in Figure 5.3. It should be noted that if the sample itself contains plasminogen, then essentially the same lysis will be seen on fibrin containing plasminogen and on plasminogen-free fibrin. This is also illustrated in Figure 5.3, where euglobulin fractions, which of course contain plasminogen, have been applied to the plates.

Fibrinogen that is free of plasminogen is easily prepared on lysine–agarose and the method is given in the Appendix. This is much more satisfactory than the older method of heating fibrin plates to destroy the plasminogen. Alternatively, plasminogen-free fibrinogen can be purchased.

Zymography

Fibrin/agarose plates can also be used as an underlay for SDS–polyacrylamide gels. This technique separates proteins on the basis of their molecular sizes. After washing the polyacrylamide gel with Triton X-100 to neutralize the SDS, it is possible to detect t-PA or u-PA activity (Booth et al 1984).

A simple adaptation of the same fibrin/agarose plate involves incorporated u-PA. The gel now lyses completely, except where inhibitors are present. The inhibitors may be applied directly into wells cut in the plate (Sprengers et al 1984) or may be present in a polyacrylamide gel that has been used to separate plasma or other biological samples (Erickson et al 1984, Booth et al 1985).

Specific assays for proteins of the fibrinolytic system

Functional assays for the proteases and inhibitors of the fibrinolytic system are commonly performed with chromogenic substrates. These are tri- or tetrapeptides with *C*-terminal *p*-nitroanilide. Reaction with proteases causes the release of *p*-nitroaniline, which can be detected spectrophotometrically at 405 nm. Various substrates with different protease specificities are commercially available.

Plasminogen

Functional plasminogen can be assayed by activating plasminogen and measuring the plasmin activity produced. Streptokinase is usually used for the activation. A chromogenic substrate sensitive to plasmin (e.g. S-2251) is employed.

Tissue plasminogen activator

The activity of t-PA cannot be measured on a direct chromogenic substrate, since no such substrate is yet available. Instead, plasminogen activation to plasmin by t-PA, and assay of the resulting plasmin, forms the basis of the method. It is necessary to include a fibrin-related stimulator for this assay, since t-PA does not activate plasminogen efficiently in the absence of fibrin.

Normal citrated plasma has very little detectable t-PA activity. As already mentioned, PAI-1 in plasma is usually present in a five-fold excess over t-PA. Any t-PA not complexed in the circulation will have sufficient time to undergo complete neutralization by PAI-1 during preparation of the plasma. Attempts to 'freeze' the in vivo situation include collection of blood onto active-site reagents, which block t-PA activity and, hence, complex formation with inhibitors (Rijken et al 1983). Collection of blood into acidified anticoagulant similarly prevents complex formation (Chmielewska & Wiman 1986).

Plasminogen activator inhibitors

Assays for protease inhibitors depend on addition of excess protease and measurement of residual protease. The assay for PAI is therefore closely related to that for t-PA (Chmielewska & Wiman 1986). It should be noted that this sometimes leads to difficulties in interpretation. For instance, in one study a rise in t-PA activity was echoed by a fall in PAI activity. Measurement of antigen showed that PAI-1 remained constant, indicating that the apparent PAI activity was strongly influenced by plasma t-PA (Hariman et al 1989).

α_2-Antiplasmin

This inhibitor is assayed by adding an excess of plasmin and then measuring the residual plasmin activity using a chromogenic substrate.

Urokinase

Direct chromogenic substrates for u-PA (e.g. S-2444) are available and these can be employed to assay u-PA. Alternatively, the assay described for t-PA can also be used for u-PA. However, the activity detected in plasma is virtually all due to t-PA; u-PA activity is not normally detectable in plasma, where it occurs as scu-PA.

Immunological methods

It is frequently helpful to assay specific components of a system by both functional and immunological assays, especially since the functional assays are not always entirely specific. The most common methods used are rocket immunoelectrophoresis and enzyme-linked immunoabsorbent assay (ELISA).

Rocket immunoelectrophoresis

This is a useful method for assaying proteins whose concentration is greater than about 30 μg/ml. Thus it can be applied to measure plasminogen, histidine-rich glycoprotein, α_2-antiplasmin and other plasma protease inhibitors. It depends on electrophoresis of samples through an agarose gel that contains specific antiserum. The antigen moves through the gel until it has achieved maximal binding of antibody, at which point it precipitates. This gives a characteristic rocket shape, the size of the rocket being proportional to the antigen concentration at a fixed antibody concentration (Laurell 1966).

The percentage of antiserum required depends on its titre. Even if data on this are available, it is advisable to check experimentally, using a range of concentrations. The aim is to achieve reasonably intense rockets with a height range of approximately 1–5 cm for the standards. At high antiserum concentrations the rockets will be small and intense; at lower antiserum concentrations they will be taller but less intense. The choice of optimal concentration depends also on the samples to be tested. These points are illustrated in Figure 5.4, where a simple range-finding experiment was set up to define the concentration of antiserum to α_2-macroglobulin for use in assays of plasma.

Enzyme-linked immunoabsorbent assay

Proteins that have plasma concentrations in the nanogram per millilitre range can only be detected by much more sensitive methods than rocket immunoelectrophoresis. Radioimmunoassay (RIA) and ELISA are the two

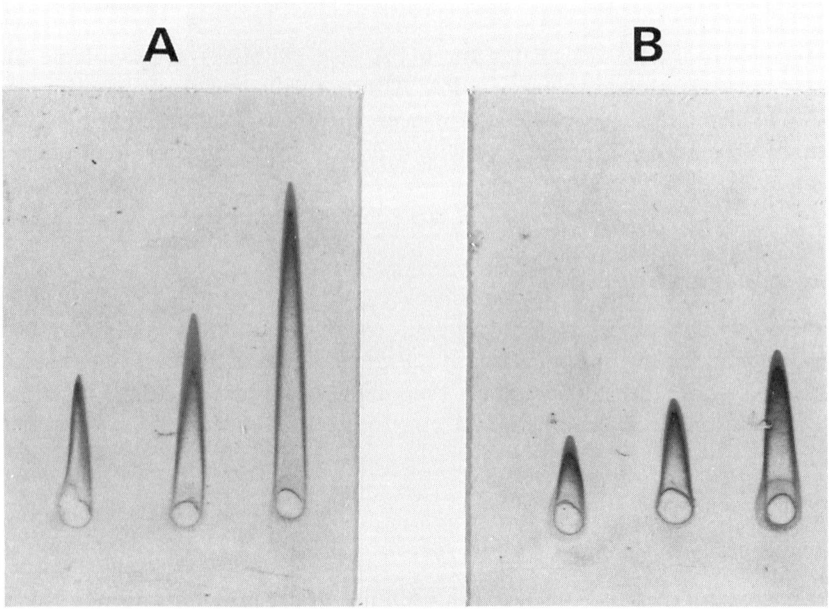

Fig. 5.4 Rocket immunoelectrophoresis for α_2-macroglobulin. Antiserum concentrations were: **A**, 0.5%; **B**, 1.0%. Samples in both panels were, left to right, normal plasma diluted 1:32, 1:16 and 1:8.

methods of choice. ELISA has the advantage of longevity of reagents and many recent immunoassays are of this type.

Several ELISA methods are now available and only their general features will be discussed in this chapter. General advice on the development of ELISAs is given by Voller et al (1979). Specific instructions provided with commercial ELISA kits should be followed with care. Most commercially available immunoassays use two or more mouse monoclonal antibodies (Mab). A typical scheme is given in Figure 5.5. One Mab is used to coat microtitre wells by passive absorption at pH 9.6. The coated plate is then reacted with a high concentration of an irrelevant protein, usually bovine serum albumin. This blocks other sites on the wells which might otherwise adsorb proteins unrelated to the antigen under assay. After thorough washing, the samples are introduced into the wells; the buffer used for the dilution of samples and standards needs to be selected carefully to promote the antibody–antigen reaction but also to minimize non-specific interactions. The washed wells are now exposed to a second Mab, conjugated to an enzyme, often horseradish peroxidase. After washing, a substrate for the enzyme is introduced. A colour change indicates product formation and is measured spectrophotometrically.

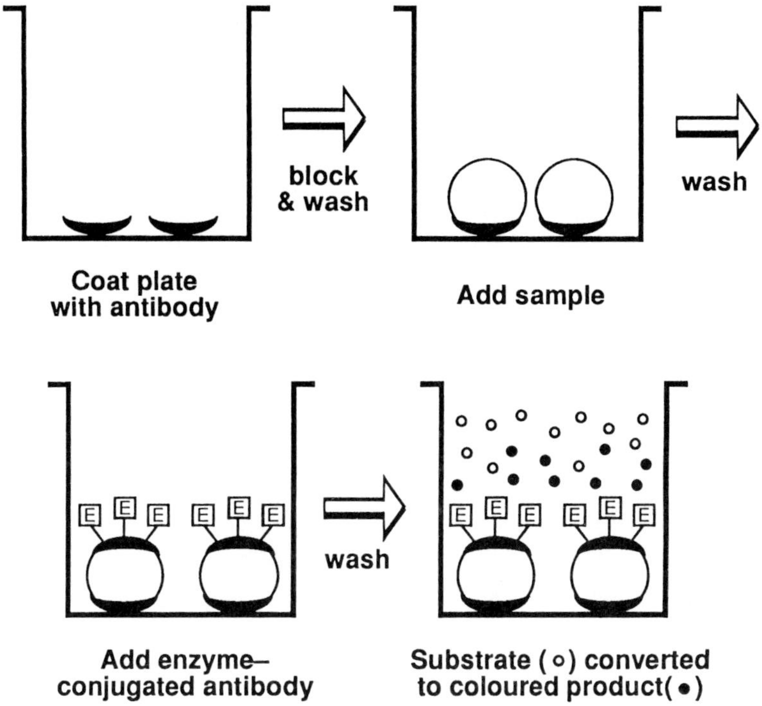

Fig. 5.5 Scheme for typical ELISA.

Two-dimensional immunoelectrophoresis

This technique is closely related to rocket immunoelectrophoresis. The sample undergoes electrophoresis in an agarose gel to separate its component proteins. The separated sample then undergoes electrophoresis in agarose containing a specific antiserum; this second electrophoresis is at right angles to the first. If only a single species of the antigen is present then a single peak, rather like a broad rocket, is seen. If two species of antigen are present a second peak will be observed (Laurell 1966).

Two-dimensional immunoelectrophoresis has been used to detect plasmin–α_2-antiplasmin complex in plasma after thrombolytic therapy (Verstraete et al 1978) and in patients with hyperfibrinolysis (Booth & Bennett 1982). It is a good, if slightly insensitive, method for following activation of the fibrinolytic system (Fig. 5.6). In situations where a more sensitive method is required, an ELISA, using antibodies to α_2-antiplasmin to coat the wells and antibodies to plasminogen to detect bound complex, can be used (Harpel 1981).

Two-dimensional immunoelectrophoresis was employed to indicate

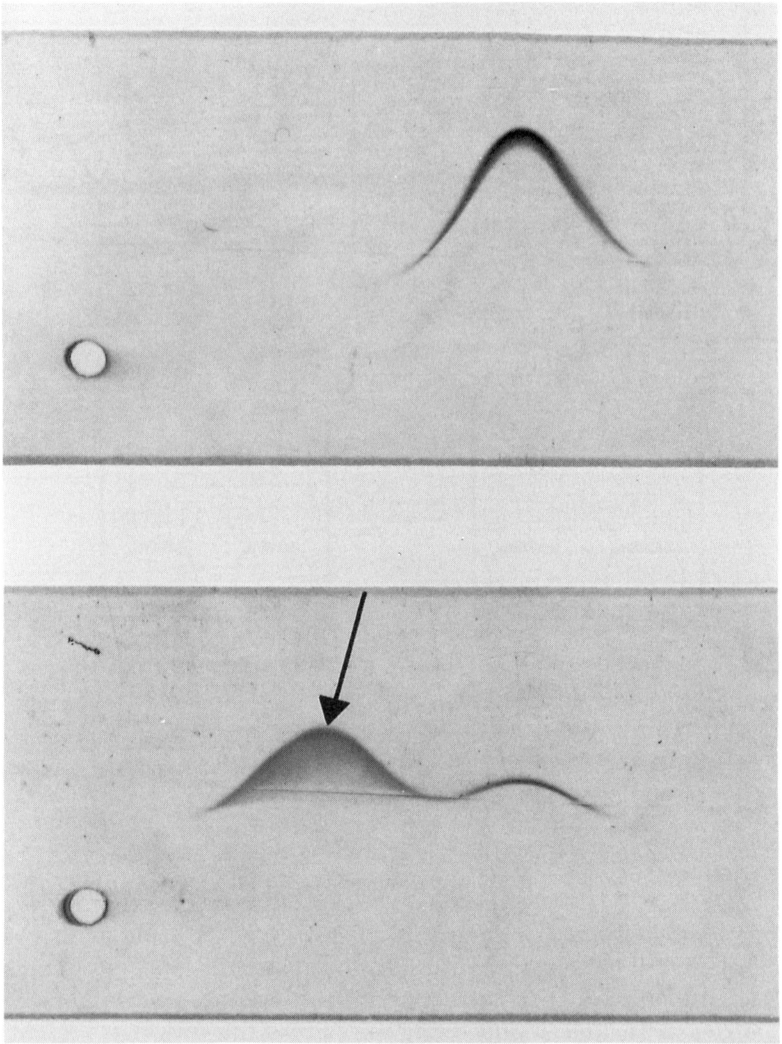

Fig. 5.6 Two-dimensional immunoelectrophoresis for α_2-antiplasmin. Upper panel, normal plasma; lower panel, DIC plasma. The arrow indicates a peak of plasmin–α_2-antiplasmin complex.

complex formation between PAI-1 and vitronectin, which has been identified as a PAI-1-binding protein (Declerck et al 1988b).

METHODS APPENDIX

Plasma preparation

Withdraw venous blood with minimal stasis and mix in a chilled tube with 0.1 volume of 0.13 M trisodium citrate (3.8 g trisodium citrate in a final volume of 100 ml distilled water). Mix and chill on ice and centrifuge as soon as possible at 1850*g* for 30 min at 4°C. This speed and duration of centrifugation is necessary in order to achieve plasma that is practically free of platelets, which is essential for any assay that might be influenced by platelet PAI-1.

If particular problems with platelet release are anticipated, plasma may be collected into 0.1 volume of ETP (78 mM EDTA, 10 mM theophylline, 0.33 μg/ml prostaglandin E_1).

For assays of t-PA activity plasma may be collected into acidified anticoagulant. This can sometimes cause problems of haemolysis but commercially available tubes (Stabilyte, Biopool) seem satisfactory.

Clot lysis assays

Blood or a fraction prepared from it can be used for the preparation of a clot. The time taken for the clot to lyse gives a measure of fibrinolytic activity.

Preparation of euglobulin fraction

Reagents.

1. *0.014% (v/v) acetic acid.* A 1% solution = 1 ml of glacial acetic acid made up to 100 ml with distilled water; a 0.014% solution = 7 ml of 1% acetic acid made up to 500 ml with distilled water. Store at 4°C.
2. *Euglobulin buffer (60 mM Tris, pH 7.4).* Dissolve 0.727 g of Tris in distilled water, adjust the pH with hydrochloric acid and make up to 100 ml. Store at 4°C.

Method.

1. Pipette 500 μl of plasma into a precooled plastic conical centrifuge tube.
2. To this add 9.5 ml of 0.014% acetic acid (cold). Mix tube and keep on ice for 15 min.
3. Centrifuge at 1000 g for 10 min at 4°C.
4. Discard supernatant (pseudoglobulin) and dry tube with filter paper.
5. Redissolve euglobulin precipitate in 500 μl of euglobulin buffer, using an orange stick to disperse it. A rotamixer may be used on a low setting. The euglobulin can then be used to test the euglobulin clot lysis time and it can also be applied to a fibrin plate, as described below.

Euglobulin clot lysis time

Reagents.

1. *Redissolved euglobulin.*

2. *Thrombin, 2 NIH units/ml.* A 5000 unit vial of bovine thrombin (Parke Davis) is made up to 50 ml with 0.9% sodium chloride solution. The stock (100 U/ml) is diluted 1:50 in 0.9% sodium chloride solution and stored frozen in small aliquots. Defrost at 37°C and keep on ice. Do not refreeze.

Method.

1. Pipette 150 µl of redissolved euglobulin into glass clotting tubes. Euglobulins from normal and from patient plasmas should be set up in duplicate.
2. To each tube add 150 µl of thrombin (2 NIH units/ml). Tilt the tube gently to mix.
3. Cover tubes with parafilm and incubate in a water bath at 37°C.
4. Examine at intervals and note time taken for lysis.

Whole blood clot lysis time

Incubate blood in a glass tube at 37°C and note the time taken for lysis. This is normally more than 48 h.

Plasma clot lysis time

Mix 0.5 ml of citrated plasma and 0.25 ml of 50 mM calcium chloride, incubate at 37°C and note the time taken for clot lysis. This is normally more than 48 h.

Fibrin plates

Reagents

1. *Fibrin plate buffer (75 mM Tris, pH 7.8; 22 mM sodium chloride).* Dissolve 9.09 g of Tris and 1.29 g of sodium chloride in distilled water, adjust pH to 7.8 with hydrochloric acid and make up to 1000 ml.
2. *1% human fibrinogen.* Dissolve 1 g Kabi L fibrinogen in 100 ml of distilled water. Store 2 ml aliquots at –20°C. Defrost quickly at 37°C.
3. *Thrombin, 10 NIH units/ml.* A 5000 unit vial of bovine thrombin (Parke Davis) is made up to 50 ml with 0.9% sodium chloride solution. The stock is diluted 1:10 and stored frozen in small aliquots. Defrost at 37°C and keep on ice. Discard after use.
4. *1% agarose (Sigma type 1) in fibrin plate buffer.* Add 40 ml of fibrin plate buffer to 0.4 g of agarose. Boil to dissolve and then keep at 56°C in a water bath until required.

Method

Standard fibrin plate in 9 cm diameter polystyrene Petri dish:

1. Insert a circle of Whatman No. 1 filter paper in the lid of the Petri dish. The bottom of the dish may be marked in quarters.

2. Defrost 2 ml of 1% fibrinogen at 37°C.
3. Add 8 ml of fibrin plate buffer.
4. Add 200 μl of thrombin (10 U/ml). Invert to mix and pour into Petri dish on a level surface. Swirl gently to cover dish but avoid introducing bubbles.
5. Place in an incubator at 37°C on a level shelf for 30 min.
6. Load 30 μl of each sample to be tested.
7. Incubate at 37°C for 24 h and measure the diameter of the zones of lysis.

Fibrin/agarose plate prepared on GelBond (10 × 7.5 cm):

1. Defrost 2 ml of 1% fibrinogen at 37°C and transfer to a water bath at 44°C for 20–30 s.
2. Transfer 8 ml of 1% agarose in fibrin plate buffer to a water bath at 44°C.
3. Add 60 μl of thrombin (10 U/ml) to agarose and then add fibrinogen. Invert to mix and pour onto the hydrophilic side of GelBond on a level surface. Leave for 1 min to set.
4. Cut 3 mm diameter holes in agarose with cutter and remove by suction
5. Load 5 μl samples into wells. Incubate at 37°C in a moist box for 24 h and measure the diameter of the zones of lysis.

Incorporating antibodies to tissue plasminogen activator or urokinase into fibrin plate

Anti-human t-PA, IgG (e.g. Biopool, raised in goat; 5 mg/ml)
Anti-human u-PA, IgG (e.g. Biopool, raised in goat; 5 mg/ml).

Add antibodies (40 μl) to fibrinogen before addition of thrombin (or thrombin/agarose), to give a final concentration in the fibrin plate of 20 μg of IgG per millilitre.

Preparation of plasminogen-free fibrinogen

Reagents

1. *Lysine–agarose, 15 g*. Equilibrate in 50 mM Tris buffer, pH 7.8, containing 20 mM sodium chloride. This is packed into a 2.5 cm diameter column; gel height about 11 cm; column volume approximately 55 ml.
2. *Fibrinogen Kabi L, 1 g*

Method. Dissolve the fibrinogen in only 25 ml of distilled water. Apply to the column at a flow rate of 50 ml/h and collect the breakthrough peak. This will be in a volume of less than 100 ml. Make up to 100 ml with 50 mM Tris buffer, pH 7.8, containing 20 mM sodium chloride and store frozen in 2 ml aliquots. Use to prepare fibrin plates as described above. The quality of the plasminogen-free fibrin can be checked by applying either u-PA or plasmin to these fibrin plates; plasmin should lyse the plates, but u-PA should not, because of the lack of fibrinogen (see Fig. 5.3).

Fibrin/agarose/urokinase plates for detection of inhibitors (Booth et al 1985)

u-PA (Leo; 100 Ploug units/ml).

Add 5 μl of u-PA to fibrinogen before addition to thrombin/agarose. Incubate at 30°C. Lysis of plate is complete in about 16 h and opaque zones due to inhibitors will be apparent.

Functional plasminogen assay

In this assay plasminogen is reacted with streptokinase to achieve total activation of the plasminogen to plasmin. The plasmin produced is then assayed using a tripeptide chromogenic substrate, with the release of *p*-nitroaniline as the end point.

Reagents

1. *50 mM Tris buffer (pH 7.4, 110 mM sodium chloride)*. Dissolve 6.1 g of Tris and 6.5 g of sodium chloride in distilled water, adjust to pH 7.4 with hydrochloric acid and make up to 1 litre.
2. *Substrate, e.g. S-2251 (H-D-Val-Leu-Lys-pNA)*. Dissolve 25 mg in 13 ml of distilled water to give a 3.5 mM solution (stable for 6 months at 2–8°C). A working substrate/buffer solution is prepared by mixing 1 volume of 3.5 mM S-2251 with 3 volumes of buffer.
3. *Streptokinase*. Reconstitute with distilled water to give a final concentration of 10 000 IU/ml.
4. *50% acetic acid*. Add 50 ml of glacial acetic acid to 50 ml of distilled water.

Method

1. Prepare a standard curve by mixing 400 μl of normal pool plasma with 3.7 ml of Tris buffer. Dilute further as follows:

Dilution	Diluted normal plasma (μl)	Buffer (ml)	Plasminogen activity (%)
0	0	1.6	0
1:164	100	1.5	25
2:164	200	1.4	50
3:164	300	1.3	75
4:164	400	1.2	100

5:164	500	1.1	125
6:164	600	1.0	150

2. Dilute 50 μl of each test plasma with 2 ml of Tris buffer.
3. Incubate 200 μl of diluted standard or test sample at 37°C for 2 min.
4. Add 100 μl of streptokinase, mix and incubate for 10 min at 37°C.
5. Add 700 μl of substrate/buffer solution, mix and incubate for exactly 3 min at 37°C.
6. Stop reaction with 100 μl of 50% acetic acid, mix and immediately place on ice.
7. Read absorbance at 405 nm, ideally within 1 h, even though the colour is believed to be stable for 4 h.
8. Draw a standard curve of absorbance at 405 nm versus percentage plasminogen activity and read the test results.

Potential sources of error are very highly coloured plasma samples, for instance in the case of liver disease. This can be overcome by setting up colour blanks for each plasma, including normal, where the substrate/buffer solution is replaced by 700 μl of buffer.

Another source of error, although rare, is where a plasma sample has endogenous protease activity. This can be corrected for by setting up a blank where no streptokinase is added; replace with 100 μl of buffer.

Functional α_2-antiplasmin

Principle

Excess plasmin is added to the sample containing α_2-antiplasmin and the residual plasmin activity is measured, using a tripeptide chromogenic substrate, with the release of *p*-nitroaniline at the end point.

Reagents

1. *50 mM Tris buffer (pH 7.4, 110 mM sodium chloride)*. Dissolve 6.1 g of Tris and 6.5 g of sodium chloride in distilled water, adjust pH to 7.4 with hydrochloric acid and make up to 1 litre.
2. *Substrate, e.g. S-2251 (H-D-Val-Leu-Lys-pNA)*. Dissolve 25 mg in 13 ml distilled water to give a 3.5 mM solution (stable for 6 months at 2–8°C).
3. *Plasmin (0.25 casein units/ml)*. To 1 vial of 25 casein units add 100 ml of a solution containing 50 ml glycerol, 40 μl of 5 M hydrochloric acid and 0.5 g of polyethylene glycol 6000. The plasmin solution is stored frozen in aliquots. It should be kept at 25°C for 1 h before use.
4. *50% acetic acid*. Add 50 ml of glacial acetic acid to 50 ml of distilled water.

Method

1. Prepare a standard curve by mixing 600 μl of normal pool plasma with 2.5 ml of Tris buffer. Dilute further as follows:

Dilution	Diluted normal plasma (μl)	Buffer (ml)	Antiplasmin activity (%)
0	0	2.4	0
1:124	100	2.3	25
2:124	200	2.2	50
3:124	300	2.1	75
4:124	400	2.0	100
5:124	500	1.9	125

2. Dilute 100 μl of each test plasma with 3 ml of Tris buffer
3. Incubate 600 μl of diluted standard or test sample at 37°C for 2 min.
4. Add 200 μl of plasmin (which has been kept for 1 h at 25°C after thawing), mix and incubate for exactly 20 s at 37°C
5. Add 200 μl of substrate, mix and incubate for exactly 2 min at 37°C.
6. Stop reaction with 100 μl of 50% acetic acid, mix and immediately place on ice.
7. Read absorbance at 405 nm, ideally within 1 h, even though the colour is believed to be stable for 4 h.
8. Draw a standard curve of absorbance at 405 nm versus percentage antiplasmin activity and read the test results from it.

Potential sources of error are very highly coloured plasma samples, for instance in the case of liver disease. This can be overcome by setting up colour blanks for each plasma, including normal, where the substrate is replaced by 200 μl of buffer.

Another source of error, although rare, is where a plasma sample has endogenous protease activity. Correction can be made by setting up a blank where no plasmin is added; replace with 200 μl of buffer.

PAI activity assay

A number of assays are available for PAI activity. It should be noted that all are correctly described as assays of PAI activity rather than of PAI-1 activity, since they are not entirely specific for PAI-1. The use of sct-PA in these assays reduces the detection of PAI-2.

Most commercially available methods depend on adding t-PA to the test sample containing inhibitors of t-PA. After a short reaction time the remaining t-PA activity is assayed. The assay depends on the generation of plasmin from plasminogen by t-PA in the presence of a fibrin stimulator. Plasmin is assayed using a tripeptide chromogenic substrate, with the release of *p*-nitroaniline at the endpoint.

Reagents

1. *50 mM Tris buffer, pH 8.3, containing 0.01% Tween 80.* Dissolve 6.1 g of Tris and 0.1 g of Tween 80 in distilled water, adjust pH to 8.3 with acetic acid and make up to 1 litre.
2. *Human plasminogen, 0.5 mg/ml in Tris buffer.* Store in aliquots at –70°C and thaw rapidly at 37°C prior to use.
3. *Plasmin chromogenic substrate S-2251.* Dissolve 25 mg in 6 ml of water to give a 7.5 mM solution (stable for 6 months at 2–8°C).
4. *Fresh plasminogen/S-2251/Tris buffer solution.* Prepare from solutions 1–3 by mixing 1 volume of plasminogen, 1 volume of S-2251 and 3 volumes of Tris buffer. Use within 1 h of preparation.
5. *0.2 M acetate buffer, pH 3.9.*
6. *Single-chain t-PA (Kabi).* Reconstitute 10 µg in 0.2 M acetate buffer, pH 3.9, to 5000 IU/ml. Keep at room temperature for approximately 10 min, mixing gently to allow complete dissolution. Store at –70°C in small aliquots. Do not refreeze. Dilution for assay: 40 µl of 5000 IU/ml stock and 4.96 ml of Tris buffer (40 IU/ml).
7. *PAI-1-depleted human plasma.* Prepare by passing over anti-PAI-1–Sepharose (Booth et al 1987a)
8. Cyanogen bromide treated fibrinogen 0.66 mg/ml (Verheijen et al 1984).
9. 20% acetic acid

Method

1. Prepare the standard curve. An arbitrary inhibitor unit is defined as inhibiting 1 IU of t-PA under the conditions of the assay. The standard curve (calibrated in AU/ml) is derived from mixtures of solutions defined as 0 AU/ml and 40 AU/ml. These are prepared as follows and mixed carefully:

	40 AU/ml	0 AU/ml
t-PA (40 IU/ml)	—	25 µl
Tris buffer	25 µl	—
PAI-1-free plasma	25 µl	25 µl
Distilled water	4 ml	4 ml

The standards are prepared from mixing these two solutions as follows:

Standard (AU/ml)	40 AU/ml (µl)	0 AU/ml (µl)
40	1000	—
30	750	250
20	500	500
10	250	750
0	—	1000

2. Incubate 25 μl plasma samples with 25 μl of t-PA (40 IU/ml) for 10 min at room temperature. Note that if plasma samples are known or expected to have high PAI activity (greater than 30 AU/ml), they should first be diluted with PAI-1-depleted plasma.
3. Add 4 ml of distilled water to each sample.
4. These dilute samples and standards are now treated identically. The assay may be performed in test-tubes or in microtitre wells.

	Test-tube	Microtitre well
Dilute sample or standard (2–8°C)	200 μl	50 μl
Plasminogen/ S-2251/Tris solution	200 μl	50 μl
Stimulator, 0.66 mg/ml	100 μl	25 μl
Incubate for 2 h at 37°C		
Stop reaction with 20% acetic acid	100 μl	25 μl.

Measure absorbance at 405 nm (reference wavelength if available should be 490 nm). Draw a standard curve of absorbance at 405 nm versus AU/ml and read test results. Correct for any dilution made to plasma before addition of t-PA.

Laurell rocket immunoelectrophoresis

Reagents

1. *Tris/barbitone buffer, pH 8.6.* Dissolve 44.3 g of Tris, 22.4 g of diethylbarbituric acid and 0.53 g of calcium lactate in distilled water and make volume up to 1 litre. Check pH is 8.6; do not adjust.
2. *1% agarose (Sigma type 1) in Tris/barbitone buffer, pH 8.6.* Add 1 g of agarose to 100 ml of Tris/barbitone buffer. Boil agarose until completely dissolved and store at 56°C until required.

Method

1. Cut GelBond sheet to required size:

5 wells	5 × 7.5 cm	4 ml agarose
12 wells	10 × 7.5 cm	8 ml agarose.

2. Set up electrophoresis apparatus. In most designs about 1 litre of buffer should be placed in each reservoir. Soak the wicks (double thickness of Whatman No. 3 filter paper) in buffer.
3. Place the required volume of agarose in a warm test-tube and replace in 56°C water bath. Add antiserum and invert gently to mix. Pour immediately onto hydrophilic side of GelBond on a level surface.
4. Stand for approximately 1 min to set. Cut the required number of wells with a 3 mm diameter cutter and remove agarose by suction.

5. Place the GelBond on the cooling plate of the electrophoresis tank and lay soaked wicks onto the edges of the agarose surface. Make sure there is a good contact between agarose plate, filter paper wicks and reservoir buffer.
6. Load samples (5 μl) carefully into wells. Standard curves consist of dilutions of a normal plasma pool. Plasma samples should be run at the same dilution as top normal pool dilution.
7. Electrophoresis is towards the anode (+). Run at 4 V/cm overnight for 18 h. The voltage should be measured across the plate. Most probes are at a fixed distance of 4 cm; in this case the setting would be 16 V (DC).

Washing and staining of immunoelectrophoresis plates

Reagents.

1. *Wash.* 0.9% (w/v) aqueous sodium chloride (9 g per litre).
2. *Stain.* 0.125% (w/v) Coomassie brilliant blue R (Cl 42660) in 45% (v/v) methanol, 9% (v/v) acetic acid. Dissolve 1.25 g Coomassie blue in 450 ml methanol. Then add water and 90 ml acetic acid to final volume of 1 litre.
3. *Destain.* 9.5% methanol, 7.5% acetic acid. Add 950 ml of methanol and 750 ml of glacial acetic acid to water and make up to 10 litres with distilled water.

Method.

1. When electrophoresis is completed, remove agarose plate from electrophoresis tank and soak in 0.9% sodium chloride for at least 1 h. If a high concentration of antiserum has been used, several changes of wash solution and longer washing times are recommended.
2. Cover the washed agarose plate with Whatman No. 1 filter paper, covered in turn by thick paper towels and a glass plate with a heavy weight. Leave for at least 15 min.
3. Remove plate and towels. Carefully peel off the filter paper. The washing/pressing procedure can be repeated if necessary to improve the clarity of the background.
4. Air-dry the plate completely and then place it in staining solution for less than 1 min. Transfer to destaining solution. Continue to transfer to fresh destain as soon as blue coloration can be seen in the solution.
5. Allow plate to dry and measure the height of the rockets.
6. Construct a standard curve from the dilutions of normal pool plasma and read unknown samples from it. Results are expressed as a percentage of normal pool plasma.

The conditions used in the author's laboratory are given below and these may be varied as appropriate if different sources of antisera are used. In some cases the antibodies specified are supplied as IgG fractions. There is no advantage in using an IgG fraction rather than an antiserum in immunoelectrophoresis.

Conditions for rocket immunoelectrophoresis

Plasminogen.
1% rabbit anti-human plasminogen IgG (DAKO code A081) or 2% antiserum (Behring)
Normal pooled plasma undiluted, 1:2 and 1:4; patient plasma undiluted.

α_2-Antiplasmin.

5% rabbit anti-human α_2-plasmin inhibitor (DAKO code A303)
Normal pooled plasma undiluted, 1:2 and 1:4; patient plasma undiluted.

α_2-Macroglobulin.

0.5% rabbit anti-human α_2-macroglobulin (DAKO code A033)
Normal pooled plasma 1:8, 1:16 and 1:32; patient plasma 1:8.

C1 inhibitor.

5% rabbit anti-human C1 esterase inhibitor (DAKO code A253) or 5% antiserum (Behring)
Normal pooled plasma undiluted, 1:2 and 1:4; patient plasma undiluted.

Histidine-rich glycoprotein.

1% rabbit anti-histidine-rich glycoprotein (Behring)
Normal pooled plasma undiluted, 1:2, and 1:4; patient plasma undiluted.

Two-dimensional electrophoresis

Reagents are as for rocket immunoelectrophoresis. Pour a plain agarose plate, using 4 ml of 1% agarose on GelBond (7.5 × 5 cm). Cut out one 3 mm well in the bottom left, as illustrated in Figure 5.7. Load the sample (5 μl) into the well and start the electrophoresis, in the direction indicated for the first dimension, at 10 V/cm for 1 h.

Remove the plate from the electrophoresis tank and cut the agarose 0.5 cm from the sample well. Scrape away the upper section of agarose and replace with agarose-containing antiserum, at the same concentration as is used for rocket immunoelectrophoresis: 2.5 ml should be sufficient to cover the upper part of the plate. Take care when pouring on the agarose/antiserum to make good contact with the original section of agarose.

Return the plate to the electrophoresis tank and run at 90° to the original electrophoresis. The electrophoresis conditions are as for rocket immunoelectrophoresis, 4 V/cm for 18 h. The washing and staining of the plates is exactly as described for rockets.

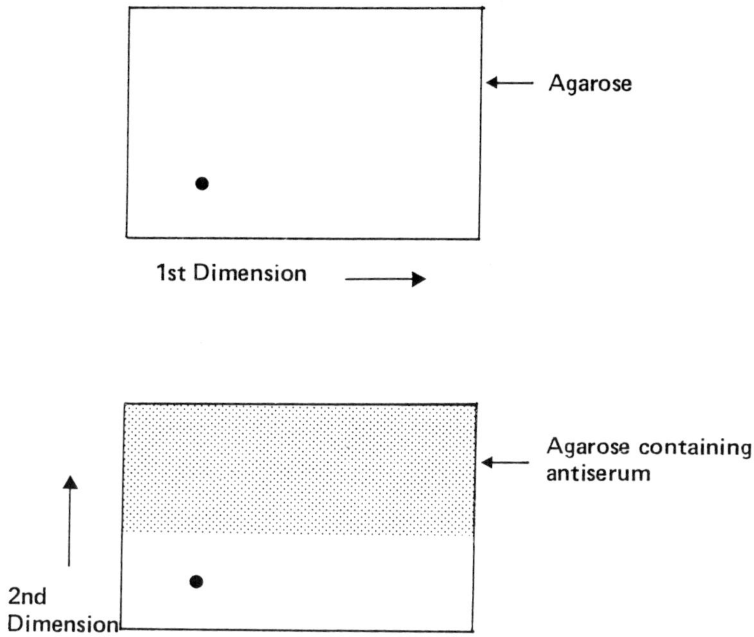

Fig. 5.7 Method for two-dimensional immunoelectrophoresis.

ACKNOWLEDGEMENTS

Alison Croll provided valuable help in compiling the Methods Appendix and in critical reading of the manuscript.

REFERENCES

Aoki N 1984 Genetic abnormalities of the fibrinolytic system. Seminars in Thrombosis and Haemostasis 10: 42–50

Astedt B, Lecander I, Ny T 1987 The placental type plasminogen activator inhibitor, PAI2. Fibrinolysis 1: 203–208

Aznar J, Estelles A, Vila V et al 1984 Inherited fibrinolytic disorder due to an enhanced plasminogen activator level. Thrombosis and Haemostasis 52: 196–200

Bennett B, Booth N A, Croll A, Dawson A A 1989 The bleeding disorder in acute promyelocytic leukaemia: fibrinolysis due to u-PA rather than defibrination. British Journal of Haematology 71: 511–517

Bennett B, Croll A, Ferguson K, Booth N A 1990 Complexing of tissue plasminogen activator with PAI-1, α_2-macroglobulin, and C1-inhibitor: studies in patients with defibrination and a fibrinolytic state after electroshock or complicated labor. Blood 75: 671–676

Blasi F, Vassalli J-D, Dano K 1987 Urokinase-type plasminogen activator: proenzyme, receptor and inhibitors. Journal of Cell Biology 104: 801–804

Booth N A, Bennett B 1982 Plasmin–α_2-antiplasmin complex as an indicator of in vivo fibrinolysis. British Journal of Haematology 50: 537–541
Booth N A, Bennett B 1984 Plasmin–α_2-antiplasmin complexes in bleeding disorders characterized by primary and secondary fibrinolysis. British Journal of Haematology 56: 545–556
Booth N A, Bennett B, Wijngaards G, Grieve J H K 1983 A new life-long hemorrhagic disorder due to excess plasminogen activator. Blood 61: 267–275
Booth N A, Anderson J A, Bennett B 1984 Plasminogen activator in alcoholic cirrhosis: demonstration of increased tissue type and urokinase type activator. Journal of Clinical Pathology 37: 772–777
Booth N A, Anderson J A, Bennett B 1985 Platelet release protein which inhibits plasminogen activators. Journal of Clinical Pathology 38: 825–830
Booth N A, MacGregor I R, Hunter N R, Bennett B 1987a Plasminogen activator inhibitor from human endothelial cells: purification and partial characterization. European Journal of Biochemistry 165: 595–600
Booth N A, Walker E, Maughan R, Bennett B 1987b Plasminogen activator in normal subjects after exercise and venous occlusion: t-PA circulates as complexes with C1-inhibitor and PAI-1. Blood 69: 1600–1604
Booth N A, Simpson A J, Croll A, Bennett B, MacGregor I R 1988 Plasminogen activator inhibitor (PAI-1) in plasma and platelets. British Journal of Haematology 70: 327–333
Booth N A, Croll A, Bennett B 1990 The activity of plasminogen activator inhibitor-1 (PAI-1) of human platelet. Fibrinolysis 4 (suppl 2): 138–140
Brogden R N, Speight T M, Avery G S 1973 Streptokinase: a review of its clinical pharmacology, mechanism of action and therapeutic uses. Drugs 5: 357–445
Carrell R W, Christey P B, Boswell D R 1987 Serpins: antithrombin and other inhibitors of coagulation and fibrinolysis. Evidence from amino acid sequences. In: Verstraete M, Vermylen J, Lijnen R, Arnout J (eds). Thrombosis and haemostasis. Leuven University Press, p 1–15
Cash J D 1978 Control mechanisms of activator release. In: Davidson J F, Rowan R M, Samama M M, Desnoyers P C (eds). Progress in chemical fibrinolysis and thrombolysis. Raven Press, New York, Vol 3, p. 65–75
Castellino F J 1984 Biochemistry of human plasminogen. Seminars in Thrombosis and Haemostasis 10: 18–23
Chmielewska J, Wiman B 1986 Determination of tissue plasminogen activator and its 'fast' inhibitor in plasma. Clinical Chemistry 32: 482–485
Chmielewska J, Ranby M, Wiman B 1983 Evidence for a rapid inhibitor to tissue plasminogen activator in plasma. Thrombosis Research 31: 427–436
Collen D 1980 On the regulation and control of fibrinolysis. Thrombosis and Haemostasis 43: 77–89
Collen D 1986 Report of the meeting of the subcommittee on fibrinolysis (ICTH), Jerusalem, Israel. Thrombosis and Haemostasis 56: 415–416
Collen D 1987 Molecular mechanisms of fibrinolysis and their application to fibrin-specific thrombolytic therapy. Journal of Cellular Biochemistry 33: 77–86
Collen D, De Maeyer L 1975 Molecular biology of human plasminogen. I Physicochemical properties and microheterogeneity. Thrombosis et Diathesis Haemorrhagica 34: 396–402
Declerck P J, Alessi M-C, Verstreken M V, Kruithof E K O, Juhan-Vague I, Collen D 1988a Measurement of plasminogen activator inhibitor I in biologic fluids with a murine monoclonal antibody-based enzyme-linked immunosorbent assay. Blood 71: 220–225
Declerck P J, de Mol M, Alessi M-C et al 1988b Purification and characterisation of a plasminogen activator inhibitor 1 binding protein from human plasma. Identification as a multimeric form of S Protein (vitronectin). Journal of Biological Chemistry 263: 15 454–15 461
Deutsch D G, Mertz E T 1970 Plasminogen: purification from human plasma by affinity chromatography. Science 170: 1095–1096
Erickson L A Ginsberg M H, Loskutoff D J 1984 Detection and partial characterisation of an inhibitor of plasminogen activator in human platelets. Journal of Clinical Investigation 74: 1465–1472
Golder J P, Stephens R W 1983 Minactivin: a human monocyte product which specifically inactivates urokinase-type plasminogen activators. European Journal of Biochemistry 136: 517–522

Hamsten A, Wiman B, De Faire U, Blomback M 1985 Increased plasma levels of a rapid inhibitor of tissue plasminogen activator in young survivors of myocardial infarction. New England Journal of Medicine 313: 1557–1563

Hamsten A, De Faire U, Walldius G et al 1987 Plasminogen activator inhibitor in plasma: risk factor for recurrent myocardial infarction. Lancet ii: 3–9

Harpel P C 1981 α_2-Plasmin inhibitor and α_2-macroglobulin–plasmin complexes in plasma. Journal of Clinical Investigation 68: 46–55

Hariman H, Grant P J, Hughes J R, Booth N A, Davies J A, Prentice C R M 1989 Effect of physiological concentrations of vasopressin on components of the fibrinolytic system. Thrombosis and Haemostasis 61: 298–300

Hashimoto Y, Kobayashi A, Yamazaki N, Sugawara Y, Takada Y, Takada A 1987 Relationship between age and plasma t-PA, PA-inhibitor and PA activity. Thrombosis Research 46: 625–633

Hauert J, Nicoloso G, Schleuning W-D, Bachman F, Schapira M 1989 Plasminogen activators in dextran sulfate-activated euglobulin fractions: a molecular analysis of factor XII- and prekallikrein-dependent fibrinolysis. Blood 73: 994–999

Heeb M J, Espana F, Geiger M, Collen D, Stump D C, Griffin J H 1987 Immunological identity of heparin-dependent plasma and urinary protein C inhibitor and plasminogen activator inhibitor–3. Journal of Biological Chemistry 262: 15 813–15 816

Hekman C M, Loskutoff D J 1985 Endothelial cells produce a latent inhibitor of plasminogen activator that can be activated by denaturants. Journal of Biological Chemistry 260: 11581–11587

Hoylaerts M, Rijken D C, Lijnen H R, Collen D 1982 Kinetics of the activation of plasminogen by human tissue plasminogen activator. Role of fibrin. Journal of Biological Chemistry 257: 2912–2919

Ichinose A, Fujikawa K, Suyama T 1986 The activation of prourokinase by plasma kallikrein and its inactivation by thrombin. Journal of Biological Chemistry 261: 3486–3489

ISIS-2 Collaborative Group 1988 Randomised trial of intravenous streptokinase, oral aspirin, both, or neither among 17 187 cases of suspected acute myocardial infarction: ISIS-2. Lancet ii: 349–360

Juhan-Vague I, Moerman B, De Cock F, Aillaud M F, Collen D 1984 Plasma levels of a specific inhibitor of tissue-type plasminogen activator (and urokinase) in normal and pathological conditions. Thrombosis Research 33: 523–530

Juhan-Vague I, Aillaud M F, De Cock F et al 1985 The fast-acting inhibitor of tissue-type plasminogen activator is an acute phase reactant protein. In: Davidson J F, Donati M B, Coccheri S (eds) Progress in fibrinolysis. Churchill Livingstone, Edinburgh, Vol VII, p 146–149

Juhan-Vague I, Valadier J, Alessi M C et al 1987 Deficient t-PA release and elevated PA inhibitor levels in patients with spontaneous or recurrent deep venous thrombosis. Thrombosis and Haemostasis 57: 67–72

Kawano T, Morimoto K, Uemura Y 1970 Partial purification and properties of urokinase inhibitor from human placenta. Journal of Biochemistry 67: 333–342

Kluft C, Brakman P 1975 Effect of flufenamate on euglobulin fibrinolysis: involvement of C1-inactivator. In: Davidson J F, Samama M M, Desnoyers P C (eds). Progress in chemical fibrinolysis and thrombolysis Raven Press, New York, Vol 1, p 375–381

Kluft C, Verheijen J H 1990 Leiden fibrinolysis working party: blood collection and handling procedures for assessment of tissue-type plasminogen activator (t-PA) and plasminogen activator inhibitor-1 (PAI-1). Fibrinolysis 4 (suppl 2): 155–161

Kluft C, Verheijen J H, Rijken D C, Chang G T G, Jie A F H, Onkelinx C 1985 Diurnal fluctuations in the activity of the fast-acting t-PA inhibitor. In: Davidson J F, Donati M B, Coccheri S (eds). Progress in fibrinolysis. Churchill Livingstone, Edinburgh, Vol VII, p 117–119

Kluft C, Dooijewaard G, Emeis J J 1987 Role of the contact system in fibrinolysis. Seminars in Thrombosis and Hemostasis 13: 50–68

Kraut J 1977 Serine proteases: structure and mechanism. Annual Reviews in Biochemistry 46: 331–358

Kruithof E K O, Ransijn A, Bachmann F 1983 Inhibition of tissue plasminogen activator by human plasma. In: Davidson J F, Bachmann F, Bouvier C A, Kruithof, E K O (eds). Progress in fibrinolysis. Churchill Livingstone, Edinburgh, vol VI, p 365–369

Kruithof E K O, Vassalli J D, Schleuning W-D, Mattaliano R J 1986 Purification and characterisation of a plasminogen activator inhibitor from the histiocytic lymphoma cell line U-937. Journal of Biological Chemistry 261: 11 207–11 212

Kruithof E K O, Gudinchet A, Bachmann F 1988 Plasminogen activator inhibitor 1 and plasminogen activator inhibitor 2 in various disease states. Thrombosis and Haemostasis 59: 7–12

Laurell C-B 1966 Quantitative estimation of proteins by electrophoresis in agarose gel containing antibodies. Analytical Biochemistry 15: 45–52

Leiper K, Booth N A, Reith A, Moore N R, Bennett B 1990 Plasminogen activator inhibitors (PAI-1, PAI-2) and t-PA–PAI-1 complex in liver disease. Fibrinolysis 4 (suppl 3): 150

Loskutoff D J, van Mourik J A, Erickson L A, Lawrence D 1983 Detection of an unusually stable fibrinolytic inhibitor produced by bovine endothelial cells. Proceedings of the National Academy of Sciences, USA 80: 2956–2960

MacGregor I R, Roberts E M, Prowse C V, Broomhead A F, Ozolins M, Litka P 1988 Fibrinolytic and haemostatic responses to desamino–D–arginine vasopressin (DDAVP) administered by intravenous and subcutaneous routes in healthy subjects. Thrombosis and Haemostasis 59: 34–39

Nilsson I M, Ljungner H, Tengborn L 1985 Two different mechanisms in patients with venous thrombosis and defective fibrinolysis: low concentration of plasminogen activator or increased concentration of plasminogen activator inhibitor. British Medical Journal 290: 1453–1456

Patthy L 1985 Evolution of the proteases of blood coagulation and fibrinolysis by assembly from modules. Cell 41: 657–663

Ranby M, Bergsdorf N, Nilsson T 1982 Enzymatic properties of the one- and two-chain forms of tissue plasminogen activator. Thombosis Research 27: 175–183

Rijken D C, Wijngaards G, Zaal de Jong M, Welbergen J 1979 Purification and partial characterization of plasminogen activator from human uterine tissue. Biochemica et Biophysica Acta 580: 140–145

Rijken D C, Hoylaerts M, Collen D 1982 Fibrinolytic properties of one-chain and two-chain human extrinsic (tissue-type) plasminogen activator. Journal of Biological Chemistry 257: 2920–2925

Rijken D C, Juhan-Vague I, Collen D 1983 Complexes between tissue-type plasminogen activator and proteinase inhibitors in human plasma, identified with an immunoradiometric assay. Journal of Clinical and Laboratory Medicine 101: 285–294

Saito H, Ratnoff O D, Waldmann R et al 1975 Fitzgerald trait: deficiency of a hitherto unrecognized agent, Fitzgerald factor, participating in surface mediated reactions of clotting, fibrinolysis, generation of kinins and the property of diluted plasma enhancing vascular permeability (PF/dil). Journal of Clinical Investigation 55: 1082–1089

Schleef R R, Higgins D L, Pillemer E, Levitt L J 1989 Bleeding diathesis due to decreased functional activity of type 1 plasminogen activator inhibitor. Journal of Clinical Investigation 83: 1747–1752

Simpson A J, Booth N A, Sewell H, MacGregor I R, Bennett B 1989 Immunochemical localization of PAI-1 in human tissues. Thrombosis and Haemostasis 62: 171

Simpson A J, Booth N A, Moore N R, Bennett B 1990 The platelet and plasma pools of plasminogen activator inhibitor (PAI-1) vary independently in disease. British Journal of Haematology 75: 543–548

Sprengers E D, Kluft C 1987 Plasminogen activator inhibitors. Blood 69: 381–387

Sprengers E D, Verheijen J H, van Hinsbergh V W M, Emeis J J 1984 Evidence for the presence of two different fibrinolytic inhibitors in human endothelial cell conditioned medium. Biochimica et Biophysica Acta 801: 163–170

Stump D, Thienpoint M, Collen D 1986 Purification and characterization of a novel inhibitor of urokinase from human urine: quantitation and preliminary characterization in plasma. Journal of Biological Chemistry 261: 12 759–12 766

Thorsen S, Philips M 1984 Isolation of tissue-type plasminogen activator–inhibitor complexes from human plasma. Evidence for a rapid plasminogen activator inhibitor. Biochimica et Biophysica Acta 802: 11–118

van Zonneveld A J, Veerman H, Pannekoek H 1986 Autonomous functions of structural domains on human tissue-type plasminogen activator. Proceedings of the National Academy of Sciences, USA 83: 4670–4674

Verheijen J H, Chang G T G, Kluft C 1984 Evidence for the occurrence of a fast-acting

inhibitor for tissue-type plasminogen activator in human plasma. Thrombosis and Haemostasis 51: 392–395
Verstraete M, Vermylen J, Schetz J 1978 Biochemical changes noted during intermittent administration of streptokinase. Thrombosis and Haemostasis 39: 61–68
Voller A, Bidwell D E, Bartlett A 1979 The enzyme linked immunosorbent assay (ELISA) Dynatech Europe, Guernsey
Wagner O F, de Vries C J M, Hohmann C, Veerman H J G, Pannekoek H 1989 Interaction between plasminogen activator inhibitor type 1 (PAI-1) bound to fibrin and either tissue-type plasminogen activator (t-PA) or urokinase-type plasminogen activator (u-PA). Journal of Clinical Investigation 84: 647–655
Wallen P 1977 Activation of plasminogen with urokinase and tissue activator. In: Paoletti R, Sherry S (eds). Thrombosis and urokinase. Academic Press, London, p 91–102
Wiman B, Chmielewska J 1985 A novel fast inhibitor to tissue plasminogen activator in plasma, which may be of great pathophysiological significance. Scandanavian Journal of Clinical and Laboratory Investigation 45 (suppl 177): 43–47
Wiman B, Collen D 1978 Molecular mechanism of physiological fibrinolysis. Nature 272: 549–550
Wun T-C, Capuano A 1987 Initiation and regulation of fibrinolysis in human plasma at the plasminogen activator level Blood 69: 1354–1362
Wun T-C, Schleuning W-D, Reich E 1982 Isolation and characterization of urokinase from human plasma. Journal of Biological Chemistry 257: 3276–3283

6. The formation, measurement and clinical value of fibrinogen derivatives

Willem Nieuwenhuizen

INTRODUCTION

The formation of a blood clot (albeit at a very low rate) is a normal physiological process. Blood clots are the products of an activated coagulation system. However, no matter how slowly blood clots are generated normally it is obvious that even such a slow process will eventually cause a blockage of the blood flow, i.e. thrombosis. Under pathophysiological conditions the coagulation system may be more active and as a consequence thrombosis might occur more rapidly.

Nature's major defence mechanism against unwanted blood clot (thrombi) formation is the fibrinolytic system. The fibrinolytic system will lyse (forming) thrombi. In most cases fibrinolysis will counterbalance coagulation. This equilibrium is known as the haemostatic balance.

Under some conditions, however, the balance is disturbed. Depending on which of the two opposing processes, coagulation and fibrinolysis, is over-active, thrombosis or bleeding will result. Thrombosis will occur when thrombi are formed at a higher rate than they are lysed by the fibrinolytic system; bleeding will result from a situation where clots are lysed more rapidly than they are generated. As a consequence of this concept, thrombosis may occur when the coagulation system functions normally but the fibrinolytic system is not sufficiently active; *and* when the fibrinolytic system functions normally but the coagulation system is over-active. Also, bleeding tendencies can be explained by two underlying mechanisms, i.e. normal coagulation in combination with over-active fibrinolysis and normal fibrinolysis in combination with defective coagulation.

The activation of the coagulation system leads to thrombin formation. This protease catalyses the first of a series of steps that eventually yield fibrin (Doolittle 1981). Fibrin is the insoluble protein matrix of a blood clot which renders the latter its mechanical stability. Activation of the fibrinolytic system leads to plasmin formation. Plasmin degrades the insoluble fibrin in a clot to soluble fibrin degradation products. As a consequence of this digestion, thrombi lose their stability and disintegrate.

It will be clear from the above that the haemostatic balance in its most elementary form can be described as the equilibrium between fibrin formation (from its soluble precursor fibrinogen) and lysis of fibrin, i.e. in a balanced situation fibrin should be formed and lysed at the same rate.

It has been realized for a long time that the activity of the fibrinolytic system may be derived from blood levels of fibrin degradation products. Due to practical limitations, the latter were assessed in serum samples and not in plasma. As will be pointed out below, the use of serum is a notorious source of artefacts and is no longer a viable proposition.

The modern assays can be performed on plasma samples. This not only enables the investigator to avoid the serum artefacts but also allows the quantification of coagulation system products in the same samples. (Coagulation products can obviously not be measured in serum.) From the limited data it will become conceivable that a much more detailed image of the status of the haemostatic balance can be derived from the simultaneous measurement of both coagulation and fibrinolytic products. Furthermore, the fibrinolytic system is not absolutely specific for fibrin. In many instances it appears to also attack fibrinogen. The latter process has been suspected previously, but could only be proven with the advent of a plasma assay specific for fibrin*ogen* degradation products. In this chapter emphasis will be on high molecular weight fibrin(ogen) derivatives which can be assessed directly in plasma without prior processing.

Formation of fibrin

Fibrinogen (Doolittle 1973, 1981, Henschen 1981), the soluble precursor of fibrin, is a symmetrical glycoprotein with a molecular weight of 340 000. It is composed of six polypeptide chains: two Aα-, two Bβ- and two γ-chains with molecular weights of approximately 67 000, 57 000 and 47 000, respectively. The six chains are kept together by multiple disulphide bonds. In electron-microscopic images fibrinogen appears to have a trinodular structure: one central, relatively small nodule connected by thin filamentous structures to two outer larger nodules. It is clear from biochemical studies that the central nodule comprises the amino terminal ends of all six fibrinogen polypeptide chains.

As stated in the introduction, activation of the coagulation system will eventually generate thrombin. Thrombin cleaves small 16 amino acid long peptides from the amino termini of the two Aα-chains (Doolittle 1973, 1981, Henschen 1981). These peptides are called fibrinopeptide A (FpA). The fibrinogen molecule devoid of FpA is designated as fibrin I or desAA fibrin. The new amino termini of the α-chains resulting from the FpA cleavage constitute sites which bind to complementary sites already pre-existing in fibrinogen. The latter sites do not require activation. At low fibrin concentration, fibrin can be kept in solution by complexing with fibrinogen. These complexes are known as soluble fibrin (Brass et al 1976, Graeff et al 1979). Beyond a certain critical (local) concentration, the fibrin I molecules will aggregate with each other to form fibrin I polymers in which the subunits will be cross-linked by coagulation factor XIIIa (Doolittle 1981). The latter is formed from its precursor by active thrombin and is a Ca^{2+}-dependent transglutaminase. The cross-links are isopeptide bonds between lysine and glutamine side chains of adjacent γ- and α-chains in the fibrin gels.

Simultaneously with FpA, but more slowly, thrombin also releases small 14 amino acid long peptides from the amino termini of the fibrinogen Bβ-chains. These peptides are designated as fibrinopeptide B (FpB). The fibrinogen without FpA and FpB is called fibrin II or desAABB fibrin. Like fibrin I, fibrin II will aggregate and become cross-linked (Hermans & McDonagh 1982).

An increase of soluble fibrin concentrations in blood indicates that the coagulation activity is increased and may not be compensated by fibrinolysis. In the latter case a thrombotic event may be impending.

Formation of fibrinogen degradation products

Plasmin, the product of an activated fibrinolytic system, is not specific for fibrin. Under special conditions it may also attack fibrinogen (Mosesson et al 1974, Holm et al 1985, Phillips 1981).

Fibrinogen occurs in the circulation in three main molecular forms: the high molecular weight form (HMW) in which both Aα-chains are virtually intact; a low molecular weight form (LMW) in which one of the two Aα- chains is shortened; and a form (LMW') in which both Aα-chains are shortened at their carboxyl terminal ends. Under normal conditions the relative amounts of HMW, LMW and LMW' fibrinogen are 70, 26 and 4% respectively. All three forms are clottable. The LMW and LMW' forms of fibrinogen are probably the result of proteolytic activity, possibly of plasmin, which affected the carboxyl terminal stretches of the Aα-chains, which are known to be extremely sensitive to proteolysis.

It is conceivable that even a low-grade increase in proteolytic activity in the blood may be reflected in an increase in the LMW'/HMW ratio.

When plasmin digestion proceeds beyond the LMW' fibrinogen formation, a product is formed, designated as fibrinogen fragment X. It is basically a slowly clottable form of fibrinogen in which approximately 70% of both Aα-chains has been removed from the carboxyl terminal ends. The amino termini of the Aα-chains are at least partly intact, i.e. FpA are still present.

Upon further digestion fragments X are cleaved asymmetrically and one so-called fragment Y and one fragment D are formed. Fragment Y is composed of the central nodule connected with one outer nodule as seen in electron-microscopic images (see above). Fragment D corresponds to the outer nodule which is missing in fragment Y and is composed of central and carboxyl terminal stretches of the Aα-, Bβ- and γ-chains of the original fibrinogen molecule. Finally, the remaining connections between fragment D and the central nodule in Y are cleaved. The central nodule is designated as fragment E, and still contains (at least some) FpA.

As will be shown below, the fibrinogen molecule fragments X, Y and E appear to undergo conformational changes (as compared with HMW, LMW and LMW' fibrinogen) which expose stretches of the Bβ-chain normally buried in the fibrinogen molecules, i.e. 'neo-epitopes'.

An interesting feature of fibrinogen degradation products, especially fragments X and Y, is their strong anticoagulant activity. The possibility to assess the concentration of fibrinogen degradation products in blood may enable the clinician to obtain a much more sophisticated understanding of possible bleeding phenomena and to design appropriate therapeutic regimens.

Formation of fibrin degradation products

Plasmin digests the different forms of fibrin, fibrin I and fibrin II (cross-linked and non-cross-linked), via a series of intermediate products comparable to those described in the previous section for fibrinogen. The reason for this appears to be that plasmin follows the same interdomainal cleavage pattern in fibrin as in fibrinogen.

Non-cross-linked fibrin I (desAA fibrin) will sequentially yield fragments X_I, Y_I, D and E_I and non-cross-linked fibrin II (desAABB fibrin), X_{II}, Y_{II}, D

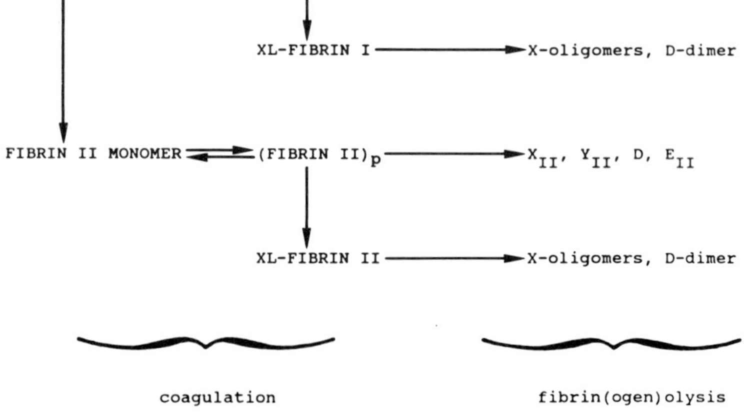

Fig. 6.1 Schematic representation of the formation of different fibrin(ogen) derivatives.

and E_{II}. The subscripts I and II indicate the absence of FpA alone and the absence of FpA *and* FpB, respectively.

Cross-linked fibrins I and II consist of very long polymers of fibrin I and II in which the subunits are cross-linked by isopeptide bonds between adjacent α- and γ-chains. Plasmin will attack the subunits in these polymeric structures in a random order. This will result in soluble fragments of the original polymers, with a range of molecular weights (Doolittle 1981, Graeff & Hafter 1982). These are collectively designated as X-oligomers (Graeff & Hafter 1982, Gaffney & Perry 1985a, Gaffney et al 1986). Extensive digestion of these X-oligomers will yield so-called fragments D-dimer and fragments E_I (or E_{II}) (Doolittle 1981, Graeff & Hafter 1982). Fragments D-dimer can be described as two fragments D covalently kept together by two isopeptide bonds (cross-links) between the γ-chain remnants of the two D-fragments. A scheme of the formation of the different fibrinogen derivatives is shown in Fig. 6.1.

The exposure of neo-epitopes (see previous section) by fibrin degradation is comparable to that induced by digestion of fibrinogen.

Molecular characteristics of fibrinogen and some of its derivatives

Some molecular features are summarized in Table 6.1 which are characteristic for fibrinogen and some of its derivatives and allow the specific recognition of these derivatives.

Table 6.1 Molecular characteristics of fibrinogen and some of its derivatives

Fibrinogen or Fibrin(ogen) derivative	Molecular features
Intact fibrinogen	FpA present; carboxyl terminal end(s) of Aα-chain(s) intact
Soluble fibrin	FpA absent; new amino terminal ends on α-chains (and possibly β-chains) are neo-epitopes (Scheefers-Borchel et al 1985). Also neo-epitopes in Aα-[148–160] (Schielen et al 1989). No cross-links present
Cross-linked fibrin	Same as soluble fibrin plus the presence of cross-links
Fibrin*ogen* degradation products (FgDP)	FpA present; no cross-links; neo-epitopes amongst others in Bβ-[58–114] (Koppert et al 1986)
X-oligomers	FpA absent; high molecular weight; cross-links present
Fibrin degradation products (FbDP)	FpA absent; neo-epitopes in Bβ-[58–114] (Koppert et al 1986); cross-links present in cross-linked FbDP
D-dimer	No FpA; cross-linked γ-chains

ASSAYS FOR FIBRINOGEN, SOLUBLE FIBRIN AND FIBRIN(OGEN) DEGRADATION PRODUCTS

Serum samples should not be used

In the majority of clinical conditions the blood concentration of the products of the two opposing systems, coagulation and fibrinolysis, will be low compared with that of fibrinogen. The former are usually present in the microgram per millilitre range, whereas the latter has a concentration of several milligrams per millilitre, i.e. is present in an excess of at least two orders of magnitude.

As a consequence, assays for FbDP or soluble fibrin have to be both sensitive and specific. Both criteria could in principle be met by immunological methods. However, until relatively recently only polyclonal antibodies were available, which cross-react virtually fully with fibrinogen. For that reason fibrinogen had to be removed completely when fibrinogen derivatives were to be assessed. The most practical method to remove fibrinogen is to prepare serum. Well-known examples of serum assays for fibrin(ogen) degradation products are the Thrombo Wellco assay and the tanned red cell haemagglutination inhibition assay (Merskey et al 1969).

It is known, however, that serum can cause a range of artefactual results. Examples are given below:

1. As stated above, the specificity of the assays is fully dependent on the effectivity of the fibrinogen removal. The latter is, however, not always complete. The test result will (partly) be due to fibrinogen remaining in the serum. This may lead to too high or false-positive results. Fibrinogen clotting may be particularly incomplete in cases of a dysfibrinogenaemia; when a patient has been treated with heparin (Connaghan et al 1986); or when anticoagulant fibrinogen degradation products are present (Haverkate et al 1979, Nieuwenhuizen & Gravesen 1981, Nieuwenhuizen et al 1982). Too high or false-positive results may be caused by fibrin degradation during serum preparation not only from the blood of hyperfibrinolytic patients, but also from blood of normofibrinolytic donors (Koopman et al 1987).
2. Too low or false-negative results may be obtained in blood. Fragments X can coagulate (Marder & Shulman 1969, Nieuwenhuizen & Gravesen 1981) and will not (completely) be recovered in the serum. Some degradation products adsorb to the clot and are removed with the latter (Gaffney & Perry 1985b, Koopman et al 1987, Niewiarowski et al 1970).

Additional major drawbacks of the use of serum are:

1. The loss of FpA from fibrinogen degradation products by thrombin activity during serum preparation. If, for example, fragments X are present in blood and their FpA are removed, they will be converted to

X_I (or X_{II}) and could no longer be identified as products of primary fibrinogenolysis but would rather be interpreted as products of lysis of non cross-linked fibrin.

2. Serum can obviously not be used to assess blood levels of products of coagulation. Since coagulation system products *in combination* with fibrinolysis products may provide valuable information on the status of the haemostatic balance, this is a serious drawback.

Most, if not all, of these artefacts and drawbacks could be avoided if plasma instead of serum could be used. Until relatively recently this was not possible. As will be shown in ensuing sections, however, recently developed enzyme immunoassays (EIA) and latex agglutination assays are based on monoclonal antibodies (MoAb) with a specificity which is compatible with the use of plasma. With the EIA products of both coagulation and fibrinolysis can be measured in the same plasma samples.

The principles of the new MoAb-based assays

The new MoAb-based assays can be divided into (quantitative) EIA and (semi quantitative) latex agglutination tests.

EIA (sandwich type)

A MoAb specific for a molecular feature of a particular (group of) fibrinogen derivative(s) is adsorbed to the wells of microtitration plates; this MoAb is the capture antibody. The capture antibody does not bind fibrinogen (with one exception, i.e. in the EIA for intact fibrinogen; see below).

In some commercially available assays the capture antibody-coated plates are supplied dried and ready for use. Examples of two such assays are given in the appendices to this chapter.

A diluted plasma sample is incubated in the MoAb-coated wells. After washing, the second antibody is added. This antibody, designated as the tagging antibody, may have a defined specificity for another molecular feature of the fibrin(ogen) derivative captured in the first step of the EIA or be a panspecific MoAb or even a polyclonal antibody. The tagging antibody is conjugated with an enzyme, usually horseradish peroxidase (HRP).

After washing, a chromogenic substrate mixture for HRP is added. During incubation a coloured product will be formed, the intensity of which is a measure of the amount of fibrin(ogen) derivative captured in the first step of the EIA.

Latex agglutination assays

These tests are based on latex particles coated with a MoAb specific for a molecular feature of one particular (group of) fibrin(ogen) derivative(s), e.g. the cross-linked area in D-dimer. Obviously, agglutination with MoAb (which bind to only *one* type of epitope) can only occur if the derivative to be assessed contains multiple (at least two) identical epitopes. Fortunately this is the case in virtually all fibrin(ogen) derivatives because they are symmetrical or polymeric

Currently described and available assays based on MoAb

As indicated previously, the EIA are all of the sandwich type in which the capture antibody recognizes a special molecular property of a fibrin(ogen) derivative and the tagging antibody may or may not be monoclonal and/or specific for another epitope in one particular derivative. Currently available EIA with their capture and tagging antibodies are listed in Table 6.2.

The EIA for fibrinogen degradation products (FgDP) and for intact fibrinogen are good examples of EIA based on two MoAb, each with a defined specificity. In FgDP EIA the capture MoAb is specific for degraded forms of both fibrin and fibrinogen (and will thus capture both FgDP and FbDp), whereas the tagging antibody binds to FpA-containing fibrinogen derivatives. Since FpA are only present in FgDP, the EIA is specific for FgDP as a result of the combined specificities.

Some of the assays are commercially available, such as the EIA for D-dimer, FgDP, FbDP and TDP. Amongst these, EIA for FgDP, FbDP and TDP are sold ready-for-use, i.e. the microtitre plates have been coated with the capture MoAb and dried by the manufacturers. Moreover, these EIA have a (very) short time-to-result (only 45 min for the FgDP, FbDP and TDP EIA and 140 min for the D-dimer EIA) which means they can be applied in emergency situations and for monitoring purposes.

The variety of MoAb-based agglutination assays is relatively limited. Only two agglutination-type assays for D-dimer are commercially available. One is based on MoAb DD3B6 (see Table 6.2) (Elms et al 1983, Rylatt et al 1983) and is available from MabCo (Brisbane, Australia); from American Diagnostica Inc. (Greenwich, USA) and from Ortho Diagnostic Systems (Beerse, Belgium). The other is available from Diagnostica Stago (Asnières, France); from Boehringer Mannheim (Mannheim, FRG) and from Organon Teknika (Turnhout, Belgium).

The only other agglutination assay for plasma concentrations of fibrin/fibrinogen degradation products is based on MoAb F_2C_5 (Mirshahi et al 1986), which is specifically reactive with a neo-epitope in the D-domain of fibrin(ogen) degradation products. It is, however, not commercially available.

The latex agglutination assays have the practical advantage that they have a very short time-to-result and they are easy to perform. The disadvantages are that they are semiquantitative and the reading of the agglutination is rather subjective.

Table 6.2 Currently described EIA for fibrinogen and its derivatives

EIA Specific for	Specificity of		Remarks	References
	Capture antibody	Tagging antibody		
Intact fibrinogen	Intact carboxyl terminus of Aα-chains (MoAb G8)	Amino terminus of Aα-chains, including FpA (MoAb Y18)	Commercially available soon. Duration of assay is only 45 min. Uses dried MoAb precoated plates	Hoegee-de Nobel et al (1988) Y18: Koppert et al (1985)
Soluble fibrin	New amino terminus of fibrin α-chain (MoAb Anti-fbn-17)	Panspecific (polyclonal)	Not (yet) commercially available	Müller-Berghaus et al (1985) Scheefers-Borchel et al (1985, 1986)
	Neo-epitope in Aα-[148–160] (MoAb Anti-Fb-1/2)	Carboxyl terminal end of α-chains (MoAb G8)	Commercially available soon. Uses dried MoAb precoated plates	Schielen et al (1989)
Fibrin*ogen* degradation products (FgDP)	Altered conformation in fibrin(ogen) degradation products (MoAB FDP-14)	Amino terminus of Aα-chains including FpA (MoAb Y18)	Commercially available[a] Duration of assay only 45 min. Uses dried MoAb precoated plates	Koppert et al (1987) FDP14: Koppert et al (1986) Y18: Koppert et al (1985)
X-oligomers	X-oligomers (MoAb NiBn52)	X-oligomers (MoAb NiBn178)	—	Gaffney & Perry (1985a) Gaffney et al (1986)
D-dimer	Cross-links in D-dimer (MoAb DD3B6)	Panspecific anti-D MoAb	Commercially available[b]	Elms et al (1983) Rylatt et al (1983)
D-dimer	Mainly for D-dimer	Panspecific antibody	Commercially available[c]	None
Fibrin degradation products (FbDP)	Altered conformation in fibrin(ogen) degradation products (MoAb FDP-14)	D-domain of both cross-linked and non-cross-linked FbDP (MoAb DD13)	Commercially available[d] Duration of assay only 45 min. Uses dried MoAb precoated plates	Koppert et al (1988) FDP14: Koppert et al (1986)
Total of degradation products (TDP) of fibrin (FbDP) plus those of fibrinogen (FgDP)	Altered conformation in fibrin(ogen) degradation products (MoAb FDP-14)	Mixture of two MoAbs (MoAb Y18 and MoAb DD13), see above	Commercially available[e] Duration of assay only 45 min. Uses dried MoAb precoated plates	Koopman et al (1987)

[a,d,e] From Organon Teknika, Turnhout, Belgium.
[b] From MabCo, Brisbane, Australia; and American Diagnostica Inc., Greenwich , USA.
[c] From Diagnostica Stago, Asnières, France, and Boehringer Mannheim, Mannheim, FRG.

Typical examples of modern MoAb-based EIA

The appendices at the end of this chapter are adapted from the texts of the inserts of the EIA kits for the determination of fibrinogen degradation products in plasma ('Fibrinostika FgDP' from Organon Teknika, Turnhout, Belgium) and of the Dimertest EIA kit of American Diagnostica Inc. They illustrate how specific, easy to perform, rapid and accurate some of the modern EIA are.

Clinical experience with the modern MoAb-based assays

The clinical experience with the new assays is rapidly growing and fibrinogen and fibrinogen derivatives have been measured in plasma samples of patients with a variety of diseases.

In the following section only a few of the most relevant findings will be described, classified according to disease. For more detailed information the reader is referred to a review on this matter (Kroneman et al 1990).

1. Disseminated intravascular coagulation (DIC)

All patients with DIC appeared to have elevated levels of D-dimer as assessed by latex agglutination assay for D-dimer (Elms et al 1986, Wilde et al 1989). This assay alone, however, does not exclude the possibility of a diagnosis of DIC when DIC is suspected (Kroneman et al 1990).

EIA for X-oligomers (Gaffney et al 1988b), D-dimer (Wilde et al 1989), FbDP, FgDP and TDP (Koopman et al 1987, Koppert et al 1987, 1988, Fabbrini et al 1989, Prisco et al 1989, Stibbe et al 1989, Tanigawa et al 1989) showed that all these fibrin(ogen) degradation products levels were higher in DIC patients than in normals. A most interesting finding in all studies was that, in DIC patients, both FbDP and FgDP levels were elevated, indicating that secondary fibrinolysis is accompanied by primary fibrinogenolysis.

Another study (Nieuwenhuizen 1987) illustrates what has been postulated implicitly in the introduction, i.e. that the status of the haemostatic balance may be derived from the (relative) concentrations of the products of coagulation and fibrinolysis. Soluble fibrin, fibrin degradation products (i.e. X-oligomers, D-dimer and FbDP) and fibrinogen degradation products were measured longitudinally in patients with all clinical symptoms of DIC; one with promyelocytic leukaemia and one who took an overdose of paracetamol. It was found that the levels of fibrin degradation products and those of soluble fibrin changed in opposite directions, i.e. when fibrin degradation products decreased, soluble fibrin increased; and vice versa. Also in this same study fibrinolysis and fibrinogenolysis were found to occur simultaneously.

2. Deep venous thrombosis (DVT) and pulmonary embolism (PE) (Kroneman et al 1990)

The diagnosis of DVT cannot be based on clinical symptoms only, and an objective diagnostic method is therefore required, usually ascending venography. The efficacy of heparin treatment is frequently assessed by repeated ascending venography. A simple laboratory screening test would be helpful to replace this invasive technique, which is not without risk.

Several studies have been performed (for a review, see Kroneman et al 1990) with the semiquantitative latex agglutination assays for D-dimer. It was concluded that used in isolation the latter are not suitable for the screening of DVT.

Using the more sensitive EIA for D-dimer it was shown that the level of D-dimer was elevated in hospitalized patients with DVT, confirmed by venography (Whitaker et al 1984, Hochstein et al 1989). No overlap was demonstrated with the D-dimer levels in normal healthy controls (cut-off value for a positive test was 0.2 μg/ml). In a group of hospitalized patients suspected to have DVT, the D-dimer EIA had a sensitivity and specificity for DVT of 100 and 23%, respectively, as assessed by venography (Rowbotham et al 1987). The cut-off value was 0.25 μg/ml. The prevalence of DVT was 52% and the negative predictive value was 100%. Similar observations were made in other studies using D-dimer EIA (Heaton et al 1987, Bounameaux et al 1989). The studies referred to above show that the diagnosis of DVT can be ruled out in hospitalized patients with clinically suspected DVT in case of normal D-dimer levels, as determined by the quantitative D-dimer EIA. As a consequence ascending venography could have been avoided in these patients.

Also in DVT patients there was a simultaneous increase in FbDP and FgDP levels, which indicates that (like in DIC) fibrinogenolysis may be linked to fibrinolysis.

Several studies have been conducted on patients with PE (Kroneman et al 1990). X-oligomer and D-dimer levels were elevated in all patients with PE. However, the D-dimer EIA alone could not exclude PE. A similar conclusion was drawn from results of the D-dimer latex assay.

The possibility of using plasma levels of FbDP or D-dimer as markers of secondary fibrinolysis to monitor thrombolytic and heparin therapy in patients with venous thromboembolism has been investigated using EIA (Mirshahi et al 1988, Faivre et al 1989a,b). It was demonstrated that a change in plasma FbDP levels was reflected in a change of thrombus size during heparin treatment. This was assessed by repeated venography based on Marder scores, a fall in FbDP level being accompanied by thrombus regression, but when the FbDP level remained constant during treatment no reduction of thrombus size could be observed (Mirshahi et al 1988). In the latter study a good correlation was found between high starting levels of plasma FbDP and thrombus size. These results suggest that FbDP measurements are useful in the monitoring of heparin treatment. More data are needed to confirm these findings.

3. *Pregnancy and (pre)eclampsia* (for review, see Kroneman et al 1990)

No increases in D-dimer levels were seen with the latex agglutination assay in normal pregnant women; whereas about 39% of the pre-eclamptic women showed elevated D-dimer levels (Trofatter et al 1989). The latter group had more clinical symptoms and a higher risk for prematurity and low birth weight. It was concluded that the semiquantitative agglutination assay for D-dimer may be a useful test to screen pre-eclamptic women in order to define a subgroup at high risk for haemostatic abnormalities.

X-oligomer levels, as assessed by EIA, were elevated in all women with clinically diagnosed pre-eclampsia; the levels did not overlap with those of women with an uncomplicated pregnancy (Gaffney et al 1988b).

Interestingly, TDP, FgDP, FbDP and D-dimer levels as assessed by EIA, were elevated in normal pregnant women, as compared with normal non-pregnant women, especially in the last trimester of the pregnancy (Rossi et al 1989a,b, Ostlund et al 1989). This shows that (despite a number of studies from which it was concluded that fibrinolysis is impaired during pregnancy (Thorsen 1973, Walker et al 1983, Gore et al 1987) fibrinolysis is not necessarily depressed during pregnancy.

The EIA for fibrin(ogen) degradation products are useful aids in the early diagnosis of pre-eclampsia and may be valuable as indicators for the start of therapy to prevent a full-blown expression of this condition.

4. *Coronary artery disease (CAD) and thrombolytic therapy* (for review, see Kroneman et al 1990)

FbDP levels in patients with unstable angina were reported to be higher than in patients with acute myocardial infarction (AMI) (Soria et al 1987). The level in patients with unstable angina was only slightly above normal and there appears to be no difference with the levels of patients with uncomplicated AMI.

During thrombolytic therapy of AMI with t-PA, FbDP and D-dimer levels increased. However, increases were also observed in normal volunteers who were infused with t-PA. These fibrin degradation products are probably derived from a (normal) body pool of fibrin showing that increases in fibrin degradation products levels cannot be considered as evidence for successful lysis of the thrombus (Seifried et al 1987, DeClerck et al 1987).

Frequently, a dramatic apparent drop in fibrinogen levels is observed during t-PA therapy even when appropriate measures are taken to prevent fibrinogenolysis in vitro (Seifried et al 1989). Interestingly, there appears to be a major discrepancy between the decreases as observed by functional assays (e.g. Clauss) and the results obtained with the EIA for *intact* fibrinogen (Seifried et al 1989).

The fall in the levels of intact fibrinogen appears to be much smaller (approximately 20%) than that of functional fibrinogen (approximately 40%). This may indicate that either FgDP in the samples prolong the clotting time in the functional assays (which is then erroneously interpreted as a decrease in fibrinogen concentration), or that a dramatic increase in LMW' fibrinogen (which clots more slowly; see above) occurs. The latter possibility is more likely since the missing 20% intact fibrinogen is not recovered as FgDP and since LMW' fibrinogen is not detected in any of the EIA as an FgDP.

Another fascinating phenomenon is observed 2–3 d after t-PA therapy. At that time the functional assays indicate a value of 140% of the pretreatment fibrinogen values, whereas the levels of immunologically intact fibrinogen are equal to the pre-values. The reason for this is not clear but it is possible that the relative concentration of HMW fibrinogen (which clots fast) has increased as compared to the pre-infusion situation. The fast-clotting HMW will yield a short clotting time which is interpreted in the Clauss method as an increase in fibrinogen concentration.

Thrombolytic therapy with streptokinase (SK) gives a strong increase both of FgDP and TDP levels. The increase in FgDP levels is approximately equal to those of TDP, indicating that virtually all degradation products are FgDP (Koopman et al 1987, Koppert et al 1987, Brommer et al 1987). This has previously been inferred from the available data but has now been demonstrated directly with the new EIA which specifically quantitates FgDP.

The monitoring of FgDP levels during thrombolytic therapy may be clinically important since an increased fibrinolytic state has been reported to be associated with severe bleeding complications (Arnold et al 1989).

5. *Liver disease and liver transplantation* (for review, see Kroneman et al 1990)

Liver cirrhosis is graded with increasing severity as Child A, Child B and Child C.

The levels of *intact* fibrinogen (HMW + LMW) decrease with the severity of liver cirrhosis and were lowest in Child C (de Maat et al 1989). The FgDP levels increased only slightly as compared to normal and did not correlate with the severity of the disease. This indicates that either fibrinogenolysis beyond the stage of LMW' formation does not occur (see above) or that the lowered level of intact fibrinogen (which may consist mainly of freshly synthesized molecules) is due to a decreased synthetic capacity of the affected liver. The levels of FbDP and TDP were elevated and the increases correlated with the severity of the disease. This indicates that secondary fibrinolysis is more active in patients with an advanced stage of liver cirrhosis, although an impaired clearance of FbDP cannot be precluded. Similar observations and conclusions were made in studies performed with the latex agglutination assays for D-dimer.

In orthotopic liver transplantation an increase was seen in FbDP and (somewhat less) in FgDP (Porte et al 1989). This indicates that both fibrinogenolysis and secondary fibrinolysis are operational during orthotopic liver transplantation.

6. *Malignancies* (for review, see Kroneman et al 1990)

D-dimer levels both in tissues and in plasma of patients with ovarian cancer were increased as compared to normal.

Elevated plasma levels of FbDP, FgDP and TDP have been reported for patients with, amongst others, carcinoma of the liver (Rossi et al 1989) and patients with acute promyelocytic leukaemia (Nieuwenhuizen 1988). This suggests that, in malignancies, fibrinolysis is accompanied by fibrinogenolysis. Elevated levels of TDP have been reported in patients with colonic as compared with breast cancer. Postoperative increases in TDP were associated with early recurrent disease (McCulloch et al 1990).

CONCLUSIONS

In this chapter the formation of fibrinogen derivatives, their molecular features and the possible clinical utility of assays for determination of degradation products of fibrin and fibrinogen have been discussed. It has been pointed out that assays based on polyclonal antibodies and performed in serum are unreliable and that their clinical use is therefore limited. Until recently, it was not possible to determine the extent of primary activation of the fibrinolytic system specifically. The new assays are performed on plasma and make it possible to quantify the extent of fibrin(ogen)olysis reliably. Furthermore, they allow discrimination between the degradation products of fibrin and of fibrinogen, since a specific assay has been developed for separate and specific determination of fibrinogen degradation products.

Fibrinolysis appears to be associated with (low grades of) fibrinogenolysis. The process of secondary fibrinolysis, as derived from FbDP and D-dimer levels, appears to predominate in DVT, PE, AMI and unstable angina. Thrombolytic therapy, especially with streptokinase, results in a pronounced fibrinogenolysis (primary fibrinolysis) as assessed by the levels of FgDP. The occurrence of an extensive fibrinogenolysis was also observed during orthotopic liver transplantation. Several diseases, such as DIC, malignancies and liver disease, exhibit both fibrinogenolysis and fibrinolysis secondary to an activated state of coagulation.

The EIA for plasma D-dimer can be used to exclude the diagnosis of

DVT in patients clinically suspected of having developed DVT, and ascending venography may not be required. The semiquantitative latex assays for D-dimer cannot be used for this purpose. Plasma FbDP levels, as detected by EIA, reflect decreases in thrombus size and may be used to monitor efficacy of heparin treatment. Low initial values of FbDP are predictive of poor thrombus dissolution in patients with DVT following SK or urokinase therapy. Elevated plasma levels of cross-linked fibrin degradation products have been measured during thrombolytic therapy of AMI. They are derived mainly from extracoronary sites and are non-predictive of recanalization following thrombolytic therapy.

Plasma fibrin degradation products levels are related to severity of liver cirrhosis. The observed increased fibrin(ogen) levels during normal and complicated pregnancy suggest that fibrinolysis is not necessarily depressed. The fibrinolytic system remains active in patients with malignancies, as demonstrated by elevated levels of D-dimers and FbDP. The following guidelines for future studies are suggested. As mentioned in the introduction, a disturbance in the haemostatic balance will presumably be reflected in the products of both coagulation and fibrinolysis. In this chapter the focus has been on fibrin(ogen)olysis. Detection of fibrin(ogen) derivatives by the monoclonal antibody-based assays provides valuable information on haemostasis in several diseases. However, it is conceivable that more clinically relevant information can be obtained when the products of the two opposing processes, coagulation and fibrinolysis, are simultaneously measured. This possibility is available. Soluble fibrin, the product of an activated coagulation system, can also be assessed by EIA in plasma (Müller-Berghaus et al 1985, Scheefers-Borchel et al 1985, 1986). In the future, studies may be performed using a combination of an EIA for a coagulation product (i.e. soluble fibrin) and an EIA for a fibrinolysis product (i.e. FbDP or D-dimer).

APPENDIX: FIBRINOSTIKA FgDP

Adapted from the kit insert of the Organon Teknika kit. For further details the reader is referred to the insert.

Principle of the test

Fibrinostika FgDP is a sandwich-type EIA. (Figure 6.2)

The wells of polystyrene Microelisa strips are coated with a murine monoclonal antibody, FDP-14 (Koppert et al 1986), which constitutes the solid phase antibody. The strips are provided dried and ready for use. FDP-14 is specific for degradation products of both fibrin and fibrinogen and does not react with intact fibrinogen or fibrin. The test sample or calibrator is added to the well; fibrin degradation products (FbDP) and fibrinogen degradation products (FgDP), if present in the sample, will bind to the

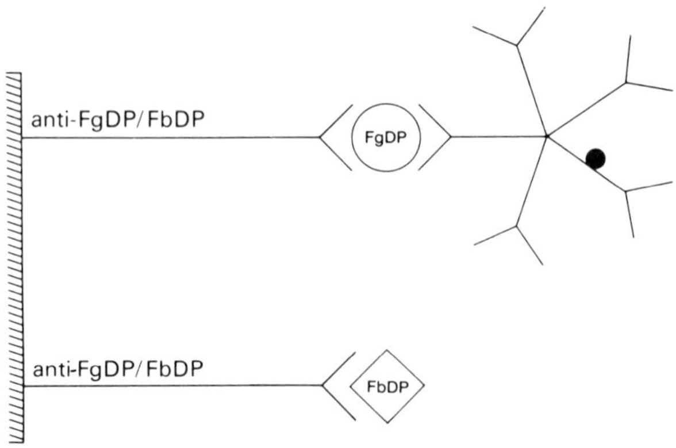

Fig. 6.2 Schematic representation of Fibrinostika FgDP.

solid phase antibody. In the next step a murine monoclonal Y-18 (Koppert et al 1985), which has been labelled with horseradish peroxidase (HRP), is added. Y-18 reacts exclusively with the captured degradation products of fibrinogen, not with those of fibrin. This labelled tagging antibody thus binds only to the solid phase antibody/FgDP complex formed in the first step. Incubation with the HRP substrate tetramethylbenzidine (TMB) produces a blue colour in the test well, which turns to yellow when the reaction is stopped by acidification with sulphuric acid. The intensity of the colour is proportional to the concentration of FgDP in the test sample. The amount of FgDP in the sample can be read from a calibration line.

Specimen collection and preparation

1. No special preparation of the patient is necessary nor is fasting required.
2. Plasma samples (derived from blood taken into citrate, heparin, oxalate or EDTA) can be used.
3. Specimens should be free of microbial contamination and may be stored at 2–8°C for 1 week. Fresh specimens may be stored for 1 year at –20°C (or lower).
4. For special applications when prolonged stability is required (e.g. samples taken after thrombolytic treatment), aprotinin at a final concentration of 100 KIU/ml and heparin at a final concentration of 50 IU/ml may be added.

Reagent preparation

Phosphate buffer

Dilute the provided phosphate buffer concentrate 1:25 with distilled water. Prepare at least 100 ml of diluted buffer for each microelisa strip used.

Peroxidase/substrate buffer

1. Dissolve the **urea peroxide** tablet in 10 ml of distilled water and mix. The solution will contain some insoluble material, but this does not affect the test results; therefore, filtration is not necessary.
2. Pipette 1.0 ml of the **urea peroxide solution** into the **substrate buffer**. This mixture is the peroxide/substrate buffer.

Tagging antibody/HRP conjugate

Pipette 6.0 ml of diluted phosphate buffer into the vial. Shake the vial gently and leave for at least 15 min before use.

Calibrator 900

Pipette 1.5 ml of diluted phosphate buffer into the vial. Shake the vial gently and leave for at least 15 min before use. This yields reconstituted calibrator **900** (concentration 900 ng FE[1]/ml).

Test procedure

1. Prepare serial three-fold dilutions (three-, nine-, 27- and 81-fold) of an aliquot of calibrator **900** with diluted **phosphate buffer** (e.g. 150 µl with 300 µl buffer and homogenize, 150 µl of this three-fold dilution with 300 µl buffer and homogenize, etc.). Calibrator **300,** calibrator **100,** calibrator **33,** and calibrator **11** are now ready for use.
2. Fit the stripholder with the required number of microelisa strips.
3. The negative control (diluted **phosphate buffer**), calibrators and test samples are first pipetted into *uncoated* wells of separate polystyrene plates. The (routinely used) 20-fold dilution of test samples can be performed in the wells (e.g. 10 µl sample with 190 µl diluted **phosphate buffer** and homogenize). After filling, transfer with a 12-channel pipette 100 µl of each well to the corresponding well of the microelisa strip.
4. Cover the strips with the adhesive plate sealer and incubate at 37°C for 15 min.
5. Wash each well four times with diluted **phosphate buffer**.
6. Pipette 100 µl **conjugate** into each well.
7. Cover the strips with a new plate sealer and incubate at 37°C for 15 min.
8. Wash each well four times with diluted **phosphate buffer**.
9. During incubation, prepare TMB substrate. Allow TMB solution to

---

[1] Fibrinogen equivalent.
tetramethylbenzidine

reach room temperature (20–25°C) and check that the **TMB** is completely melted (m.p. 18°C). The **TMB substrate** for four strips is prepared as follows: pipette 0.5 ml of **peroxide/substrate buffer** into 5.0 ml of distilled water contained in a new disposable vial and mix, then add 100 µl of **TMB solution** and mix.

10. Pipette 100 µl **TMB substrate** into each well.
11. Incubate at 37°C for 10 min. Strips should **not** be covered with a plate sealer.
12. Stop the reaction by pipetting 100 µl of 1 mol/l (2 N) sulphuric acid into each well (maintain the same sequence and time intervals used for **TMB substrate** addition). Plates should be read within 1 h.
13. Read the absorbance of the solution in each well at 450 nm.

Calculation of the test results

Calculations should be made separately for each stripholder.

Plot the optical density values on semi-logarithmic paper. Draw straight lines through the points. Read the sample concentration from this broken line. Multiply with the dilution factor (usually 20) to obtain the FgDP concentration in the original sample. A typical curve is shown in Fig. 6.3.

Remark. If needed for evaluation, samples with absorbances exceeding the instrument's linear measuring range should be retested in a higher dilution.

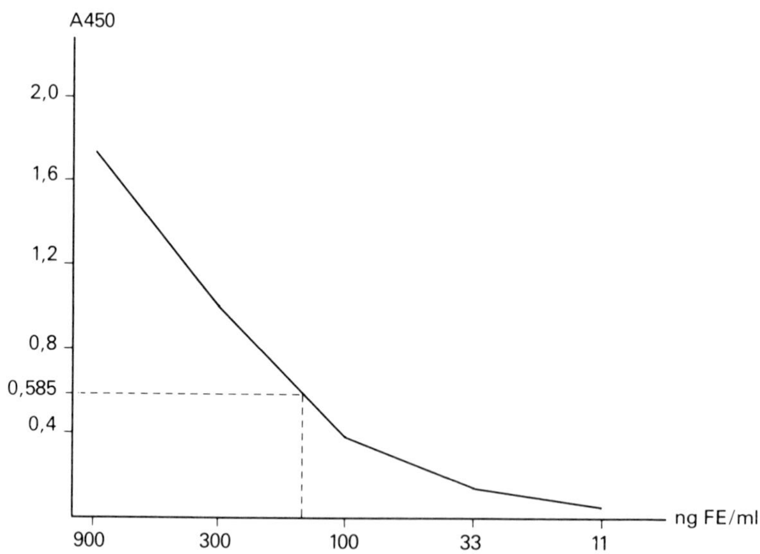

Fig. 6.3 Typical example of a calibration line to convert absorbances to ng FE/ml. Sample reading, 0.585. Result, concentration 144 × 20 = 2880 ng FE/ml.

Performance characteristics

Specificity

The catching antibody FDP-14 (Koppert et al 1986) reacts equally well with all fragment E-containing plasmin degradation products of fibrinogen and fibrin but not with intact fibrinogen and fibrin. The tagging antibody, Y-18 (Koppert et al 1985), reacts exclusively with fibrinopeptide A-containing degradation products. Addition of FbDP to plasma in concentrations as high as 1 mg/ml does not show any response in the assay. Because the catching antibody FDP-14 cannot discriminate between FgDP and FbDP, high levels of FbDP over FgDP may interfere with the assay. Experiments have shown that this interference occurs when the weight ratio of FbDP to FgDP (fragment Y) is above 7.5 (Koppert et al 1987). The assay quantitates fragments X, Y and E, which all contain the central E-domain as in fibrinogen. The level of these various types of FgDP is therefore expressed in terms of fibrinogen concentration (i.e. in fibrinogen equivalents).

Use of plasma samples is imperative because the cleavage of fibrinopeptides from fibrinogen degradation products by thrombin during serum preparation will convert FgDP, if present, to FbDP and makes it impossible to discriminate between FgDP and FbDP. Furthermore, the level of degradation products in serum is not a true reflection of the plasma concentration in vivo and numerous data indicate too high or too low results in serum.

Reproducibility

1. Standard curve (15 runs in duplicate):

Calibrator (ng FE/ml)	CV[1] within run (%)	CV between run (%)
0	3.3	25.1
11	3.8	12.5
33	4.1	13.2
100	3.9	12.1
300	3.4	10.6
900	3.2	9.2

[1] CV, coefficient of variation.

2. Clinical samples (three runs in triplicate):

Sample	Concentration (ng FE/ml)	CV within run (%)	CV between run (%)
1	6785	15.7	19.3
2	3176	7.0	12.5
3	1341	8.1	14.0
4	257	3.3	8.9

Expected values

Analysis of 42 healthy individuals in an outside laboratory showed an upper limit for FgDP of 250 ng FE/ml.

APPENDIX: D-DIMER EIA

Partly adapted from the kit insert of American Diagnostika Inc. For full details the reader is referred to the insert.

Principle of the test

The test is a sandwich-type EIA for cross-linked fibrin degradation products containing the D-dimer configuration (Elms et al 1983).

Plates are provided filled with coating solution containing a murine monoclonal antibody which binds to D-dimer, D-dimer-E and high-molecular-weight derivatives. These products, if present in the sample, bind in the first step of the EIA to the solid phase monoclonal antibody. In the second step a tagging antibody (mouse monoclonal anti-FDP) conjugated with HRP is added. Incubation with a HRP substrate produces a coloured product. The intensity of the colour is proportional to the amount of antigen present in the test sample.

Specimen collection

Both serum and plasma samples may be assayed. However, serum XDP (cross-linked fibrin degradation products) values are generally lower than plasma XDP values (Whitaker et al 1984). *PLASMA IS THE PREFERRED SAMPLE.* Blood may be collected in citrate, heparin or EDTA tubes. XDP levels in ascitic fluid can also be measured. Plasma or serum samples may be kept at 20 –25°C for 8 h, at 2–8°C for 4 d or stored frozen for at least 4 months. Frozen plasma samples must be thawed at 37°C and mixed well and centrifuged before assay.

Preparation

Buffer reagent

Add the contents of the phosphate buffer salts bottle (provided in the kit) and the contents of the Tween 20 vial (5 mls) to a beaker containing 1 litre of distilled water. Mix until dissolved. This produces a final Tween concentration of 0.2% (v/v).

D-dimer standard preparation

Reconstitute the vial of standard with diluent according to the instructions on the vial to give a concentration of 5 μg/ml. Leave for 10 min, then mix gently until complete dissolution is obtained. Prepare, using the diluent provided in the kit, serial two-fold dilutions of the reconstituted standard to give concentrations of 5, 2.5, 1.25, 0.625, 0.312, 0.156 and 0.078 μg/ml. Diluent is used as the blank.

Washing of the coated plates

Just before use, unwrap the microtitre plate and remove the tape from the upper surface. Invert the plate and shake out plate contents, wash by flooding the plate with buffer reagent. Leave 2 min, then empty. Blot the plate by inverting on absorbent material to remove excess liquid.

Test procedure

1. Pipette 100 μl of buffer reagent into each well.
2. Add 25 μl of serial dilutions of the calibrator and unknown plasmas.
3. Mix gently and incubate for 1 h at room temperature.
4. Reconstitute (no more than 15 min before use) the tagging antibody conjugate by adding 6.0 ml of buffer reagent, mix well by inverting the bottle several times and avoid frothing.
6. Add 50 μl of reconstituted tagging antibody to each well. Incubate for 1 h at room temperature. Invert the plate to remove contents. Wash three times with buffer reagent.
7. Add 10 μl of the hydrogen peroxide provided to the ABTS 2,2-azinobis (3-ethylbenzothiazoline sulphonic acid) substrate vial. Mix thoroughly.
8. Pipette 100 μl of this activated substrate into each well.
9. Incubate for 20 min at room temperature to allow colour development.
10. Pipette 50 μl of stopping reagent (provided with the kit) into each well to stop the reaction.
11. Read the absorbance of each well at 405–450 nm (optimum 420 nm).

Calculation of the test results

Results can be plotted by log–linear or log–log data reduction.

1. Plot the optical density against the D-dimer concentrations of the calibrators.
2. Read the D-dimer concentrations of the unknown samples from the calibration curve.
3. Samples outside the measuring range should be retested after further dilution.

Specificity

The cross-linked fibrin degradation products, D-dimer, D-dimer-E, and high molecular weight derivatives are all recognised by the Dimertest monoclonal antibodies. No binding was found to the fibrinogen degradation products X, Y, D, E up to 20 μg/ml or to fibrinogen up to 1 mg/ml.

Reproducibility

A panel of plasma samples with a concentration of less than 2 μg/ml was assayed repeatedly. The intra-assay (within) variability was calculated to be less than 5% , and the inter-assay (between) variability was calculated to be less than 10%.

The insert gives no information as to the actual concentration of the samples and whether these variabilities refer to the optical density or to the concentrations.

REFERENCES

Arnold A E R, Brouwer R W, Collen D, Van Es G A, Lubsen J, Serruys P W, Simoons M L, Verstraete M 1989 Increased serum levels of fibrinogen degradation products due to treatment with recombinant tissue-type plasminogen activator for acute myocardial infarction are related to bleeding complications, but not to coronary patency. Journal of the American College of Cardiology 14: 581–588

Bounameaux H, Schneider P A, Reber G, De Moerloose P, Krahenbuhl B 1989 Measurement of plasma D-dimer for diagnosis of deep venous thrombosis. American Journal of Clinical Pathology 91: 82–85

Brass E P, Forman W B, Edwards R V, Lindan O 1976 Fibrin formation: the role of the fibrinogen–fibrin monomer complex. Thrombosis and Haemostasis 36: 36–48

Brommer E J P, Engbers J, Van de Laarse A, Nieuwenhuizen W 1987 Survival of fibrinogen degradation products in the circulation after thrombolytic therapy for acute myocardial infarction. Fibrinolysis 1: 149–153

Connaghan D G, Francis D W, Ryan D H, Marder V J 1986 Prevalence and clinical implications of heparin-associated false positive tests for serum fibrin(ogen) degradation products. American Journal of Clinical Pathology 86: 304–310

DeClerck P, Mombaerts P, Holvoet P, Collen D 1987 Plasma levels of fragment D-dimer of cross-linked fibrin during thrombolytic therapy with recombinant tissue-type plasminogen activator. Thrombosis and Haemostasis 58 (abstract 853)

De Maat M P M, Nieuwenhuizen W, Knot E A R 1989 Discrepancies between levels of intact

and functional fibrinogen in patients with liver cirrhosis. Thrombosis and Haemostasis 62 (abstract 225)
Doolittle R F 1973 Structural aspects of the fibrinogen to fibrin conversion. Advances in Protein Chemistry 27: 1–109
Doolittle R F 1981 Fibrinogen and fibrin. Scientific American 245: 92–101
Elms M J, Bunce J H, Bundesen P G, Rylatt D B, Webber A J, Masci P P, Whitaker A N 1983 Measurement of cross-linked fibrin degradation products — an immunoassay using monoclonal antibodies. Thrombosis and Haemostasis 50: 591–594
Elms M J, Bunce I A, Bundesen B G, Rylatt D B, Webber A J, Masci P P, Whitaker A N 1986 Rapid detection of cross-linked fibrin degradation products in plasma using monoclonal antibody-coated particles. American Journal of Clinical Pathology 85: 360–364
Fabbrini N, Hoppensteadt D, Walenga J M, Schumacher H, Fareed J 1989 Diagnostic efficacy of specific fibrinogen and fibrin related degradation products measured by ELISA methods. Thrombosis and Haemostasis 62 (Abstract 738)
Faivre R, Mirshahi M, Ducellier D, Soria C, Soria J, Mirshahi M, Kieffer Y, Bassand J P, Caen J, Maurat J P 1989a Evolution of plasma specific fibrin degradation products during thrombolytic therapy in patients with thrombo-embolism. Thrombosis Research 50: 583–589
Faivre R, Ducellier D, Neuhart E, Mirshahi M, Soria C, Caen J, Bassand J P, Maurat J P 1989b How long must be given thrombolytic therapy for massive venous thromboembolism? Thrombosis and Haemostasis 62 (abstract 546)
Gaffney P J, Perry M J 1985a 'Giant' fibrin fragments and thrombosis. Thrombosis and Haemostasis 54: 931 (abstract)
Gaffney P J, Perry M J 1985b Unreliability of current serum fibrin degradation products (FDP) assays. Thrombosis and Haemostasis 53: 301–302
Gaffney P J, Creighton L C, Harris R, Perry M J 1986 Monoclonal antibodies (MABS) to crosslinked fibrin fragments. Their characterization and potential clinical use. In: Müller-Berghaus G, Sheefers-Borchel U, Selmayer E, Henschen A (eds) Fibrinogen and its derivatives. Biochemistry, physiology and pathophysiology. Excerpta Medica, Amsterdam p 273–284
Gaffney P J, Creighton L J, Perry M J, Callus M, Thorpe R, Spitz M 1988a Monoclonal antibodies to crosslinked fibrin degradation products (XL-FDP). I. Characterization and preliminary evaluation in plasma. British Journal of Haematology 68: 83–90
Gaffney P J, Creighton L J, Callus M, Thorpe R 1988b Monoclonal antibodies to crosslinked fibrin degradation products (XL-FDP). II. Evaluation in a variety of clinical conditions. British Journal of Haematology 68: 91–96
Gore M, Eldon S, Trofatter K F, Soong S J, Pizzo S V 1987 Pregnancy induced changes in the fibrinolytic balance: evidence for defective release of tissue plasminogen activator and increased levels of fast acting tissue plasminogen activator inhibitor. American Journal Obstetrics and Gynecology 156: 674–680
Graeff H, Hafter R 1982 Detection and relevance of crosslinked fibrin derivatives in blood. Seminars on Thrombosis and Haemostasis 8: 57–68
Graeff H, Hafter R, von Hugo R 1979 On soluble fibrinogen–fibrin complexes. Thrombosis Research 16: 575–576
Haverkate F, Timan G, Nieuwenhuizen W 1979 Anticlotting properties of fragments D from human fibrinogen and fibrin. European Journal of Clinical Investigation 9: 253–255
Heaton D C, Billings J D, Hickton C M 1987 Assessment of D-dimer assay for the diagnosis of deep vein thrombosis. Journal of Laboratory and Clinical Medicine 110: 588–591
Henschen A 1981 Fibrinogen — Blutgerinnungsfaktor I. Biochemische Aspekte. Hämostaseologie 1: 49-61
Hermans J, McDonagh J 1982 Fibrin: structure and interactions. Seminars on Thrombosis and Haemostasis 8: 11–24
Hochstein B E, Johns A S, Ockelford P A 1989 D-dimers (Dimertest): a screening for the diagnosis of venous thrombosis. Thrombosis and Haemostasis 62 (abstract 124)
Hoegee-de Nobel E, Voskuilen M, Briët E, Brommer E J P, Nieuwenhuizen W 1988 A monoclonal antibody-based quantitative enzyme immuno assay for the determination of plasma fibrinogen concentrations. Thrombosis and Haemostasis 60: 415–418
Holm B, Nilsen D W T, Kierulf P, Godal H C 1985 Purification and characterization of 3 fibrinogens with different molecular weights obtained from normal human plasma. Thrombosis Research 37: 165–176

Koopman J, Haverkate F, Koppert P W, Nieuwenhuizen W, Brommer E J P, Van der Werf W G C 1987 New enzyme immunoassay of fibrin–fibrinogen degradation products in plasma using a monoclonal antibody. Journal of Laboratory and Clinical Medicine 109: 75–84
Koppert P W, Huijsmans C M G, Nieuwenhuizen 1985 A monoclonal antibody, specific for human fibrinogen, fibrinopeptide A-containing fragments and not reacting with free fibrinopeptide A. Blood 66: 503–507
Koppert P W, Koopman J, Haverkate F, Nieuwenhuizen W 1986 Production and characterization of a monoclonal antibody reactive with a specific neoantigenic determinant (comprising Bβ 54–118) in degradation products of fibrin and of fibrinogen. Blood 68: 437–441
Koppert P W, Kuipers W, Hoegee-de Nobel E, Brommer E J P, Koopman J, Nieuwenhuizen W 1987 A quantitative enzyme immunoassay for primary fibrinogenolysis products in plasma. Thrombosis and Haemostasis 57: 25–28
Koppert P W, Hoegee-de Nobel E, Nieuwenhuizen W 1988 A monoclonal antibody-based enzyme immunoassay for fibrin degradation products in plasma. Thrombosis and Haemostasis 59: 310–315
Kroneman H, Nieuwenhuizen W, Knot E A R 1990 Monoclonal antibody-based plasma assays for fibrinogen and derivatives, and their clinical relevance. Blood Coagulation and Fibrinolysis 1: 91–111
McCulloch P, Nieuwenhuizen W, Douglas J, Lowe G D O, George W D 1990 Coagulation disturbances in cancer of the breast and colon measured with specific monoclonal antibody enzyme immunoassay for fibrin–fibrinogen degradation products. Haemostasis 20: 73–80
Marder V J, Shulman N R 1969 High molecular weight derivatives of human fibrinogen produced by plasmin. II. Mechanism of their anticoagulant activity. Journal of Biological Chemistry 244: 2120–2124
Merskey C, Lalezazi P, Johnson A J 1969 A rapid simple sensitive method for measuring fibrinolytic split products in human serum. Proceedings of the Society of Experimental Biological Medicine, New York 131: 871–875
Mirshahi M, Soria J, Soria C, Perrot J-Y, Boucheix C 1986 A latex immunoassay of fibrin/fibrinogen degradation products in plasma using a monoclonal antibody. Thrombosis Research 44: 715–728
Mirshahi M, Soria C, Soria J, Mirshahi M, Faivre R, Kieffer Y, Bassand J P, Toulemonde F, Caen J 1988 Changes in plasma fibrin degradation products as marker of thrombus evolution in patients with deep venous thrombosis. Thrombosis Research 51: 295–302
Mosesson M W, Galanakis D K, Finlayson J S 1974 Comparison of human plasma fibrinogen subfractions and early plasmic fibrinogen derivatives. Journal of Biological Chemistry 249: 4656–4664
Müller-Berghaus G, Scheefers-Borchel U, Fuhge P, Eberle R, Heimburger N 1985 Detection of fibrin in plasma by a monoclonal antibody against the amino-terminus of the alpha-chain of fibrin. Scandinavian Journal of Clinical and Laboratory Investigations 45(suppl 178): 145–151
Nieuwenhuizen W 1987 A double blind comparative study of six monoclonal antibody-based plasma assays for fibrinogen derivatives. In: Lowe G D O, Douglas J T, Forbes C D, Henschen A (eds) Fibrinogen 2. Biochemistry, physiology and clinical relevance. Excerpta Medica, Amsterdam p 181–186
Nieuwenhuizen W 1988 New strategies in the determination of fibrin and fibrin(ogen) derivatives by monoclonal antibodies. Blut 57: 285–291
Nieuwenhuizen W, Gravesen M 1981 Anticoagulant and calcium-binding properties of high molecular weight derivatives of human fibrinogen, produced by plasmin (fragments X). Biochimica et Biophysica Acta 668: 81–88
Nieuwenhuizen W, Voskuilen M, Hermans J 1982 Anticoagulant and calcium-binding properties of high molecular weight derivatives of human fibrinogen (plasmin fragments Y). Biochimica et Biophysica Acta 708: 313–316
Niewiarowski S, Stewart G J, Marder V J 1970 Formation of highly ordered polymers from fibrinogen and fibrin degradation products. Biochimica et Biophysica Acta 221: 326–341
Ostlund E, Almqvist I, Blombäck M, Bremme K, Wallin M 1989 Activation of coagulation and fibrinolysis during normal pregnancy. Thrombosis and Haemostasis 62 (abstract 236)
Phillips H M 1981 Isolation of six homogeneous preparations of high molecular weight and low molecular weight fibrinogen. Canadian Journal of Biochemistry 59: 332–342

Porte R J, Bontempo F A, Knot E A R, Lewis J H, Kang Y G 1989 Systemic effects of tissue plasminogen activator associated fibrinolysis and the relation with thrombin generation in orthotopic liver transplantation. Transplantation 47: 978–984
Prisco D, Paniccia R, Bonechi F, Francalanci I, Abbate R, Gensini G F 1989 Evaluation of new methods for the selective measurement of fibrin and fibrinogen degradation products. Thrombosis Research 56: 547–551
Rossi L, Felloni L, Vannini F, Lechinni L, Panicucci F 1989a Evaluation of fibrinogen and fibrin degradation products in physiological and pathological conditions using monoclonal antibodies. Thrombosis and Haemostasis 62 (abstract 232)
Rossi L, Vannini F, Felloni L, Bartolai S, Lechinni L, Panicucci F 1989b Evaluation of D-dimer with monoclonal antibodies and its clinical importance. Thrombosis and Haemostasis 62 (abstract 236)
Rowbotham B J, Carroll P, Whitaker A N, Bunce I A, Cobcroft R G, Elms M J, Masci P P, Bundesen P G, Rylatt D B, Webber A J 1987 Measurement of crosslinked fibrin derivatives — use in the diagnosis of venous thrombosis. Thrombosis and Haemostasis 57: 59–61
Rylatt D B, Blake A S, Cottis L E, Massingham D A, Fletcher W A, Masci P P, Whitaker A M, Elms M, Bunce J, Webber A, Wyatt D, Bundesen P G 1983 An immunoassay for human D-dimer using monoclonal antibodies. Thrombosis Research 31: 767–778
Scheefers-Borchel U, Müller-Berghaus G, Fuhge P, Eberle R, Heimburger N 1985 Discrimination between fibrin and fibrinogen by a monoclonal antibody against a synthetic peptide. Proceedings of the National Academy of Sciences, USA 82: 7091–7095
Scheefers-Borchel U, Müller-Berghaus G, Fuhge P, Heimburger N 1986 Discrimination between fibrin and fibrinogen by a monoclonal antibody against a synthetic hexapeptide representing the amino-terminus of the alpha-chain of fibrin. In: Lane D A, Henschen A, Jasani M K (eds) Fibrinogen, fibrin formation and fibrinolysis. Walter de Gruyter, Berlin p 253–260
Schielen W J G, Voskuilen M, Tesser G I, Nieuwenhuizen W 1990 The sequence Aα-[148–160] in fibrin, but not in fibrinogen, is accessible to monoclonal antibodies. Proceedings of the National Academy of Sciences, USA 86: 8951–8954
Seifried E, Tanswell P, Rijken D C, Kluft C, Hoegee E, Nieuwenhuizen W 1987 Fibrin degradation products are not specific markers for thrombolysis in myocardial infarction. Lancet ii: 334–335
Seifried E, Hoegee-de Nobel E, Haere W, Ellbruck D, Tanswell P, Nieuwenhuizen W 1989 Intact fibrinogen and fibrin(ogen) degradation products in the evaluation of fibrin specificity of tissue-type plasminogen activator. Thrombosis and Haemostasis 62 (abstract 965)
Soria C, Soria J, Mirshahi M, Mirshahi M, Dunnica S, Boucheix C, Beaufils R, Slama R, Caen J P 1987 Dynamic coronary fibrinolysis evaluation in patients with myocardial infarction and unstable angina by specific plasma fibrin degradation product determination. Thrombosis Research 45: 383–392
Stibbe J, Gomes M, De Oude A 1989 Management of chronic DIC. Evaluation of separate measurements of fibrin (FbDP) and fibrinogen (FgDP) degradation products concomitant with fibrin monomers (FM). Thrombosis and Haemostasis 62 (abstract 1165)
Tanigawa M, Takagi M, Wada H, Deguchi K, Shirakawa S, Suzuki H, Tanaka I 1989 Coagulation study before onset of intravascular coagulation. Thrombosis and Haemostasis 62 (abstract 1155)
Thorsen S 1973 The inhibition of tissue plasminogen activator and urokinase induced fibrinolysis by some natural proteinase inhibitors and by plasma and serum from normal and pregnant subjects. Scandinavian Journal of Clinical and Laboratory Investigation 31: 51–59
Trofatter K P, Howell M L, Greenberg C S, Hage M L 1989 Use of the fibrin D-dimer in screening for coagulation abnormalities in preeclampsia. Obstetrics and Gynecology 73: 435–439
Walker J E, Gow L, Cambell D M, Ogston D 1983 The inhibition by plasma of urokinase and tissue activator induced fibrinolysis in pregnancy and puerperium. Thrombosis and Haemostasis 49: 21–23
Whitaker A N, Elms M J, Masci P P, Bundesen P G, Rylatt D B, Webber A J, Bunce I H 1984 Measurement of cross-linked fibrin derivatives in plasma: an immunoassay using monoclonal antibodies. American Journal of Clinical Pathology 37: 882–887
Wilde J T, Kitchen S, Kinsey S, Greaves M, Preston P E 1989 Plasma D-dimer levels and their relation to serum fibrinogen/fibrin degradation products in hypercoagulable states. British Journal of Haematology 71: 65–70

7. Laboratory aspects of thrombolytic therapy

Gordon D. O. Lowe   Ann Rumley

INTRODUCTION

The balance of haemostasis and thrombosis

There is increasing evidence for a physiological balance between haemostasis and thrombosis (Fig. 7.1). Following vascular injury, the normal interactions of platelets and coagulation factors upon the damaged vessel wall result in the formation of a stable, platelet–fibrin haemostatic plug. The endogenous fibrinolytic system (Fig. 7.2) subsequently removes this fibrin layer. In parallel, tissue repair processes restore vascular architecture. Bleeding disorders arise from congenital or acquired abnormalities of blood vessels, platelet number or function, or coagulation factors. Less commonly, bleeding may arise from localized or generalized over-active fibrinolysis which lyses haemostatic plugs prematurely.

The burden of thrombosis

With increasing age, thrombosis becomes a more important threat to life and limb in Western countries than bleeding, accounting for over 50% of deaths (Table 7.1). Each year in the UK, about half a million people suffer a heart attack due to coronary artery thrombosis. Half of these die suddenly (sudden coronary death) from a disturbance of heart rhythm (ventricular

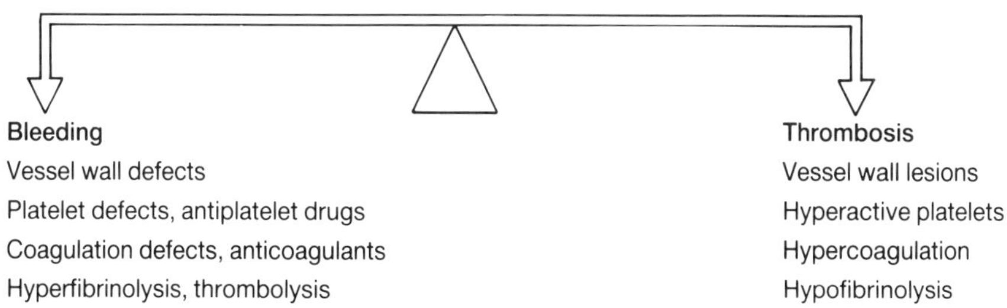

Fig. 7.1 The physiological balance between haemostasis and thrombosis. Thrombolytic therapy lyses thrombi, but also increases the risk of bleeding by lysing recently formed haemostatic plugs in vessel wall defects, and also by its systemic effects on platelets and coagulation.

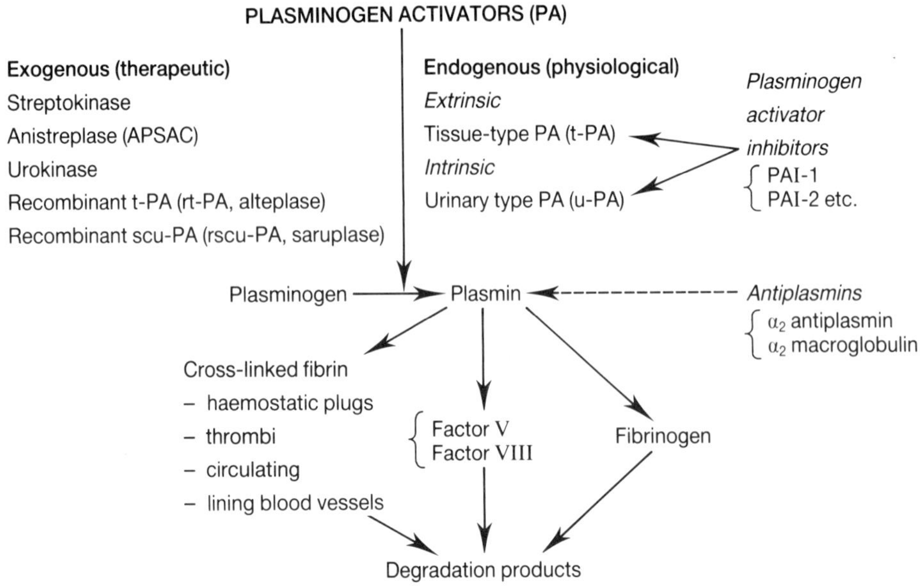

Fig. 7.2 The fibrinolytic system.

Table 7.1 Common types of thrombi and role of thrombolytic therapy

Site and syndrome	Thrombolytic therapy
Coronary arteries	
Sudden death	Not applicable
Myocardial infarction	Intravenous therapy considered routinely; intracoronary therapy used occasionally
Unstable angina	Experimental
Cerebral arteries	
Cerebral infarction	Experimental
Limb arteries (or grafts)	
Critical limb ischaemia → Limb infarction (gangrene)	Local intra-arterial therapy considered in selected cases
Deep vein thrombosis of limbs ↓	Intravenous therapy considered in selected cases (e.g. impending venous gangrene)
Pulmonary thromboembolism	Intravenous or pulmonary artery infusions considered in selected cases (e.g. shock)

fibrillation): most of these people die before they see a doctor. In others, thrombotic occlusion causes persistent chest pain, with necrosis of part of their heart (myocardial infarction). A third group have recurrent or persistent chest pain without losing the blood-starved (ischaemic) heart muscle (unstable angina). Patients with myocardial infarction or unstable angina have an increased risk of death, usually from rhythm disorders or heart failure. This increased risk is highest in the first few days, but continues in subsequent years.

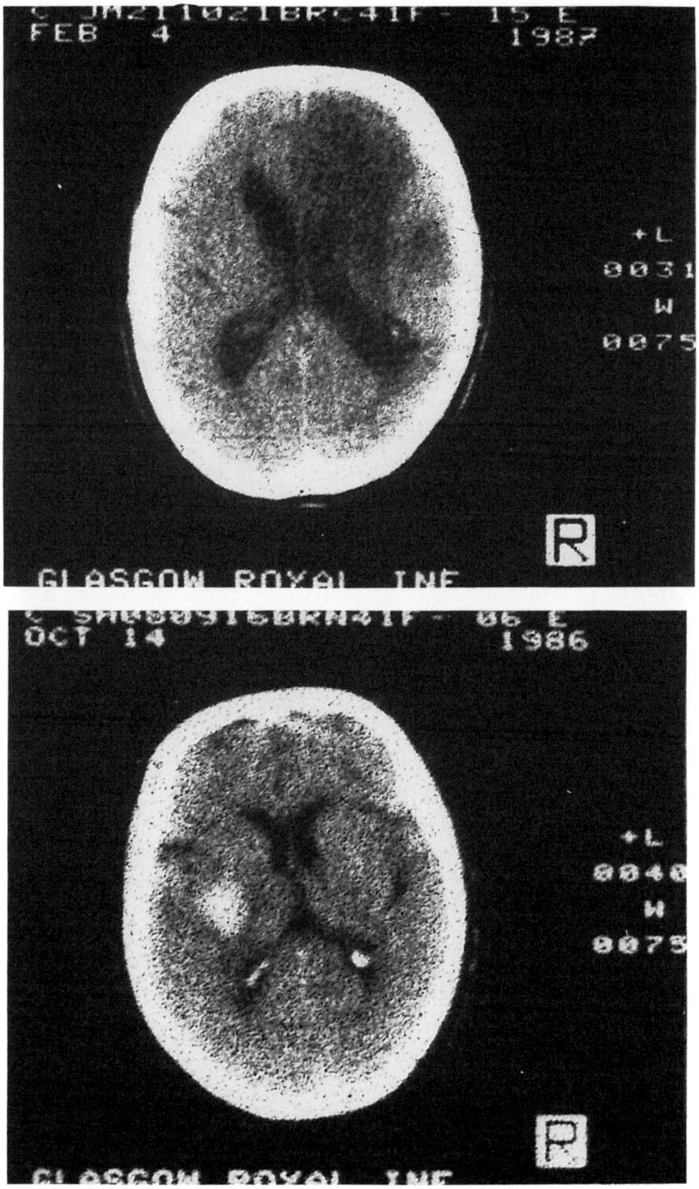

Fig. 7.3 **a** Cerebral infarction due to thrombotic occlusion of a cerebral artery, shown as a dark area on CT brain scanning. A theoretical indication for thrombolytic therapy.
b Intracerebral haemorrhage due to blood vessel rupture, shown as a white area on CT brain scanning. This can be a complication of thrombolytic therapy.

In the UK an additional 100 000 people suffer a stroke each year. Most strokes are due to blockage of an artery supplying the brain, either by local thrombus in the artery, or by a fragment of thrombus which detaches upstream from the heart or from a larger artery (embolism). As in the heart, the blood-starved part of the brain supplied by the artery may become necrosed (cerebral infarction). However, about 15% of strokes are due not to cerebral infarction, but to cerebral haemorrhage. Both types of stroke cause a similar clinical picture (usually paralysis of the one side of the body). A brain scan, using computerized X-ray tomography (CT scanning) to build up a picture of slices of the brain, is required to distinguish the two types of stroke (Fig. 7.3). Following a major stroke, about one-third of patients die, one-third live but are dependent on others for their care and one-third regain independence.

The third commonest site of arterial thrombosis is in the legs, causing a cold, painful leg which may eventually become gangrenous. This affects about 50 000 people each year in the UK, of whom about 10% require amputation of the leg. In others bypass grafting of the artery may save the leg but such grafts commonly thrombose, causing recurrent symptoms.

Thrombosis in the leg veins deep within the calf muscles is also common, especially in sick patients lying in hospital beds. Many such thrombi cause no symptoms until the thrombus detaches and blocks an artery in the lungs (pulmonary embolism). One in every 100 patients admitted to hospital in the UK dies of pulmonary embolism; usually they die before a doctor can make the diagnosis or initiate treatment. In other patients, life-threatening pulmonary embolism causes shock, breathlessness and chest pain but the doctor has a chance to intervene with antithrombotic therapy. Some deep vein thrombi cause a painful swollen leg by obstructing the return of blood through the major leg veins. Again, the doctor has a chance to intervene with antithrombotic therapy before the patient develops either a pulmonary embolism; a block in the leg circulation so severe that the leg may perish (venous gangrene); or a chronically swollen, aching leg with varicose veins and sometimes leg ulcers (post-thrombotic syndrome) which the patient must endure for life.

Antithrombotic therapy: a double-edged sword

Thrombi, whether in arteries or veins, are composed of similar platelets and fibrin to those which occur in haemostatic plugs. It is therefore logical to prevent or treat thrombosis with antiplatelet or anticoagulant drugs. In hospital patients, the risk of deep vein thrombosis and pulmonary embolism can be reduced by subcutaneous injections of low-dose heparin (Collins et al 1988) or by antiplatelet drugs such as aspirin (Antiplatelet Trialists' Collaboration Meeting 1990). Aspirin also reduces mortality in patients with acute myocardial infarction (ISIS-2 Collaborative Group 1988, Hennekens et al 1989). Anticoagulant drugs are effective in treatment of acute myocardial infarction, deep vein thrombosis and pulmonary embolism (Meade 1984, Poller 1987, Anonymous 1988).

On the other hand, the benefits of antiplatelet or anticoagulant therapy are, to some extent, balanced by an increased risk of bleeding. These drugs not only reduce the extension of platelet–fibrin arterial and venous thrombi but also reduce the formation of platelet–fibrin haemostatic plugs. Hence aspirin or anticoagulants increase the risk of bleeding into the brain (Fig. 7.3) from the stomach, or after injury, surgery (from the wound) or tooth extraction (from the socket). Doctors must therefore carefully evaluate each patient for both thrombotic and bleeding tendency, to see if their risk of thrombosis justifies making them an 'acquired haemophiliac' by prescribing aspirin or anticoagulant drugs. The coagulation laboratory can help them in two ways:

1. In selected patients, by screening for a pre-existing haemostatic defect (e.g. thrombocytopenia, liver disease, haemophilia) before they commence anticoagulant therapy.
2. By careful control of full-dose anticoagulant therapy.

Enhancement of endogenous fibrinolysis

Growth of fibrin thrombi may be favoured by an imbalance between overactive coagulation and underactive fibrinolysis (Astrup 1958). This concept is supported by an increased ratio of thrombin activity to plasmin activity in the plasma of persons at increased risk of thrombosis, as shown by measurement of fibrinogen derivatives of thrombin or plasmin action (Lowe et al 1991). High levels of fibrinogen and of the major plasminogen activator inhibitor (PAI-1; Fig. 7.2) are found with increased frequency in patients with thrombosis, or who are at increased risk of thrombosis, and are also predictive of thrombosis in follow-up studies (Lowe 1987, Kruithof 1988). Several groups of drugs have been shown to stimulate the endogenous fibrinolytic system, notably anabolic steroids, which reduce plasma levels of fibrinogen and PAI-1 and increase plasma levels of plasmin activity (Lowe & Small 1988, Small et al 1989). Unfortunately, few controlled trials of anabolic steroids have been performed to assess their efficacy in prevention of thrombosis and published studies in prevention of venous thrombosis show no benefit (Lowe and Small 1988). Furthermore, the same authors also showed that the long-term adverse effects of anabolic steroids preclude their use in most patients. On the other hand, reduction in risk factors such as obesity and high levels of blood fat by diet appears to stimulate endogenous fibrinolysis, without adverse effects, and should be positively encouraged as part of health education.

Thrombolytic therapy: a larger double-edged sword

Antithrombotic therapy with aspirin or anticoagulants may stop thrombi extending while the endogenous fibrinolytic system breaks them down. However, in some patients with thrombi threatening life or limb, such treatment may not be effective in time. Thrombolytic therapy may then be indicated, to break down the thrombus and restore blood flow more rapidly.

Some early studies used infusions of direct thrombolytic enzymes such as plasmin or Brinase. However, all currently used thrombolytic drugs are plasminogen activators, which convert endogenous circulating plasminogen to plasmin (Fig. 7.2). Plasmin then digests fibrin thrombi.

Streptokinase, a plasminogen activator produced by streptococci, was first infused systemically into arm veins in 1959 by Sherry and colleagues in St Louis, USA (Fletcher et al 1959). Streptokinase was infused locally through a catheter into a thrombosed leg artery 4 years later by McNicol and colleagues in Glasgow Royal Infirmary (McNicol et al 1963). Repeated visualization of the thrombus by injection of radiographic contrast medium into the blood vessel (angiography) showed rapid lysis of the thrombus (Fig. 7.4). Since then, numerous angiographic studies have shown that thrombolytic therapy lyses both arterial and venous thrombi more frequently, and to a greater extent than either no therapy or else anticoagulation with heparin. Why then has it taken so long to establish thrombolytic therapy as a routine treatment in patients with thrombosis?

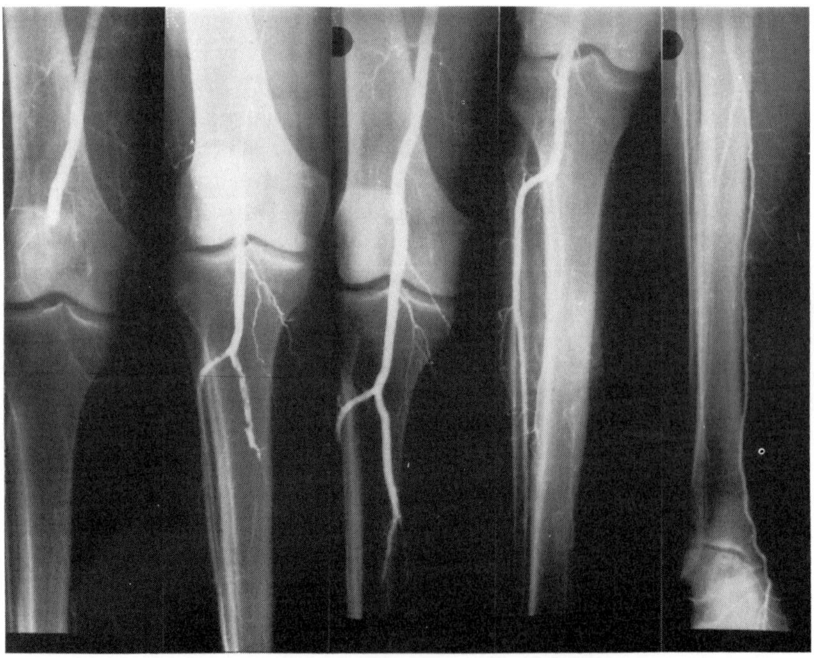

Fig. 7.4 Serial angiograms showing progressive reperfusion following local infusion of streptokinase in a patient with recent peripheral arterial thromboembolism. (Reproduced from Lowe (1991), with permission, and with kind permission of Dr A. Reid, Dr O. Reid and Dr J. G. Pollock.)

One reason is that it has taken a long time to show by large trials, that thrombolytic therapy benefits patients (see below). Secondly, thrombolytic therapy is expensive. Thirdly, streptokinase is a foreign protein which can cause allergic reactions. However, the major adverse effect of thrombolytic therapy is bleeding. Nobody has yet discovered a plasminogen activator which will digest fibrin in thrombi, while sparing fibrin in haemostatic plugs. It seems likely that nobody ever will.

Antiplatelet or anticoagulant therapy increases the risk of bleeding by reducing the formation of new haemostatic platelet–fibrin plugs. However, it does not digest existing haemostatic plugs as thrombolytic therapy does. Some patients receiving thrombolytic therapy will in the previous 10–14 days have suffered a leaking blood vessel somewhere, which is sealed with a fibrin plug which has not yet been stabilized by tissue repair. This could be a scab on cut skin, a bruised gum from vigorous tooth-brushing the previous morning, or a fibrin plug in a stomach ulcer or brain aneurysm. In such patients thrombolytic therapy can break down the fibrin plugs, causing bleeding which, in the case of the stomach or brain, can be life threatening. The longer the duration of thrombolytic therapy, the greater the risk of bleeding.

Doctors must therefore balance the individual patient's risk from persistent thrombosis against the risk of bleeding during thrombolytic therapy. A careful history and examination is required to detect contraindications to thrombolytic therapy (Table 7.2). Most of these contraindications are situations in which recently formed haemostatic plugs may be lysed by thrombolytic therapy, causing bleeding. Unfortunately, some patients have lesions liable to bleed which even the most careful history and examination will not reveal.

Thrombolytic therapy increases the risk of bleeding not only by lysing haemostatic fibrin plugs but also by causing systemic hyperplasminaemia which digests circulating fibrinogen and other clotting factors, giving rise to high levels of fibrinogen degradation products (FDP) (Fig. 7.2). These changes have both antiplatelet and anticoagulant effects (Fig. 7.5). While they may be useful in preventing recurrent thrombosis, they may also increase the risk of bleeding. The antiplatelet effects of thrombolytic therapy will be enhanced by current antiplatelet drugs (e.g. aspirin). The anticoagulant effects of thrombolytic therapy will be enhanced by current anticoagulant drugs (e.g. heparin). Complex haemostatic defects therefore exist during thrombolytic therapy. They are considered in more detail later in the chapter.

The role of the laboratory in thrombolytic therapy

The role of the laboratory can be summarized as follows:

1. Prior to initiation of thrombolytic therapy, a standard coagulation

Table 7.2 Some contraindications to thrombolytic therapy

Risk of bleeding
Current or recent (within 6 months) internal bleeding or stroke
Bleeding disorder (e.g. thrombocytopenia, haemophilias, severe liver or kidney disease)
Possible aortic dissection, acute pericarditis or oesophagitis
Oesophageal varices, active peptic ulcer, ulcerative colitis, gastrointestinal neoplasm, acute pancreatitis
Previous intracranial haemorrhage (at any time)
Severe hypertension (risk of intracranial haemorrhage)
Haemorrhagic retinopathy, bacterial endocarditis
Active genitourinary lesion, lung cavitation or intracranial disease
Recent (within 2–4 weeks) surgery or trauma (especially cranial or ocular), organ biopsy, puncture of non-compressible vessels, prolonged cardiopulmonary resuscitation, abortion or obstetric delivery
Pregnancy (risk of retroplacental haemorrhage)
Age over 75 years
Risk of embolism
Left heart thrombus
Contraindications to streptokinase or anistreplase
Known hypersensitivity
Recent streptococcal infection
Recent (within 6–12 months) treatment with either drug (unless clinical situation can await measurement of streptokinase resistance)

Note. Many contraindications are relative rather than absolute: e.g. life-threatening pulmonary embolism in a pregnant (or elderly) patient may well justify thrombolytic therapy despite the increased risk of placental (or intracranial) bleeding.

From Lowe (1991) with permission.

screen can be performed to exclude a systemic bleeding disorder which may contraindicate thrombolytic therapy, e.g. thrombocytopenia, liver failure or haemophilias (Cairns et al 1989). However, the time delay involved will reduce the clinical benefit of early treatment in acute myocardial infarction, where even an hour's delay may be important. It is useful to perform not only a platelet count, prothrombin time and activated partial thromboplastin time (APTT), but also a thrombin clotting time. The latter gives a most useful, rapid measure of fibrinogen depletion and FDP formation during thrombolytic therapy. A baseline thrombin time is therefore advised.

2. Prior to initiation of streptokinase therapy, performance of a streptokinase resistance test (Amery et al 1963, Hirsh et al 1970, Jalihal & Morris 1990) estimates the titre of antistreptococcal antibodies in the patient's plasma, which have to be neutralized before a sufficient level of plasma streptokinase exerts a plasminogen activating effect (Fig. 7.3). Such a test allows titration of an appropriate loading dose.

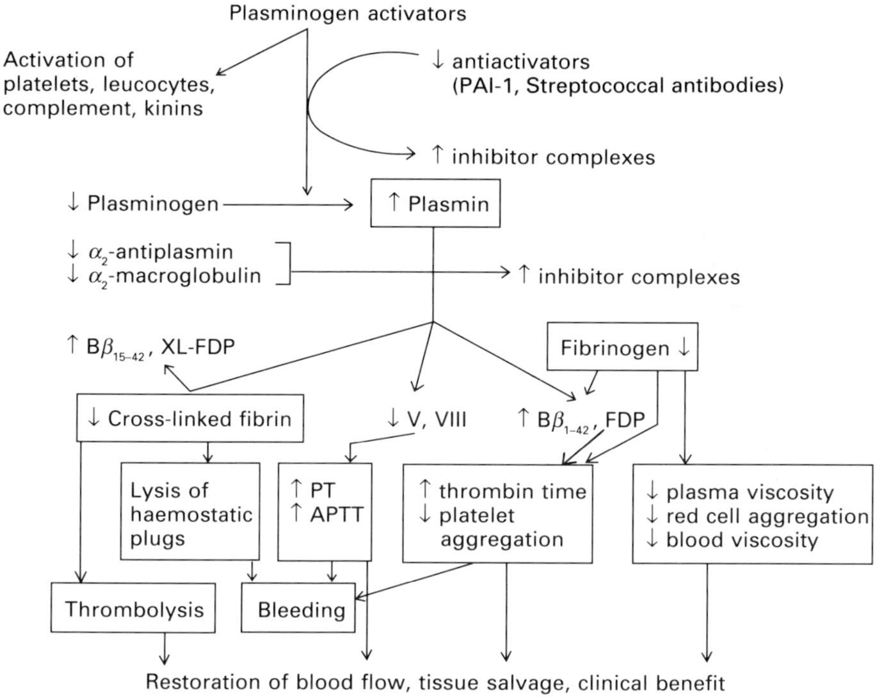

Fig. 7.5 Systemic effects of thrombolytic therapy. (Reproduced from Lowe (1991), with permission.)

However, once again the time delay involved will reduce the clinical benefit of treatment in acute myocardial infarction, in which a short-term, high-dose intravenous infusion (1.5 million units over 1 h) is highly beneficial (Schroeder et al 1983, ISIS-2 Collaborative Group 1988, Cairns et al 1989, International Study Group 1990). In venous thromboembolism treated by traditional long-duration, low-dose intravenous infusion, a loading dose of 250 000 units appears safe even if streptokinase antibody titres exceed this dose: systemic hyperplasminaemia may be delayed by several hours in this situation (Hirsh et al 1970, Chesterman 1987).

3. During prolonged thrombolytic therapy (e.g. for venous thromboembolism), the development of systemic hyperplasminaemia can be rapidly confirmed by repeating the thrombin clotting time (which measures the combined effect of fibrinogen depletion and FDP formation on the clotting of plasma fibrinogen and its derivatives by thrombin), and subsequently by measurement of fibrinogen and FDP levels. About 10% of patients treated with streptokinase or urokinase do not develop significant changes in fibrinogen or FDP levels: such patients appear to have a lower incidence of thrombolysis (Marder and Sherry 1988), hence changes in thrombolytic therapy may be indicated.

4. After cessation of thrombolytic therapy, monitoring of coagulation times (e.g the APTT) can be used to determine the timing of initiation of maintenance anticoagulant therapy with heparin (if required) or, alternatively, to determine the risk of bleeding prior to surgical procedures.
5. If serious bleeding occurs during or after thrombolytic therapy, a coagulation screen will act as a guide to appropriate replacement therapy with fresh frozen plasma, cryoprecipitate or platelets.
6. In patients whose thrombolytic therapy is followed by full-dose heparin, daily platelet counts are useful to detect heparin-induced thrombocytopenia.

INDICATIONS AND CONTRAINDICATIONS FOR THROMBOLYTIC THERAPY

Acute myocardial infarction

Streptokinase was first used in the treatment of myocardial infarction in 1959 (Fletcher et al 1959), but it took another 30 years before it was accepted as routine treatment (Cairns et al 1989). Its lack of acceptance by cardiologists probably reflected their doubts about the causal role of coronary thrombosis in myocardial infarction; the reporting of 'negative' as well as 'positive' trials; the cost and complications of streptokinase; and their interest in other aspects of myocardial infarction. In the last 10 years, interest in thrombosis and thrombolysis was renewed by evidence that thrombosis was present in most cases of myocardial infarction and played a causal role (Davies et al 1979, DeWood et al 1980). Furthermore, coronary angiography combined with intracoronary thrombolysis showed a high incidence of reperfusion of the infarct-related artery (Rentrop et al 1981). Because acute cardiac catheterization is expensive, wastes time and is not available in most hospitals treating patients with myocardial infarction, high-dose, short-term intravenous infusions of streptokinase (1.5 million units over 1 h) were then studied and were shown to be effective in lysing coronary thrombi (Schroeder et al 1983). Subsequently, this regimen was shown to reduce mortality in acute myocardial infarction by about 20% (GISSI 1986, ISAM Study Group 1986, ISIS-2 Collaborative Group 1988). The last study also showed that the old, established simple aspirin tablet, chewed on admission to hospital then taken daily for a month, reduced mortality as effectively as streptokinase; furthermore, the combination of streptokinase and aspirin had additive effects in reducing mortality (ISIS-2 Collaborative Group 1988, Hennekens et al 1989).

Streptokinase and aspirin probably reduce mortality in myocardial infarction by lysing fibrin-rich coronary thrombi and also by lowering plasma fibrinogen which reduces blood viscosity (Fig. 7.5): these two actions restore blood flow to the blood-starved area of the heart and reduce

Table 7.3 Comparison of hospital mortality and clinical events in a randomized trial of alteplase versus streptokinase in 20 981 patients with suspected acute myocardial infarction of less than 6 h duration. Alteplase was associated with higher risks of stroke and total bleeding, and with lower risks of major bleeds, allergic reactions and hypotension. Mortality was similar with either drug

	Alteplase %	Streptokinase %	Relative risk (95% C I)
Death	8.9	8.5	1.05 (0.95–1.16)
Stroke	1.3	0.9	1.41 (1.09–1.83)
All bleeds	4.2	3.3	1.26 (1.09–1.45)
Major bleeds	0.6	0.9	0.67 (0.49–0.91)
Allergic reactions	0.2	1.7	0.20 (0.15–0.27)
Hypotension	1.7	3.8	0.45 (0.38–0.53)

Data from International Study Group Trial (1990). CI = Confidence Intervals

the size of the part of the heart which dies (infarct size): consequently less patients die of heart failure (Lowe 1991). Their anticoagulant and anti-platelet effects also reduce the risk of rethrombosis in the affected coronary artery (Fig. 7.5). Streptokinase and aspirin is now the standard treatment of evolving myocardial infarction. A reduction in mortality is maintained for at least 1 year after infarction. It is also the cheapest thrombolytic regimen (the cost of the standard dose of 1.5 million units of streptokinase in the UK in 1990 was about £80, and the cost per life 'saved' was about £3000). The newer thrombolytic agents, anistreplase and alteplase, also reduce mortality in acute myocardial infarction (Wilcox et al 1988, AIMS Trial Study Group 1990) but are more expensive. A recent, large comparative study found similar mortality in patients treated with streptokinase or alteplase (International Study Group 1990; Table 7.3). A further study (the ISIS-3 Study) comparing streptokinase, anistreplase and alteplase, with and without early heparin therapy, should clarify the question of the optimal thrombolytic agent in acute myocardial infarction.

Thrombolytic therapy should be considered in all patients with suspected evolving acute myocardial infarction (Cairns et al 1989). Its benefits are greatest when given early (less than 6 h from the onset of symptoms); hence every effort should be made to educate the public about the symptoms and to admit patients as soon as possible to coronary care units for initiation of treatment. Baseline coagulation screens are not usually performed as they cause delay and reduce the benefit of early therapy. However they may be requested quite reasonably when a pre-existing haemostatic defect is suspected. Its confirmation or exclusion may decide the balance of risk and benefit for thrombolytic therapy in an individual patient.

Unstable angina

Patients with unstable angina frequently have non-occlusive thrombi in their coronary arteries and are at risk of complete thrombotic occlusion, myocardial infarction and sudden death. It is therefore logical to treat such patients with thrombolytic therapy (Gold 1989). However, antiplatelet therapy with aspirin reduces the risks of myocardial infarction and death (Hennekens et al 1989), and heparin infusions also appear clinically effective (Theroux et al 1988, Neri Serneri et al 1990). Thus, while several studies of thrombolytic therapy in unstable angina have been performed there is as yet no evidence that thrombolysis is superior to antiplatelet or anticoagulant treatment which may be sufficient to inhibit further platelet–fibrin thrombosis in the coronary artery (Gold 1989, Neri Serneri et al 1990).

Stroke

As previously noted, thromboembolism causes about 85% of strokes. There is no proven specific treatment for such strokes (Lowe 1990). Several studies of thrombolytic therapy in thromboembolic stroke are in progress (Sloan et al 1989, Anonymous 1990), some of which have shown promising initial results (i.e. lysis of cerebral thrombi, clinical improvement). However there are many problems, including the need for rapid admission of patients with evolving stroke to hospital, rapid differentiation of thrombotic from haemorrhagic stroke by CT brain scanning (Fig. 7.3), the risk of bleeding into the damaged brain and the risk of fatal brain swelling after the occluded artery is reopened. At present, therefore, the use of thrombolytic therapy in stroke remains experimental.

Occlusion of limb arteries or bypass grafts

Intravenous thrombolytic therapy in patients with thromboembolism of limb arteries was first reported in 1959 (Fletcher et al 1959) and may be successful in about 50% of cases. However, it is associated with a high mortality and risk of bleeding, especially into the brain, therefore it is now seldom used (Graor and Olin 1989). It has been replaced by local infusion of the thrombolytic agent into the occluded artery, close to the thrombus. Repeated angiography can be performed through the infusion catheter, to detect thrombolysis and reperfusion of the limb (Fig. 7.4). The advantage of local infusion is that lower doses can be used (e.g. 5000 units of streptokinase per h), thus minimizing the risk of generalized bleeding. However, systemic effects are often observed in practice, especially after reperfusion which increases the systemic circulation of the infused thrombolytic agent. Bleeding at the site of insertion of the catheter is common but can usually be controlled. Careful selection of patients is required, with close cooperation between surgeons, radiologists and angiologists (Anonymous 1990). With such selection, limb artery patency can be restored in about 80% of patients (Graor and Olin 1989). A baseline coagulation screen should be performed and repeated at least daily if thrombolytic therapy is continued for more than a few hours, in the event of major bleeding or in patients requiring urgent surgery.

Venous thromboembolism

The use of thrombolytic agents in deep vein thrombosis of the leg or in pulmonary embolism varies widely between doctors. This partly reflects the lack of large trials showing clinical benefit from such therapy (Hyers et al 1989). There is no doubt that thrombolytic therapy increases both the occurrence and the extent of lysis of both deep vein thrombi and pulmonary emboli, compared to conventional anticoagulation with heparin and warfarin. Patients receiving intravenous streptokinase for deep vein thrombosis were 3.7 times more likely to show significant lysis of their thrombi at repeat venography than patients receiving heparin (95% confidence intervals 2.5–5.7) (Goldhaber et al 1984). In the Urokinase Pulmonary Embolism Trial (1973), patients receiving urokinase had significantly greater reduction in their pulmonary emboli after 24 h, as shown by both repeat pulmonary angiography and measurement of arterial pressures. However, the clinical significance (symptoms, mortality) of such increased thrombolysis is at present not known (Hyers et al 1989). Many clinicians therefore feel that in most cases of venous thromboembolism, anticoagulant therapy is adequate and that the additional cost and bleeding risks of thrombolytic therapy are not justified.

On the other hand, thrombolytic therapy is often justified in the minority of patients who have severe symptoms due to massive venous thromboembolism which threatens life or limb, e.g. impending venous gangrene, or massive pulmonary embolism causing shock. The clinical response to thrombolytic therapy in such patients is often impressive, although there is a lack of controlled trials for several reasons (Lowe 1991). A baseline coagulation screen is indicated prior to initiation of treatment, followed by monitoring to establish the presence of systemic fibrinogenolysis which is associated with lysis of thromboemboli (Marder and Sherry 1988).

Other indications for thrombolytic therapy

The place of thrombolysis in rarer types of thromboembolism is considered by Marder and Sherry (1988) and by Kwaan and Samama (1989).

Contraindications to thrombolytic therapy

These are summarized in Table 7.2.

THROMBOLYTIC AGENTS

Streptokinase

Streptokinase is produced by β-haemolytic streptococci. It forms a 1:1 stoichiometric complex with plasminogen, in which it exposes an active site, conferring plasminogen activator activity upon the complex. It is the current 'gold standard' drug in thrombolytic therapy because (a) it has been the most widely used clinically, (b) it is the cheapest and (c) it is clinically as effective as newer thrombolytic agents (e.g. International Study Group 1990). Its disadvantages are a higher risk of allergic reactions and hypotension, as well as antibody formation which may complicate further thrombolytic therapy in the subsequent year (Jalihal and Morris 1990).

Anistreplase

Anistreplase (anisoylated streptokinase – plasminogen activator complex, APSAC) is a pro-enzyme, whose catalytic serine active site is temporarily masked by an anisoyl group. Following intravenous infusion it is slowly activated by sustained deacylation and release of the anisoyl group. It has a half-life in vivo of about 90 min (compared to about 25 min for streptokinase). Unlike streptokinase, it can be given as a bolus injection intravenously over 5 min (the dose is 30 units). Bolus dosage offers the potential for earlier administration prior to hospital admission in patients with evolving myocardial infarction (e.g. by trained general practitioners or ambulancemen). The benefits and risks of such out-patient administration are currently under evaluation. The systemic effects, adverse effects and coronary reperfusion rates in acute myocardial infarction appear comparable to streptokinase, as do its effects on the blood (Hoffmann et al 1987). The cost in the UK in 1990 was about five times higher than streptokinase. Anistreplase significantly reduces mortality in acute myocardial infarction compared to placebo (AIMS Trial Study Group 1990). Its risks and benefits relative to streptokinase and alteplase are currently being assessed in the ISIS-3 Study.

Alteplase

Alteplase (recombinant tissue-type plasminogen activator, rt–PA) is produced by recombinant biotechnology for pharmaceutical use: endogenous t-PA is a serine protease plasminogen activator of physiological importance (Fig. 7.2). The dose of single-chain alteplase is 100 mg (or 1.5 mg/kg for patients weighing under 67 kg), infused over 3 h in a decreasing dosage schedule. The half-life in the circulation is about 5 min. However, as it binds specifically to fibrin and activates plasminogen at the fibrin surface several hundred times more efficiently than in the circulation, its effects on fibrin thrombi (or on fibrin haemostatic plugs) may be prolonged for several hours. Possibly because of its relative 'fibrin specificity' relative to streptokinase, it produces higher early coronary artery patency rates in acute myocardial infarction (Verstraete et al 1985, Cheseboro et al 1987). However 24 h patency rates are similar for the two drugs (Cheseboro et al 1987) and in a large recent study comparing alteplase with streptokinase their effects on mortality and overall adverse effects were comparable (International Study Group 1990). Its cost in the UK in 1990 was about 10 times higher than streptokinase. Alteplase causes less hypotension and allergic reactions than streptokinase and is not inactivated by antistreptococcal antibodies. It may therefore be preferred in patients known to be allergic to streptokinase or anistreplase and in patients requiring repeat thrombolytic therapy within a year of treatment with streptokinase or anistreplase, who are likely to have high antistreptococcal antibody titres (Jalihal and Morris 1990). Its risks and benefits relative to streptokinase and anistreplase are being assessed in the ISIS-3 study of acute myocardial infarction, which should also answer the question as to whether early intravenous heparin should be given following thrombolytic therapy. This question may be especially important for alteplase, which causes less depletion of plasma fibrinogen and less systemic anticoagulation (which may prevent rethrombosis) than other thrombolytic agents. Alteplase is also being assessed as an alternative to streptokinase or urokinase in the treatment of limb artery thromboembolism and in venous thromboembolism.

Urokinase

Urokinase has been produced commercially, initially from human urine and latterly from tissue culture of kidney cells: both forms have similar activities and are less antigenic than streptokinase in man. The systemic effects of urokinase are similar to those of streptokinase, but slower in onset. It is more expensive than streptokinase, but as with alteplase may be indicated in patients known to be allergic to streptokinase or anistreplase and in patients recently treated with such agents.

Saruplase

Saruplase (recombinant single-chain urinary-type plasminogen activator, rscu-PA) is produced by recombinant biotechnology for pharmaceutical use. Endogenous scu-PA is another plasminogen activator of physiological importance (Fig 7.2). Like alteplase, it shows enhanced plasminogen activation in the presence of fibrin, although the mechanisms are different. Saruplase is not yet licensed for clinical use but is currently under evaluation in treatment of acute myocardial infarction (PRIMI Trial Study Group 1989). It produces slightly less fibrinogen depletion and FDP formation than streptokinase (PRIMI Trial Study Group 1989).

LABORATORY MONITORING OF THROMBOLYTIC THERAPY

Thrombolytic therapy should not be undertaken unless local laboratory facilities are available for monitoring its systemic effects. In the event of major bleeding or the need for urgent surgery, assessment of such effects is required to guide appropriate replacement therapy with fresh frozen plasma, cryoprecipitate or platelet transfusions. The minimum requirement is for a routine haemostatic screen (platelet count, APTT, prothrombin time, thrombin time and bleeding time) as well as measurements of plasma fibrinogen and FDP. Other tests which change during thrombolytic therapy are of interest in research studies but are of little practical help in patient management.

Blood sampling and handling

In view of the risk of bruising from multiple venepunctures, it is desirable to insert a large venous cannula in each arm, which is kept flushed with dilute heparin–saline. One cannula is used for blood sampling (ensuring that the initial few millilitres of blood drawn is discarded to clear the heparin–saline flush and that a new syringe is used to take the second sample for coagulation studies). The other cannula is used for intravenous medication, including the thrombolytic drug, heparin, etc. Samples taken through an indwelling cannula may be influenced by activation of platelets and coagulation in the cannula (Thomson 1985). However, if samples are carefully taken such influences are usually minimal compared to the systemic effects of thrombolytic therapy. If adequate samples cannot be obtained through the cannula, or if test results are surprising, then sampling via separate venepunctures is required. Care should then be taken to minimize bleeding at venepuncture sites by prolonged compression.

The routine anticoagulant for coagulation and fibrinolytic studies is 3.2% (0.109 M) trisodium citrate; 9 volumes of blood are added to 1 volume of anticoagulant (Thomson 1985). After careful mixing, blood samples should be transferred directly into a container of crushed melting ice, transported to the laboratory without delay, and centrifuged (4°C; 15 min at 2000 *g* or 30 min at 1500 *g*) within 30 min of sample collection to obtain platelet-poor plasma (Thomson 1985). Aliquots of plasma should either be kept on melting ice for immediate testing, or else snap frozen and stored at –70°C for subsequent assays. These conditions of speed and temperature are required to minimize deterioration of the labile clotting factors, V and VIII (Thomson 1985), which are consumed during thrombolytic therapy in vivo; and also to minimize in vitro digestion of factors V, VIII and fibrinogen by high plasma concentrations of the therapeutic plasminogen activator.

To further minimize in vitro digestion of fibrinogen, some authorities recommend addition of fibrinolytic inhibitors to the citrate anticoagulant. Such inhibitors include ε-aminocaproic acid (EACA, 0.07 M; Hoffmann et al 1987), aprotinin (Trasylol; 150–500 U/ml; Graor et al 1986, Verstraete et al 1986, Brommer et al 1987, Siegfried and Tanswell 1987, Rao et al 1988, Loscalzo et al 1989) and the synthetic serine protease active site blocking agent, PPACK (D-Phe-Pro-Arg-CH_2Cl; Tiefenbrunn et al 1986,

Siegfried and Tanswell 1987). Both polyclonal (Siegfried and Tanswell 1987) and monoclonal (Douglas et al 1988) antibodies to recombinant t-PA (alteplase) have also been used as fibrinolytic inhibitors. Samples containing such inhibitors cannot be used for measurements of plasminogen activator activity, plasminogen activity, or antiplasmin activity (Siegfried and Tanswell 1987). Aprotinin also prolongs the APTT; while PPACK prolongs the APTT, prothrombin time and thrombin time (Siegfried and Tanswell 1987). Antibodies to rt-PA are probably ideal but are expensive and not widely available, hence are currently limited to research studies.

At present, therefore, for routine laboratory monitoring of thrombolytic therapy with coagulation screens, the addition of aprotinin or PPACK to the citrate anticoagulant is not recommended in view of their interference with coagulation times. Rapid cooling and handling of samples is recommended, to minimize in vitro degradation of fibrinogen, factor V and factor VIII. If samples are to be stored for fibrinogen measurement the addition of EACA, aprotinin, PPACK or anti-rt-PA (with alteplase only) to a separate blood sample is recommended. The addition of aprotinin to citrate does not appear to alter FDP levels (Brommer et al 1987).

Coagulation screens

As previously discussed, a standard coagulation screen should be performed prior to thrombolytic therapy to exclude systemic bleeding disorders which may contraindicate such treatment. The exception is acute myocardial infarction, where time is of the essence in achieving clinical benefit. Delaying treatment for an hour while a coagulation screen is obtained may be clinically unacceptable. In other situations (peripheral arterial thrombosis, deep vein thrombosis, pulmonary embolism, stroke) a coagulation screen should be obtained. This should comprise a platelet count, APTT, prothrombin time and thrombin time. A streptokinase resistance test (Amery et al 1963, Hirsh et al 1970, Jalihal and Morris 1990) may also be indicated. Plasma aliquots should be stored deep frozen in case subsequent measurement of fibrinogen or other factors is required (if fibrinogen is not included in the routine coagulation screen).

During prolonged thrombolytic therapy (i.e. more than the 1–3 h, which is sufficient in acute myocardial infarction), it is useful to establish the presence of systemic hyperplasminaemia and fibrinogenolysis by repeating coagulation times (e.g. at 2–4 hours after the initiation of therapy). The thrombin time is most sensitive to the combined effect of fibrinogen depletion and FDP formation on the clotting of plasma fibrinogen and its derivatives. Digestion of factors V and VIII will also prolong the prothrombin time and APTT, respectively (Fig. 7.5). Subsequent measurement of fibrinogen and FDP can be performed to quantitate changes from baseline, as can the euglobulin clot lysis time to confirm high plasma plasminogen activator levels.

In about 10% of patients receiving standard doses of intravenous streptokinase or urokinase, tests of coagulation and fibrinolysis show no significant changes (e.g. clotting times less than 1.5 times baseline). These patients are at risk of thrombotic extension (Marder and Sherry, 1988). In such a situation, the clinician's choices are:

1. To repeat the coagulation test after a short interval (perhaps using a fresh venepuncture, if artefactual shortening of clotting times by coagulation activation in a sample taken through an indwelling cannula is suspected)
2. To increase the dose of the thrombolytic agent (perhaps after performing a streptokinase resistance test in the case of streptokinase or anistreplase), then to repeat the coagulation tests
3. To change to a different thrombolytic agent, then to repeat the coagulation tests, or
4. To stop thrombolytic therapy and substitute heparin, which will at least reduce the risk of thrombotic extension.

In local intra-arterial thrombolytic therapy (e.g. for limb artery or graft thromboembolism, or for pulmonary embolism confirmed by pulmonary angiography), a substantial percentage of patients will show systemic effects on coagulation and fibrinolysis, but some will not. In such patients, repeated arteriography may show progressive thrombolysis and in such cases the clinician may understandably be guided by the angiogram rather than by the lack of a systemic 'lytic state'.

In most patients undergoing intravenous thrombolytic therapy, and also in a substantial percentage of those undergoing intra-arterial thrombolytic therapy, coagulation times are prolonged to a similar degree (1.5–3-fold) as 'therapeutic' levels of heparin therapy. It is reasonable to suppose that such anticoagulation is of similar efficacy to heparin in preventing thrombotic extension or rethrombosis. It is also reasonable to suppose that more marked prolongation of coagulation times may increase the risk of bleeding, although bleeding may be related more to digestion of haemostatic plugs than to systemic anticoagulation (see above). There is little published data to support this supposition. Bovill (1990) recently reported that in the TIMI-II study of alteplase in myocardial infarction, a APTT greater than 90 s was associated with a relative risk of bleeding of 1.7 (95% confidence intervals 1–2.9). What action should be taken if coagulation times are markedly prolonged during sustained thrombolytic therapy? Our policy has been to discontinue thrombolytic therapy should the thrombin time be prolonged more than five-fold (Lowe and Prentice 1980), recommencing at a lower dosage when the thrombin time approaches twice the control value. However, other authors (e.g. Raskob and Hull 1989) recommend that the dose of streptokinase be *increased*, in order to complex the excess plasmin in a streptokinase–plasmin(ogen) complex. Further studies are required to establish the optimal handling of greatly prolonged clotting times during prolonged thrombolytic therapy.

After cessation of thrombolytic therapy, maintenance anticoagulation with heparin is commonly practised. This seems eminently reasonable in venous thromboembolism, where anticoagulation is the mainstay of treatment (Poller 1987, Anonymous 1988) as well as in peripheral arterial thromboembolism. However, the place of maintenance anticoagulation after thrombolytic therapy in acute myocardial infarction remains to be established by future controlled trials: maintenance antiplatelet therapy with aspirin may be sufficient (ISIS-2 Collaborative Group 1988, Cairns et al 1989, Hennekens et al 1989, International Study Group 1990). If heparin is to be used, the APTT should be monitored and heparin should not be started until the APTT falls to about twice the control value. Heparin should then be monitored at least daily using the APTT. Daily platelet counts are also advisable in heparinized patients, to detect heparin-induced thrombocytopenia (which appears particularly common in North America). In the TIMI-II study of alteplase in myocardial infarction, Bovill (1990) found that a platelet count less than 100×10^9/litre was associated with a relative risk of bleeding of 7.5 (95% confidence intervals 2.3–24).

In the event of serious bleeding during or after thrombolytic therapy, or the need for urgent surgery, a coagulation screen (including fibrinogen level) should be obtained urgently as a guide to the need for replacement therapy. The infusion of the thrombolytic agent should be stopped. However, plasminogen activators which are highly fibrin bound (e.g. alteplase) may continue to exert local lytic effects on fibrin haemostatic plugs for several hours. Circulating plasmin can be inhibited by infusions of aprotinin or tranexamic acid (de Bono 1989). In patients receiving heparin, the heparin infusions may be stopped and reversal of heparin guided by the APTT. Marked prolongation of the thrombin time, or fibrinogen depletion (under 1 g/l), should lead to consideration of replacement of fibrinogen (with fresh frozen plasma or cryoprecipitate). Thrombocytopenia (platelet count under 100×10^9/litre) or platelet dysfunction (bleeding time over 10 min with platelet count over 100×10^9/litre) should lead to consideration of platelet transfusion. Despite large doses of fresh frozen plasma, cryoprecipitate and platelets, there is a high risk of bleeding and a high mortality in patients undergoing surgery within 12 h of intravenous streptokinase therapy (Lee et al 1988). This may reflect the haemorrhagic effects of thrombolytic therapy on haemostatic plugs, in contrast to its systemic effects.

In this context, Gimple et al (1989) correlated prolongation of the skin bleeding time with clinical bleeding during alteplase therapy of myocardial infarction. The role of platelets in bleeding during and after thrombolytic therapy may have been neglected (Coller 1990). However, in practical terms, aspirin has an additive beneficial effect with streptokinase on mortality in myocardial infarction, with little excess bleeding (ISIS-2 Collaborative Group 1988). Moreover, monitoring of the bleeding time is not practical during routine thrombolytic therapy.

Fibrinogen

Most patients treated with thrombolytic therapy develop a degree of systemic hyperplasminaemia, with digestion of circulating plasma fibrinogen to degradation products (Fig. 7.5). As noted in the previous section, measurement of the plasma fibrinogen level is useful to confirm a lytic state during prolonged thrombolytic therapy and is also of value in patients with major bleeding or in those who require urgent surgery, to assess the need for replacement with fresh frozen plasma or cryoprecipitate. Precautions with sample handling to minimize in vitro degradation of fibrinogen by plasma plasminogen activators have also been noted.

The type of assay used to measure plasma fibrinogen can also markedly affect the results and is one reason for discrepant reports in the literature. Clotting assays, such as the Clauss (1957) method which is most widely used in the UK and the USA, measure clottable fibrinogen and are therefore affected in a downwards direction by high levels of thrombin inhibitors such as FDP and heparin. In contrast, physical or chemical precipitation assays or immunological assays measure non-clottable FDP and hence overestimate fibrinogen levels (Cowley et al 1983, Graor et 1986). The standard Ratnoff–Menzie assay (Ratnoff and Menzie 1951) is probably most accurate, measuring clottable fibrinogen while being minimally affected by FDP, especially if the concentration of plasma relative to saline is increased (Alving and Bell 1976). While useful in research studies, for example evaluation of new thrombolytic agents (Clauss et al 1990), the Ratnoff–Menzie assay is time consuming and therefore not practical in routine monitoring of patients. For the latter purpose, the Clauss (1957) method is recommended because it is rapid, widely available and shows reasonable inter-laboratory agreement. In addition, assay of clottable fibrinogen is probably a more reliable index of haemostatically effective fibrinogen than other rapid assays (i.e. precipitation or immunological assays) which overestimate fibrinogen levels.

Thrombolytic therapy with intravenous streptokinase usually causes early, profound falls in plasma fibrinogen. For example, within 20 min of starting the standard dose of streptokinase in acute myocardial infarction (1.5 million units over 1 h) the mean plasma fibrinogen level (measured by the Clauss assay) falls to about 20% of baseline. Fibrinogen levels slowly return to normal over the subsequent 24–48 h (Collen et al 1986, Mentzer et al 1986). Similar changes are observed following anistreplase, urokinase or saruplase therapy (Marder et al 1987, PRIMI Trial Study Group 1989). Alteplase therapy causes a lesser degree of fibrinogen depletion (Collen et al 1986, Rao et al 1988), the mean plasma level falling to about 40% of baseline with current dosage regimens. However, this lesser degree of fibrinogen depletion may be falsely reassuring in terms of bleeding risk. Marder and Sherry (1988) suggest that following alteplase infusion all of the normal circulating fibrinogen has indeed been degraded, but largely to early degradation products such as fragment X which are still clottable and which therefore account for much of the residual assay of plasma 'fibrinogen'. Although thus counting as 'fibrinogen' in the laboratory, fragment X forms clots of weaker tensile strength than native fibrinogen and also has anticoagulant and antiplatelet effects, all of which may impair haemostasis in vivo (Marder and Sherry 1988).

A fall in plasma fibrinogen may also be beneficial in several respects. Firstly, it causes reductions in plasma viscosity and red cell aggregation and therefore reductions in whole blood viscosity (Fig. 7.5), which may increase blood flow in addition to lysis of thrombi. Secondly, fibrinogen depletion and increased levels of FDP result in systemic antiplatelet and anticoagulant effects which, while potentially impairing haemostasis, also are potentially antithrombotic and may prevent thrombotic extension or rethrombosis (Figs 7.1 and 7.5).

In practice, it has been difficult to show relationships between the degree of fall in plasma fibrinogen and either the success of thrombolytic therapy, or the incidence of bleeding (Marder and Sherry 1988, Lowe and Douglas 1991). In prolonged treatment of venous thromboembolism or peripheral arterial thromboembolism, there has generally been little correlation between fibrinogen depletion and the success of thrombolysis although, as previously noted, thrombolysis appears less common in the 10% of patients who have no evidence of systemic fibrinogen digestion (Marder and Sherry 1988). In acute myocardial infarction, some studies have related the fall in plasma fibrinogen to reperfusion on serial angiography (Burkett et al 1985, Gold et al 1986, Lew et al 1986, Kakkar and Stringer 1987) but others have not (Reduto et al 1981, Rao et al 1988, Douglas et al 1990a). We have recently found that the *baseline* fibrinogen level was higher in patients who did not reperfuse their occluded coronary artery following streptokinase or anistreplase therapy (Douglas et al 1990a); however, this difference was of little clinical value. A recently reported, large, randomized study of alteplase versus streptokinase in acute myocardial infarction found similar mortality in the two groups (International Study Group 1990; Table 7.3). Hence, while alteplase produces a higher incidence of angiographic coronary reperfusion than streptokinase, the greater systemic fibrinogenolytic effect of streptokinase (with its rheological, antiplatelet and anticoagulant consequences) may have a compensatory effect in preventing rethrombosis and increasing myocardial blood flow. Therefore, the overall benefit to the heart and circulation may be similar with the two drugs (Fig. 7.5).

In regard to the relationship between plasma fibrinogen levels and bleeding, there is little evidence for any relationship during treatment with streptokinase or urokinase (Marder and Sherry 1988, Rao et al 1988,

Fennerty et al 1989). Three reports from the TIMI studies of alteplase in acute myocardial infarction have shown some relationship between fibrinogen depletion and bleeding. Fibrinogen levels less than 1.5 g/l (Clauss assay; Clauss 1957) were five times more likely (Rao et al 1988) or 2.6 times more likely (Mueller et al 1987) to occur in patients who bled, compared to those who did not bleed. In the TIMI-II study, Bovill (1990) recently reported that the relative risk of bleeding was 1.8 in patients whose plasma fibrinogen fell below 2 g/l compared to those whose fibrinogen level stayed above this level. However, the 95% confidence intervals were wide (0.7–5.2). In part, this relationship between bleeding and fibrinogen level may simply reflect the dose of alteplase per kilogram of body weight. Reduction in plasma fibrinogen following alteplase therapy is dose dependent. For example, the currently used total dose of 100 mg produces a mean plasma fibrinogen level of about 2 g/l, whereas the previously used dose of 150 mg (now abandoned because of a high risk of intracranial bleeding; Braunwald et al 1987) produces a mean plasma fibrinogen level of about 1 g/l (Bovill 1990). In the TIMI-II studies, low body weight (and hence a higher dose per kilogram of body weight with a standard dose) was associated with increased risk of bleeding (Bovill 1990).

It should be noted that in the large randomized trial of alteplase versus streptokinase in acute myocardial infarction, the risk of bleeding was similar, despite the difference in mean plasma fibrinogen levels between the two drugs (International Study Group 1990; Table 7.3). This may reflect the imperfect, degraded nature of the higher residual plasma 'fibrinogen' level during alteplase therapy (Marder and Sherry 1988), as discussed above, as well as the increasing evidence that dissolution of haemostatic fibrin plugs is the most important cause of bleeding during and after thrombolytic therapy (Marder and Sherry 1988). Such evidence includes the poor relationship of anticoagulant effects of thrombolytic therapy to bleeding, the lesser risk of bleeding with anticoagulant or defibrinogenating drugs than with thrombolytic therapy and the strong relationship of bleeding after thrombolytic therapy to invasive procedures, which should be minimized where possible (de Bono et al 1989, Fennerty et al 1989).

In summary, while measurement of plasma fibrinogen levels is indicated during prolonged thrombolytic therapy, and in those who have major bleeding or require urgent surgery, there is little evidence that its routine measurement during short-term treatment of acute myocardial infarction is worthwhile.

Fibrinogen degradation products

Most patients treated with thrombolytic therapy develop raised levels of degradation products, which originate from both fibrinogen and cross-linked fibrin (Fig. 7.5). As with fibrinogen assays, measurement of FDP can confirm a 'lytic state'; however, there is at present little evidence that their routine measurement is of value in predicting either successful thrombolysis, or risk of bleeding.

Traditionally, *measurements of serum FDP* have been employed, for example by the tanned red cell haemagglutination immunoassay (Merskey et al 1969) (e.g. Wellcome FDP kit; Rao et al 1988). Such tests are more sensitive to low molecular weight, incoagulable FDP which are present in serum. Alteplase treatment, which produces high molecular weight, coagulable FDP (Marder and Sherry 1988), therefore produces smaller elevations than streptokinase treatment (Verstraete et al 1985, Collen et al 1986). More recently, the development of monoclonal antibodies against neoantigens has allowed *measurement in plasma of specific types of FDP*. Examples include D-dimer, a measure of cross-linked fibrin degradation products (XL-FDP) (Lew et al 1986, Eisenberg et al 1987, Douglas et al 1990a) and the combined measurement of total fibrinogen and fibrin degradation products (TDP) along with FDP (Brommer et al 1987) (see also Chapter 6). Studies with the latter tests showed that following streptokinase therapy, the majority of FDP are derived from fibrinogen rather than fibrin; that the disappearance curves were not influenced by persistent fibrinolytic activity of the blood; and that collection of blood in citrate with aprotinin, compared to citrate alone, did not result in lower TDP or FDP levels (Brommer et al 1987).

Because some degradation products of cross-linked fibrin originate from thrombi (Fig. 7.5), there has been recent interest in the possibility that lysis of thrombi in vivo might be assessed by serial measurement of such products in plasma as an alternative to serial angiography. Potential markers of thrombolysis include the Bβ-[15–42] peptide (Kudryk et al 1983, Eisenberg et al 1987, Douglas et al 1990a) and D-dimer (Lew et al 1986, Eisenberg et al 1987, Douglas et al 1990a). Eisenberg et al (1987) observed that patients with acute myocardial infarction treated with alteplase (which produces higher early coronary reperfusion rates than streptokinase) had higher levels of both Bβ-[15–42] and D-dimer than patients treated with streptokinase. However, Douglas et al (1990a) observed no relationship of either Bβ-[15–42] or D-dimer to angiographic reperfusion in patients treated with streptokinase or anistreplase. Previous studies have also failed to correlate XL-FDP levels with coronary reperfusion (Francis et al 1986, Samama et al 1986, Soria et al 1987). Jespersen et al (1990a) calculated that the increase in fibrin degradation products following alteplase treatment in acute myocardial infarction corresponded to lysis of fibrin generated from all the fibrinogen present in 9 ml of normal plasma. Because most occlusive coronary thrombi have volumes much less than 1 ml, it appears that the majority of fibrin degradation products following thrombolytic therapy in acute myocardial infarction originate from sites other than thrombi. Such fibrin may be present in haemostatic plugs, as an endo-endothelial fibrin lining of blood vessels, or be circulating in plasma (Fig. 7.5). It is perhaps therefore not surprising that plasma levels of cross-linked fibrin degradation products do not correlate with thrombolysis in vivo.

As with fibrinogen assays, there is little evidence that FDP levels correlate with bleeding after thrombolytic therapy with streptokinase or urokinase (Marder and Sherry 1988, Rao et al 1988, Fennerty et al 1989). Three reports from the TIMI studies of alteplase in acute myocardial infarction have shown some relationship between serum FDP elevation and bleeding. FDP levels greater than 400 μg/ml were three times more likely (Rao et al 1988) or 4.1 times more likely (Mueller et al 1987) to occur in patients who bled, compared to patients who did not bleed. In the TIMI-II study, Bovill (1990) recently reported that the relative risk of bleeding was 1.7 in patients whose peak FDP level exceeded 300 μg/ml compared to those with lower levels; however, the 95% confidence intervals were wide (0.95–3.1). As with fibrinogen levels, this relationship between bleeding and FDP level may simply reflect the dose of alteplase per kilogram of body weight.

In summary, there is little evidence that routine measurement of FDP during thrombolytic therapy is of clinical utility.

Plasminogen activator and anti-activator levels

During thrombolytic therapy, plasma levels of the infused activator can be measured with global plasminogen activator assays, such as the plasma euglobulin clot lysis time (ECLT) or the area of lysis on a fibrin plate produced by a volume of plasma or the plasma euglobulin fraction (see p. 136). The ECLT is most practical for monitoring during thrombolytic therapy as the result is rapidly available (Lowe and Prentice 1980). In the absence of evidence of systemic fibrinogenolysis during prolonged thrombolytic therapy, the ECLT can be used to determine whether the plasminogen activator infusion has not overcome inhibition by circulating inhibitors, either because there has been some problem with infusion of the drug or because of high levels of inhibitors (Fig. 7.5). In the case of streptokinase or anistreplase, these inhibitors are usually antistreptococcal antibodies, e.g. from recent streptococcal infection or recent treatment with one of these therapeutic agents. A streptokinase resistance test (Amery et al 1963, Hirsh et al 1970, Jalihal and Morris 1990) can be used to quantitate the antibody titre and thus to calculate a dose which will saturate the inhibitors. Alternatively, another thrombolytic agent which is not inhibited by streptococcal antibodies (e.g. urokinase or alteplase) can be substituted.

Specific antigenic assays of newer thrombolytic agents, such as alteplase, are available for use in research or pharmacokinetic studies (Verstraete et al 1986, Booth et al 1990). t-PA is inhibited by plasminogen activator inhibitors (predominantly PAI-1) which form inhibitor complexes (Fig. 7.5), and PAI-1 levels are elevated in patients with acute myocardial infarction or venous thromboembolism (Kruithof 1988). However, the usual therapeutic doses of alteplase (rt-PA) are sufficient to swamp such PAI-1 levels. Also, there is no rapid increase in plasma PAI-1 levels following alteplase treatment in acute myocardial infarction (Booth et al 1990).

Plasminogen and antiplasmins

During thrombolytic therapy, plasma plasminogen is activated to plasmin. Plasma concentrations of the primary antiplasmin, α_2-antiplasmin (~1 μM) are sufficient to complex with and neutralize the plasmin formed from about two-thirds of plasma plasminogen (plasma concentration, ~1.5 μM). Thereafter, further plasmin is neutralized by the 'first reserve', less specific plasma protease inhibitor, α_2-macroglobulin (Fig. 7.5; Collen 1980). Intravenous thrombolytic therapy (and in many cases, local intra-arterial thrombolytic therapy) with streptokinase, anistreplase, urokinase or alteplase is followed by profound falls in plasma plasminogen, α_2-antiplasmin and α_2-macroglobulin (Collen et al 1986, Mentzer et al 1986), e.g. to 20% of baseline levels within 30 min of starting treatment of acute myocardial infarction. Plasma levels slowly rise to normal over the next 24–48 h. While total plasminogen depletion may limit the delivery of fresh plasminogen to the thrombus surface, and hence limit thrombolysis, there is as yet little evidence that monitoring plasma levels of plasminogen, α_2-antiplasmin, α_2-macroglobulin or plasmin–antiplasmin complexes is clinically useful in assessing either thrombolytic efficacy or bleeding risk.

Blood rheology

The plasma fibrinogen level is an important determinant of both plasma viscosity (resistance to flow) and of red cell aggregation, which occurs under low shear conditions (such as occur during low blood flow states, e.g. in arterial and venous thrombosis). Hence the fibrinogen level is an important determinant of whole blood viscosity, and thereby of blood flow, especially in low-flow states (Lowe 1987, 1988, Rampling 1988). Depletion of plasma fibrinogen during thrombolytic therapy therefore reduces plasma viscosity, red cell aggregation (including the erythrocyte sedimentation rate, which therefore cannot be used as an index of disease activity) and whole blood viscosity (Fig. 7.5), especially when the latter is measured at low shear rates (Theiss et al 1980, Arnitz et al 1985, Jan et al 1985, Douglas et al 1988, 1990a,b, Moriarty et al 1988). These rheological changes may be less marked during treatment with alteplase than with streptokinase (Jan et al 1985, Douglas et al 1990a,b) because of the lesser degree of plasma 'fibrinogen' depletion and the high circulating levels of high molecular weight FDP, which may complex with fibrinogen forming high molecular weight complexes (Rampling 1988). As previously discussed, such rheological differences may partly explain why streptokinase shows similar clinical benefits to alteplase in treatment of acute myocardial infarction, although it produces a lower early coronary reperfusion rate (International Study Group 1990). We have not found any correlation between reduction in plasma viscosity and coronary reperfusion during thrombolytic treatment of myocardial infarction with streptokinase or anistreplase (Douglas et al 1990a), and at present there is little evidence that monitoring of blood rheology during thrombolytic therapy is of clinical value.

Other effects of thrombolytic therapy

The effects of thrombolytic therapy on blood platelets are complex (Coller 1990). On the one hand, fibrinogen depletion and FDP formation inhibit platelet aggregation (Fig. 7.5) and prolong the skin bleeding time; these effects may contribute to both bleeding at sites of trauma (Gimple et al 1989) and to prevention of rethrombosis. On the other hand, there is evidence for marked *in vivo activation* of platelets following streptokinase treatment in acute myocardial infarction, which may be relevant to rethrombosis and dysrhythmias (Fitzgerald et al 1988). The additive effects of aspirin and streptokinase in reducing mortality after myocardial infarction (ISIS-2 Collaborative Study 1988) may partly reflect reduction by aspirin of platelet activation by streptokinase.

Recent studies have also suggested that the effects of thrombolytic therapy on the coagulation system are also more complex than the anticoagulant effects of coagulation factor depletion and FDP formation. Plasma levels of fibrinopeptide A (Rapold et al 1989) and thrombin–antithrombin complexes (Gulba et al 1988, Jespersen et al 1990b) are elevated after thrombolytic therapy and correlate with coronary artery reocclusion following successful thrombolytic treatment of acute myocardial infarction. Such increased thrombin formation may result from activation of platelets or from endothelial effects, with exposure of subendothelium and tissue thromboplastin and activation of factor VII (Jespersen et al 1990a).

Finally, it should be noted that thrombolytic therapy with streptokinase activates leucocytes, kinins and the complement system (Fig. 7.5): the latter effects may be responsible for the hypotension which commonly follows treatment.

LABORATORY METHODS

Standard assays of coagulation (APTT, prothrombin time, thrombin time, fibrinogen) and fibrinolysis (ECLT, plasminogen, antiplasmin, FDP) are sufficient for monitoring of thrombolytic therapy. Suitable methods are described elsewhere in this volume and also in previous editions (Thomson 1980, 1985).

Streptokinase resistance test and calculation of titrated initial dose of streptokinase (Amery et al 1963, Collen 1980)

Principle

The minimal amount of streptokinase required to induce lysis of a blood clot in 20 min is proportional to the amount of streptokinase antibodies present in the blood.

Reagents

1. *Streptokinase.* This should be preferably from the same batch as will be used for thrombolytic therapy.
2. *10 ml of anticoagulated blood from the patient.* For example, 9 ml of blood collected into 1 ml of 3.2% (0.109 M) trisodium citrate.
3. *Thrombin solution.* 100 NIH units/ml in saline, diluted with an equal volume of 0.05 M calcium chloride.
4. *Isotonic saline.*

Method

1. To a series of test-tubes add 0.2 ml of saline. Add 0.2 ml of streptokinase solution (concentration 20 000 U/ml) to the first tube and make doubling dilutions by transferring 0.2 ml to the next tube. The concentrations of streptokinase in the tubes are 10 000, 5 000, 2 500, 1 250, 625, 312, 156, 78 and 39.
2. Transfer 0.1 ml from each tube to another series of test-tubes and add 0.7 ml of blood and 0.2 ml of thrombin–calcium chloride mixture. Start a stopwatch, mix by inversion and incubate at 37°C.
3. Tilt the tubes gently and examine for lysis at 1 min intervals during the first 30 min and at 15 min intervals during the following 90 min.

Calculation of the titrated initial dose

The lysis time in minutes is plotted versus the logarithm of the streptokinase concentration in the tubes. A concave curve will be obtained with a minimum lysis time of 3–6 min. At lower streptokinase concentrations the lysis time is longer due to neutralization by antibodies. At higher streptokinase concentrations the lysis time prolongs due to consumption of plasminogen by formation of plasmin(ogen)–streptokinase complexes.

The minimal amount of streptokinase which will induce lysis in 20 min is read from the curve and the titrated initial dose calculated by multiplying this amount with 110 times the patient's body weight in kilograms (0.63 ml of undiluted blood used in the test; approximately 70 ml blood per kilogram of body weight). The titrated initial dose is less than 352 000 units in over 95% of patients, but may vary from 25 000 to 3 000 000 units.

REFERENCES

AIMS Trial Study Group 1990 Long-term effects of intravenous anistreplase in acute myocardial infarction: final report of the AIMS Study. Lancet 335: 427–431

Alving B M, Bell W R 1976 Methods for correcting inhibitory effects of fibrinogen degradation products in fibrinogen determinations. Thrombosis Research 9: 1–8

Amery A. Maes H, Vermylen J et al 1963 The streptokinase reactivity test. I. Standardization. Thromb Diath Haemorrh 9: 175–188

Anonymous 1988 Management of venous thromboembolism. Lancet i:

Anonymous 1990 Non-coronary thrombolysis. Lancet 335: 691–693

Antiplatelet Trialists' Meeting, Oxford 1990 Personal communication

Arnitz R, Haltz J, Schafer H et al 1985 Hemorheology in acute myocardial infarction: effects of high dose intravenous streptokinase. Circulation III: 417

Astrup T 1958 The haemostatic balance. Thromb Diath Haemorrh 2: 347

Booth N A, Moore N R, Gemmill J D et al 1990 Plasma t-PA after bolus injection in myocardial infarction: complex formation with PAI-1 and other inhibitors. Fibrinolysis 4(suppl 3): 68

Bovill E G 1990 Laboratory monitoring of thrombolytic therapy: experience from the TIMI trials. Fibrinolysis 4(suppl 3): 111

Braunwald E, Knatterud G L, Passamani E et al 1987 Update from the Thrombolysis in Myocardial Infarction Trial. Journal of the American College of Cardiologists 10: 970

Brommer E J P, Engbers J, van der Laarase A et al 1987 Survival of fibrinogen degradation products in the circulation after thrombolytic therapy for acute myocardial infarction. Fibrinolysis 1: 149–153

Burket M W, Smith M R, Walsh T E et al 1985 Relation of the effectiveness of intracoronary thrombolysis in acute myocardial infarction to systemic lytic state. American Journal of Cardiology 56: 441–444

Cairns J A, Collins R, Fuster V et al 1989 Coronary thrombolysis. Chest 95(suppl): 73S–87S

Cheseboro J H, Knatterud G, Roberts R et al 1987 Thrombolysis in myocardial infarction (TIMI) trial, phase I: a comparison between intravenous tissue plasminogen activator and intravenous streptokinase. Circulation 76: 142–154

Chesterman C 1987 Thrombolytic therapy. In: Bloom A L, Thomas D P (eds) Haemostasis and thrombosis, 2nd edn. Churchill Livingstone, Edinburgh, p 829–848

Claus G, Gulba D C, Barthels M et al 1990 Monitoring of fibrinogen levels during thrombolytic therapy — which assay should be selected. Fibrinolysis 4(suppl 3): 31

Clauss A 1957 Gerinnungsphysiologische Schnellmethode zur Bestimmung des Fibrinogens. Acta Haematologica 17: 237–246

Collen D 1980 Inhibitors of fibrinolysis. In: Thomson J M (ed) Blood coagulation and haemostasis. A practical guide, 2nd edn. Churchill Livingstone, Edinburgh, p 261–278

Collen D, Bounameaux H, De Cock F et al 1986 Analysis of coagulation and fibrinolysis during intravenous administration of recombinant human tissue-type plasminogen activator (rt-PA) in patients with acute myocardial infarction. Circulation 73: 511–517

Coller B S 1990 Platelets and thrombolytic therapy. New England Journal of Medicine 322: 33–42

Collins R, Scrimgeour A, Yusuf S et al 1988 Reduction in fatal pulmonary embolism and venous thrombosis by perioperative administration of subcutaneous heparin. New England Journal of Medicine 318: 1162–1173

Cowley M J, Hastillo A, Vetrovec G W et al 1983 Fibrinolytic effects of intracoronary streptokinase administration in patients with acute myocardial infarction and coronary insufficiency. Circulating 67: 1031–1038

Davies M J, Fulton W F M, Robertson W B 1979 The relation of coronary thrombus to ischaemic myocardial necrosis. Journal of Pathology 127: 99–110 de Bono D 1989 Problems in thrombolysis. In: Julian D, Kübler W, Norris R M, Swan H J C, Collen D, Verstraete M (eds) Thrombolysis in cardiovascular disease. Marcel Dekker, Basel p 279–292

De Wood M A, Spores J, Notske R et al 1980 Prevalence of total coronary occlusion during the early hours of transmural myocardial infarction. New England Journal of Medicine 303: 897–902

Douglas J T, Hillis W S, Dunn F G et al 1988 Coagulation, fibrinolysis and viscosity during thrombolytic therapy of acute myocardial infarction with recombinant tissue plasminogen activator (rt-PA), APSAC and streptokinase. Fibrinolysis 2(suppl 1): 85

Douglas J T, Hogg K J, Gemmill J D et al 1990a Relationship of coronary artery patency to plasma fibrinogen, viscosity and plasmin activity following thrombolytic therapy with streptokinase or anistreplase in acute myocardial infarction. Fibrinolysis 4(suppl 3): 134

Douglas J T, Gemmill J D, Hogg K J et al 1990b Haemostatic and haemorheological changes and coronary reperfusion following bolus injection of rt-PA in acute myocardial infarction. Fibrinolysis 4(suppl 3): 68

Eisenberg P R, Sherman L A, Tiefenbrunn A J et al 1987 Sustained fibrinolysis after administration of t-PA despite its short half-life in the circulation. Thrombosis and Haemostasis 57: 35–40

Fennerty A G, Levine M N, Hirsh J 1989 Hemorrhagic complications of thrombolytic therapy in the treatment of myocardial infarction and venous thromboembolism. Chest 95(suppl): 88S–97S

Fitzgerald D J, Catella F, Roy L et al 1988 Marked platelet activation in vivo after intravenous streptokinase in patients with acute myocardial infarction. Circulation 77: 142–150

Fletcher A P, Sherry S, Alkjaersig N et al 1959 Maintenance of a sustained thrombolytic state in man. II. Clinical observations on patients with myocardial infarction and other thromboembolic disorders. Journal of Clinical Investigation 38: 1111–1119

Francis C W, Connaghan D G, Marder V J 1986 Assessment of fibrin degradation products during fibrinolytic therapy for acute myocardial infarction. Circulation 74: 1027–1036

Gimple L W, Gold H K, Leinbach R C et al 1989 Correlation between template bleeding times and spontaneous bleeding during treatment of acute myocardial infarction with recombinant tissue-type plasminogen activator. Circulation 80: 581–588

GISSI (Gruppo Italiano per Lo Studio della Streptochinasi nell' Infarto Miocardio) 1986 Effectiveness of intravenous thrombolytic treatment in acute myocardial infarction. Lancet i: 397–402

Gold H K 1989 Thrombolysis in patients with unstable angina pectoris. In: Julian D, Kübler W, Norris R M, Swan H J C, Collen D, Verstraete M (eds) Thrombolysis in cardiovascular disease. Marcel Dekker, Basel p 325–335

Gold H K, Leinbach R C, Garabedian H O et al 1986 Acute coronary reocclusion after thrombolysis with recombinant human tissue-type plasminogen activator: prevention by a maintenance infusion. Circulation 73: 347–352

Goldhaber S Z, Buring J E, Lipnick R J et al 1984 Pooled analyses of randomized trials of streptokinase and heparin in phlebographically documented acute deep venous thrombosis. American Journal of Medicine 76: 393–397

Graor R A, Olin J W 1989 Regional thrombolysis in peripheral arterial occlusions. In: Julian D, Kübler W, Norris R M, Swan H J C, Collen D, Verstraete M (eds) Thrombolysis in cardiovascular disease. Marcel Dekker, Basel p 381–395

Graor R A, Risius B, Lucas F V et al 1986 Thrombolysis with recombinant human tissue-type plasminogen activator in patients with peripheral artery and bypass graft occlusions. Circulation 74(suppl 1): I-15–I-20

Gulba D C, Barthels M, Reil G H et al 1988 Thrombin–antithrombin III complex level as early predictor of reocclusion after successful thrombolysis. Lancet ii: 97

Hennekens C H, Buring J E, Sandercock P, Collins R, Peto R 1989 Aspirin and other antiplatelet agents in the secondary and primary prevention of cardiovascular disease. Circulation 80: 749–756

Hirsh J, O' Sullivan E F, Martin M 1970 Evaluation of a standard dosage schedule with streptokinase. Blood 35: 341–349

Hoffmann J J M L, Bonnier J J R M, De Swart J B R M 1987 Systemic effects of thrombolytic drugs in acute myocardial infarction: comparison of intravenous APSAC (BRL 26921) and intracoronary streptokinase. Fibrinolysis 1: 225–230

Hyers T M, Hull R D, Weg J G 1989 Antithrombotic therapy for venous thromboembolic disease. Chest 95(suppl): 37S–51S
ISAM Study Group 1986 A prospective trial of intravenous streptokinase in acute myocardial infarction (ISAM). New England Journal of Medicine 314: 1465–1471
International Study Group 1990 In-hospital mortality and clinical course of 20 981 patients with suspected acute myocardial infarction randomised between alteplase and streptokinase with or without heparin. Lancet 336: 71–75
ISIS-2 (Second International Study of Infarct Survival) Collaborative Group 1988 Randomised trial of intravenous streptokinase, oral aspirin, both, or neither among 17 187 cases of suspected acute myocardial infarction: ISIS-2. Lancet ii: 349–360
Jalihal S, Morris G K 1990 Antistreptokinase titres after intravenous streptokinase. Lancet 335: 184–185
Jan K M, Reinhart W, Chien S et al 1985 Altered rheological properties of blood following administrations of tissue plasminogen activator and streptokinase in patients with acute myocardial infarction. Circulation III: 417
Jespersen J, Munkvad S, Gram J 1990a Thrombolytic therapy with t-PA induces systemic degradation of fibrin and activation of prothrombin. Fibrinolysis 4(suppl 3): 95
Jespersen J, Munkvad S, Gram J 1990b Induction of coagulant activity and increase of t-PA and PAI-1 in plasma after thrombolysis of patients with myocardial infarction. Fibrinolysis 4(suppl 3): 95
Kakkar V V, Stringer M D 1987 Are the 'clot-selective' agents truly clot-selective? In: Kakkar V V, Kennedy J W, Mettinger K L (eds) Coronary thrombolysis: current answers to critical questions. Current Medical Literature, London, p 23–35
Kruithof E K O 1988 Plasminogen activator inhibitor type 1: biochemical, biological and clinical aspects. Fibrinolysis 2(suppl 2): 59–70
Kudryk B, Rohoza A, Ahadi M et al 1983 Specificity of a monoclonal antibody for the NH_2-terminal region of fibrin. Molecular Immunology 20: 1191–1200
Kwaan H C, Samama M M (eds) 1989 Clinical Thrombosis. C R C Press, Boca Raton
Lee K F, Mandell J, Rankin J S et al 1988 Immediate versus delayed coronary grafting after streptokinase treatment: postoperative blood loss and clinical results. Journal of Thoracic and Cardiovascular Surgery 95: 216–222
Lew A S, Cerecek B, Laramee P et al 1986 The time interval from initiation of IV streptokinase is directly related to the residual fibrinogen level and is shortened by pretreatment with heparin. Journal of the American College of Cardiologists 7: 17
Loscalzo J, The Pro-urokinase for Myocardial Infarction Study Group 1989 Clot-selective coronary thrombolysis with pro-urokinase. Circulation 79: 776–782
Lowe G D O (ed) 1987 Blood rheology and hyperviscosity syndromes. Baillière's Clinical Haematology 1: 597–867
Lowe G D O (ed) 1988 Clinical blood rheology. CRC Press, Boca Raton
Lowe G D O 1990 Drugs in cerebral and peripheral arterial disease. British Medical Journal 300: 524–528
Lowe G D O 1991 Clinical and laboratory aspects of thrombolytic therapy. In: Poller L (ed) Recent advances in blood coagulation, vol 5. Churchill Livingstone, Edinburgh 265–291
Lowe G D O, Douglas J T 1991 Haematological aspects of thrombosis and thrombolysis. In: Hillis W S, Dunn F (eds) Thrombolytic therapy in acute myocardial infarction. M T P Press, Lancaster (in press)
Lowe G D O, Prentice C R M 1980 The laboratory investigation of fibrinolysis. In: Thomson J M (ed) Blood coagulation and haemostasis. A practical guide, 2nd edn. Churchill Livingstone, Edinburgh p 222–260
Lowe G D O, Small M 1988 Stimulation of endogenous fibrinolysis. In: Kluft C (ed) Tissue-type plasminogen activator (t-PA): physiological and clinical importance, vol II. C R C Press, Boca Raton p 129–169
Lowe G D O, Wood D A, Douglas J T et al 1991 Relationships of plasma viscosity, coagulation and fibrinolysis to coronary risk factors and angina. Thrombosis and Haemostasis (in press)
McNicol G P, Reid W, Bain W H et al 1963 Treatment of peripheral arterial occlusion by streptokinase perfusion. British Medical Journal i: 1508–1509
Marder V J, Sherry S 1988 Thrombolytic therapy: current status. New England Journal of Medicine 318: 1512–1520, 1585–1595

Marder V J, Kinsella P A, Brown M J 1987 Fibrinogen concentration and coronary artery reperfusion after intravenous anisoylated plasminogen streptokinase activator complex or intracoronary streptokinase therapy. Drugs 33(suppl 3): 237–241
Meade T W (ed) 1984 Anticoagulants in myocardial infarction. A reappraisal. Wiley, Chichester
Mentzer R L, Budzynski A Z, Sherry S 1986 High-dose, brief-duration intravenous infusion of streptokinase in acute myocardial infarction: description of effects in the circulation. American Journal of Cardiology 57: 1220–1226
Merskey C, Lalezari P, Johnson A J 1969 A rapid, simple sensitive method for measuring fibrinolytic split products in human serum. Proceedings of the Society for Experimental Biology and Medicine 131: 871–875
Moriarty A J, Highes R, Nelson S D et al 1988 Streptokinase and reduced plasma viscosity: a second benefit. European Journal of Haematology 41: 25–36
Mueller H S, Rao A K, Forman S A et al 1987 Thrombolysis in myocardial infarction (TIMI): comparative studies of coronary reperfusion and systemic fibrinogenolysis with two forms of recombinant tissue type plasminogen activator. Journal of the American College of Cardiologists 10: 479–490
Neri Serneri G G, Gensini G F, Poggesi L et al 1990 Effect of heparin, aspirin, or alteplase in reduction of myocardial ischaemia in refractory unstable angina. Lancet 335: 615–618
Poller L 1987 Oral anticoagulant therapy. In: Bloom A L, Thomas D P (eds) Haemostasis and thrombosis, 2nd edn. Churchill Livingstone, Edinburgh p 870–885
PRIMI Trial Study Group 1989 Randomised double-blind trial of recombinant pro-urokinase against streptokinase in acute myocardial infarction. Lancet i: 863–868
Rampling M 1988 Red cell aggregation and yield stress. In: Lowe G D O (ed) Clinical blood rheology, vol I. C R C Press, Boca Raton p 45–65
Rao A K, Pratt C, Berke A et al 1988 Thrombolysis in myocardial infarction (TIMI) trial, phase 1: hemorrhagic manifestations and changes in plasma fibrinogen and the fibrinolytic system in patients treated with recombinant tissue plasminogen activator and streptokinase. Journal of the American College of Cardiologists 11: 1–11
Rapold H J, Kuemmerli H, Weiss M et al 1989 Monitoring of fibrin generation during thrombolytic therapy of acute myocardial infarction with recombinant tissue-type plasminogen activator. Circulation 79: 980–989
Raskob G E, Hull R D 1989 Venous thrombosis. In: Kwaan H C, Samama M M (eds) Clinical thrombosis. C R C Press, Boca Raton p 59–90
Ratnoff O D, Menzie C 1951 A new method for the determination of fibrinogen in small samples of plasma. Journal of Laboratory and Clinical Medicine 37: 316–320
Reduto L A, Freund G C, Gaeta J M et al 1981 Coronary artery reperfusion in acute myocardial infarction: beneficial effects of intracoronary streptokinase on left ventricular salvage and performance. American Heart Journal 102: 1168–1175
Rentrop P, Blanke H, Karsch K R et al 1981 Selective intracoronary thrombolysis in acute myocardial infarction and unstable angina. Circulation 63: 307–317
Samama M, Verdy E, Conard J et al 1986 Activateur tissulaire du plasminogene (tPA) dans l 'infarctus du myocardial infarction. Archieves des Maladies du Coeur et des Vaisseaux 11: 618–624
Schroeder R, Biamino G, Leitner E R et al 1983 Intravenous short-term infusion of streptokinase in acute myocardial infarction. Circulation 67: 536–548
Siegfried E, Tanswell P 1987 Comparison of specific antibody, D-Phe-Pro-Arg-Ch_2Cl and aprotinin for prevention of in vitro effects of recombinant tissue-type plasminogen activator on haemostasis parameters. Thrombosis and Haemostasis 58: 921–926
Sloan M A, del Zoppo G J, Brott T G 1989 Thrombolysis and stroke. In: Julian D, Kübler W, Norris R M, Swan H J C, Collen D, Verstraete M (eds) Thrombolysis in cardiovascular disease. Marcel Dekker, Basel p 361–380
Small M, Kluft C, MacCuish A, Lowe G D O 1989 Tissue plasminogen activator inhibition in diabetes mellitus. Diabetes Care 12: 655–658
Soria J, Soria C, Mirshahi M et al 1987 Specific determination and identification of cross-linked fibrinogen degradation products in patients under thrombolytic therapy for myocardial infarction. Seminars in Thrombosis and Haemostasis 13: 223–228
Theiss W, Volger E, Wirtzfeld A et al 1980 Coagulation studies and rheological measurements during streptokinase treatment of myocardial infarction. Klinische Wochenschrift 58: 607–611

Theroux P, Ouimet H, McCans J et al 1988 Aspirin, heparin or both to treat acute unstable angina? New England Journal of Medicine 319: 1105–1111
Tiefenbrunn A J, Graor R A, Robison A K et al 1986 Pharmacodynamics of tissue-type plasminogen activator characterized by computer-assisted simulation. Circulation 73: 1291–1299
Thomson J M (ed) 1980 Blood coagulation and haemostasis. A practical guide, 2nd edn. Churchill Livingstone, Edinburgh
Thomson J M (ed) 1985 Blood coagulation and haemostasis. A practical guide, 3rd edn. Churchill Livingstone, Edinburgh
Urokinase Pulmonary Embolism Trial 1973 A national cooperative study. Circulation 47(suppl 2): 1–108
Verstraete M, Bernard R, Bory M et al 1985 Randomised trial of intravenous recombinant tissue-type plasminogen activator versus intravenous streptokinase in acute myocardial infarction. Lancet i: 842–847
Verstraete M, Su C A P F, Tanswell P et al 1986 Pharmacokinetics and effects on fibrinolytic and coagulation parameters of two doses of recombinant tissue-type plasminogen activator in healthy volunteers. Thrombosis and Haemostasis 56: 1–5
Wilcox R G, Olsson C G, Skene A M et al 1988 Trial of tissue plasminogen activator for mortality reduction in acute myocardial infarction (ASSET). Lancet ii: 525–530

8. An approach to the infant with impaired haemostasis

Maureen Andrew   Marilyn Johnston

Introduction

Newborn infants with haemorrhagic or thrombotic complications present challenges to both clinical and laboratory physicians for several reasons. (1) The dynamic physiological state of the haemostatic system in newborns necessitates multiple reference ranges of normal values that are dependent on gestational and postnatal age. (2) The infants' small size presents a technical challenge to laboratory physicians since large volumes of blood cannot be obtained for testing and microtechniques must be used. (3) Although the haemostatic system must be considered physiological in healthy infants, it is immature with little reserve capacity to respond to pathological insults related to the birth process or the immediate postnatal period. (4) Acquired haemostatic problems occur in great excess over congenital problems. However the latter need to be considered because they frequently first present in otherwise healthy infants who are bleeding in the first week of life. The differentiation of inherited deficiencies from physiological values can be difficult. (5) Certain diseases are only encountered in newborns and failure to consider these diseases may delay institution of effective therapy. The clinical presentation of some haemostatic disorders may have features unique to newborns. The following discussion provides a practical clinical and laboratory approach for the investigation, diagnosis and management of congenital and acquired haemostatic abnormalities in newborn infants. The laboratory assays described are those used by the authors.

PLATELET VESSEL WALL INTERACTION

1. Physiological process

(i) General

Under physiological conditions the vessel wall provides an important antithrombotic surface. There are hints in the literature that vessel wall function differs in newborns compared to children or adults and that the vessel wall undergoes an ageing process beginning in the fetus (Aballi & de Lamerens 1962, Stuart & Breeze 1973, Jacqz & Barrows 1985). However, due to the difficulty of investigating the physiology of the vessel wall in newborns, many aspects of vessel wall structure and function have not been studied. In contrast to the vessel wall, the number and functions of newborn plateletes have been extensively studied (Mull & Hathaway 1970, Whaun 1973, Stuart 1979, Stuart & Allen 1982, Gill 1983, Andrew & Kelton 1984, Andrews et al 1985, Barradas & Mikhailidis 1986). Healthy infants have platelet counts in the range of normal adult values, although the average values may be slightly lower than for adults (normal range: 150–450 × 10^9/litre) (Gill 1983, Andrew & Kelton 1984). Platelet counts within the adult range are achieved early in fetal life and remain constant after approximately 18 weeks' gestation (Daffos et al 1985). Similarly, the mean platelet volume of newborn platelets is similar to adults with values between 7–9 fl (Kipper & Sieger 1982, Arad et al 1986, Castle et al 1986).

There are many similarities and some well-characterized differences in platelet function between newborns and adults. Platelet adherence has not been assessed in newborns using sensitive assays; however, there is no evidence that a clinically significant defect is present. Von Willebrand factor (vWF) is the plasma component which acts as a bridge between the subendothelial surface and glycoprotein Ib on platelet surfaces (Nachman et al 1971, Jenkins et al 1976, Okomura & Jamieson 1976). Levels of vWF are increased in newborns over adults and an enhanced reactivity is present due to increased concentrations of the functionally high molecular weight forms of vWF (Katz et al 1989, Weinstein et al 1989). Glycoprotein Ib is present on newborn platelets early in fetal life in amounts similar to adults (Gruel et al 1986). Following stimulation by a variety of platelet agonists, newborn platelets undergo normal shape change.

For platelet aggregation to occur, plasma fibrinogen binds to glycoprotein IIb/IIIa receptors on platelets and serve as a bridge between platelets (Gogstad et al 1982). Glycoproteins IIb/IIIa are present on newborn platelets early in gestation (Gruel et al 1986), and fibrinogen is present in adult amounts from early fetal life (Aballi & de Lamerens 1962). The process of platelet aggregation, as assessed in vitro following stimulation with platelet agonists, is consistently altered in newborns compared to adults for the agonists adrenalin and ristocetin (Mull & Hathaway 1970, Whaun 1973, Ts'ao et al 1976, Alebouyeh et al 1978, Stuart 1979, Corby & Barr 1981, Stuart & Allen 1982, Ahlsten et al 1983, Stuart et al 1984, Andrew et al 1985, Jones et al 1985, Barradas et al 1986, Gader et al 1988, Corrigan et al 1989). The decreased response to adrenalin is likely due to a decrease in functional adrenalin receptors on newborn platelets (Alexander et al 1978, Grant & Scrutton 1980, Corby & Barr 1981, Corby & O'Barr 1981, Daiguji et al 1981, Jones et al 1985). The enhanced response to ristocetin reflects elevated concentrations of vWF as well as increases in reactive high molecular weight forms of vWF (Ts'ao et al 1976, Katz et al 1989, Weinstein et al 1989). The response of newborn platelets to other agonists such as ADP, collagen, thrombin and arachidonic acid is variable and may be moderately decreased or in some studies similar to adult platelets (Mull & Hathaway 1970, Whaun 1973, 1980, Corby & Zuck 1976, Ts'ao et al 1976, Stuart 1977, 1978, 1979, Alebouyeh et al 1978, Koztalanyi et al 1980, Corby & Barr 1981, Stuart & Allen 1982, Stuart et al 1984, Andrews et al 1985, Jones et al 1985, Ahlsten et al 1985, Stuart & Dusse 1985, Barradas & Mikhailidis 1986, Gader et al 1988, Walenga et al 1988). The contractile activity of newborn platelets is normal (Israels et al 1987).

There are several plausible explanations for variable aggregation results in newborns. These include the study of platelets from cord blood rather than newborns, the speed with which samples are processed, the influence of labour and differences in concentrations and composition of platelet agonists used (Ts'ao et al 1976, Suarez et al 1984, 1988, Landolfi et al 1988). From studies published to date, it is clear that neither a significant storage pool defect nor an aspirin like platelet defect is present in newborn platelets (Weiss et al 1968, Corby & Zuck 1976, Stuart 1977, Corby & Barr 1981, Corby & O'Barr 1981, Stuart & Allen 1982, Ahlsten et al 1985, Andrews et al 1985, Jones et al 1985, Stuart & Dusse 1985, Walenga et al 1988). The explanation for differences in aggregation between newborn and adult platelets is still not apparent. More importantly, the physiological significance, if any, has not been elucidated. Probably the most important in vivo test of platelet interaction with the vessel wall is the bleeding time, which is consistently normal or short in newborns compared to adults (Harker & Slichter 1972, Feusner 1980, Andrew et al 1987b, 1989b, 1990b).

2. Thrombocytopenia

(i) Clinical

The most common haemostatic abnormality encountered in a neonatal intensive care unit is thrombocytopenia (Pearson & McIntosh 1978, Mehta et al 1980, Feusner et al 1983, Gill 1983, Andrew & Kelton 1984, Castle et al 1987). The definition of thrombocytopenia is a platelet count less than 150×10^9 litre (Pearson & McIntosh 1978, Mehta et al 1980, Feusner et al 1983, Gill 1983, Andrew & Kelton 1984, Castle et al 1987). Approximately one-quarter of infants admitted to a tertiary-care intensive care unit will develop thrombocytopenia, and for over half of these infants the platelet count will reach a nadir below 100×10^9/litre (Castle et al 1986, Andrew et al 1987b). Approximately 20% of thrombocytopenic infants will have a platelet count less than 50×10^9/litre at some time during their hospital stay. The natural history of thrombocytopenia in sick infants is very consistent. Thrombocytopenia is present by day 2 of life, reaches a nadir by day 4 of life and recovers to normal values by day 10 of life for the vast majority of infants (Castle et al 1986, Andrew et al 1987b).

Thrombocytopenia is secondary to either decreased platelet production, increased platelet destruction, pooling in an enlarged spleen, or any combination of these. Characterization of the mechanism responsible for the thrombocytopenia has practical implications in the management of these infants. Thrombocytopenia secondary to increased platelet destruction is characterized by increased platelet size, decreased platelet survival and normal or increased numbers of megakaryocytes in the bone marrow. Other cell lines are usually unaffected. In contrast, thrombocytopenia secondary to decreased platelet production is characterized by platelets of normal size and normal platelet survivals. Numbers of megakaryocytes are decreased in the bone marrow and other cell lines are frequently affected.

For the vast majority of thrombocytopenic infants in tertiary-care units, the platelet survival is short, the mean platelet volume is high and megakaryocytes are present in the bone marrow (Castle et al 1986, 1987, Andrew et al 1987b). These findings are indicative of a destructive process. The aetiology of the increased platelet consumption can be categorized as immune mediated or non-immune mediated. The immune thrombocytopenias are characterized by elevated platelet-associated IgG (PAIgG) thought to be of maternal origin. For most infants, the elevated PAIgG does not signify the presence of maternal autoimmune disorders such as idiopathic thrombocytopenic purpura (ITP) nor alloimmune thrombocytopenia (Castle et al 1986). Rather, the PAIgG is associated with a variety of underlying pathological disorders in the perinatal period such as sepsis and pre-eclampsia (Tate et al 1981, Castle et al 1986, Samuels et al 1987). The most frequent causes of non-immune thrombocytopenia are disseminated intravascular coagulation (DIC) and exchange transfusions (Podolsak 1973, Castle et al 1986). Exchange transfusions cause thromboctyopenia by a dilutional effect which is dependent upon the volumes exchanged (Podolsak 1973, Castle et al 1986). Many disease states are associated with increased platelet destruction and are listed in Table 8.1 (Pearson & McIntosh 1978, Mehta et al 1980, Feusner et al 1983, Gill 1983, Andrew & Kelton 1984, Ballin et al 1987).

Thrombocytopenia secondary to decreased platelet production is very rare, accounting for less than 5% of thrombocytopenic infants. This is a group comprised of bone marrow replacement disorders as well as disorders of bone marrow aplasia (Table 8.1). (Pearson & McIntosh 1978, Mehta et al 1980, Andrew & Kelton 1984). The most common bone marrow disorders are the thrombocytopenia absent radii (TAR) syndrome and isolated amegakaryocytic thrombocytopenia (Hall et al 1969, Homans et al 1988, Hedberg & Lipton 1988, Lecompte 1988).

Finally, for some infants hypersplenism contributes to the presence and persistence of thrombocytopenia. The hypersplenism is itself a secondary problem related to other diseases processes which cause thrombocytopenia. Numerous case reports and case series draw our attention to the pathological states associated with neonatal thrombocytopenia (Andrew & Kelton 1984) (Table 8.1).

Table 8.1 Mechanisms of neonatal thrombocytopenia: associated pathological states

1. Increased clearance
a. Associated with thrombin generation
asphyxia
perinatal aspiration
necrotizing enterocolitis
haemangiomas
neonatal thrombosis
respiratory distress syndrome
b. Associated with increased platelet associated IgG
maternal autoimmune disorders (i.e. ITP, SLE)
maternal drugs
maternal pre-eclampsia
maternal alloantibody
c. Unknown
hyperbilirubinaemia
phototherapy
polycythaemia
Rh haemolytic anaemia
Congenital TTP
total parenteral nutrition
inborn errors of metabolism
Wiskott–Aldrich syndrome
multiple congenital anomalies
2. Decreased production
a. Bone marrow hypo/aplasia
thrombocytopenia absent radii
amegakaryocytic thrombocytopenia
Fanconi's anaemia
other rare hypo/aplastic disorders
b. Bone marrow replacement disorders
congenital leukaemia
congenital leukaemoid reactions
neuroblastoma
histiocytosis
osteopetrosis
3. Hypersplenism

ITP, idiopathic thrombocytopenic purpura; SLE, systemic lupus erythematosus; TTP, thrombotic thrombocytopenic purpura.

(ii) Clinical management

The need to intervene therapeutically when thrombocytopenia is present is dependent upon the underlying diagnosis, the degree of thrombocytopenia, the mechanism responsible for the thrombocytopenia and the presence of concurrent platelet dysfunction. Most importantly, the evidence for clinical bleeding or an anticipated haemostatic challenge will influence the decision to treat. Bleeding at any given platelet count is more likely to occur in patients who have an added deficit in platelet function (i.e. indomethacin, renal failure) and if the thrombocytopenia is secondary to decreased production of platelets.

Platelet counts less than approximately 30–50 × 10^9/litre clearly place otherwise healthy infants at some risk of serious bleeding including intracranial haemorrhage (ICH). The data to support this statement comes both from the risk of ICH in infants with the TAR syndrome (Hall et al 1969, Hedberg & Lipton 1988) as well as the risk of ICH in infants with an immune-mediated thrombocytopenia secondary to a maternal autoantibody or alloantibody (Hedge 1985). Choosing a platelet number at which to intervene is somewhat arbitrary and will vary depending upon the clinical situation. However, a value of 50 × 10^9/litre leaves some reserve capacity for most infants thereby allowing time for the appropriate institution of therapy. Platelet counts greater than 50 × 10^9/litre in an otherwise well, full-term infant do not appear to place the infant at risk for spontaneous serious bleeding. The importance of platelet counts between 50–100 × 10^9/litre in sick premature infants is still unclear (Andrew et al 1987, Lupton et al 1988).

If an infant is bleeding or the platelet count is less than 50 × 10^9/litre, a trial of platelet concentrates is indicated using 10–15 ml/kg. The platelet count usually increases to a safer level although not to the number or for the duration expected if there was no destructive process present (Andrew et al 1987). Because the natural history is short, platelet transfusions are helpful over the period during which most infants are thrombocytopenic (Shulman et al 1964, Castle et al 1986, Andrew et al 1987b). Infants with obvious evidence of bleeding secondary to the thrombocytopenia should be treated with random donor platelets unless a more specific form of therapy is indicated and immediately available.

(iii) Alloimmune thrombocytopenia

The immune thrombocytopenias are secondary to an IgG antiplatelet autoantibody or alloantibody produced in the mother. This antibody crosses the placenta into the newborn causing neonatal thrombocytopenia (Shulman et al 1964, Morell et al 1971, Hedge 1985). The continued presence of the antibody in the infant's circulation depends upon the quantity of maternal IgG and the rate of clearance. Normally this would be several months, because the half-life of IgG is approximately 21 d; however, since the antibody binds to platelets its lifespan is dependent upon the lifespan of the sensitized platelets and therefore can be as short as hours. Autoimmune thrombocytopenia must be differentiated from alloimmune thrombocytopenia since the management and severity of these disorders are quite different.

In alloimmune thrombocytopenia the mothers have normal platelet counts and no bleeding history although they may have had a previously affected child (Pearson et al 1964, Brockmeier et al 1983, Katz et al 1984, Mueller-Eckhardt et al 1989). The maternal alloantibody is directed against a specific paternally derived antigen on the infant's platelets which is absent on maternal platelets. The most frequently implicated alloantigen is the PLA_1 (Zw^a) antigen that is present on platelets of 98% of the general population (Shulman et al 1962, von dem Borne et al 1981, McFarland et al 1989). Other less common alloantigens may also be the immunological stimulus for maternal alloantibody production (von dem Borne et al 1980, Kieffer et al 1984, Friedman & Aster 1985, Mueller-Eckhardt et al 1986, Shibata et al 1986a,b, Kiefel et al 1989, McGrath et al 1989).

Alloimmune thrombocytopenia presents clinically as a severe isolated thrombocytopenia in otherwise healthy infants (Blanchette 1988, Reznikoff-Etieant et al 1988, Mueller-Eckhardt et al 1989). Most infants have evidence of minor bleeding in the form of petechiae, gastrointestinal tract haemorrhage or haematuria. As many as 15% of infants may develop the serious complication of ICH. Unfortunately, ICH may occur prenatally as well as postnatally and in either case can result in the presence of hydrocephalus, porencephalic cysts and/or epilepsy (Lam & Shulman 1985, Herman et al 1986, Burrows et al 1988). It is likely that the severity of bleeding in infants with alloimmune thrombocytopenia reflects not only the low platelet count but platelet dysfunction induced by an antibody directed against the glycoprotein IIb/IIIa complex which functions as an integral part of platelet aggregation.

The diagnosis of alloimmune thrombocytopenia is based on the clinical presentation and the severity of the thrombocytopenia. Specific therapy should be instituted immediately followed by serologic testing for confirmation. The laboratory tests which are useful in confirming the presence of a platelet alloantibody include platelet typing the mother to determine which platelet alloantigen she is missing and determining the specificity of the antiplatelet alloantibody in her serum (Kelton et al 1980, McFarland et al 1989). Occasionally, the alloantibody can be demonstrated in maternal sera by reacting the sera against paternal platelets.

An infant with alloimmune thrombocytopenia should receive washed, irradiated compatible platelets (von dem Borne et al 1981, Blanchette 1988, Reznikoff-Etieant et al 1988, Editorial 1989). Matched platelets from an unrelated donor can be used, particularly if the infant is known to be at risk for alloimmune thrombocytopenia and the typing of the alloantibody has been performed previously (Adner et al 1969). However, maternal platelets are usually used because of their certain compatibility, availability and safety. A unit of whole blood is removed from the mother (prenatally if the infant is likely to be affected or postnatally if the disorder was not suspected prenatally). The maternal platelets are washed to remove maternal alloantibody and radiated to prevent graft-versus-host disease caused by maternal lymphocytes (Martin et al 1983). Frozen maternal platelets have also been used (McGill et al 1987). Other forms of therapy, including the use of corticosteroids and exchange transfusions, are not likely to be effective (McIntosh et al 1973). An infant with clinically significant bleeding should receive random donor platelets while awaiting maternal platelets. In addition, intravenous IgG may be effective in raising the platelet count either in the absence of maternal platelets, if these are not available, or in addition to maternal platelets if the response has not been sufficient (Sidiropoulos & Straume 1984, Derycke et al 1985, Massey et al 1987).

Because ICH may occur in utero in an infant with alloimmune thrombocytopenia, therapeutic management of the infant now begins prenatally. If a previous sibling was affected, there is a high probability that subsequent infants will be similarly affected. All potentially affected fetuses should be monitored by ultrasound after approximately 20 weeks' gestational age for evidence of ICH. Cordocentesis can be performed by a skilled operator in order to confirm the presence of thrombocytopenia as well as providing a route for the therapeutic administration of compatible platelets to the affected fetuses (Daffos et al 1984, 1985, Kaplan et al 1988, Nicolini et al 1988). An alternative approach is the weekly administration of IV IgG to the mother in the latter part of the pregnancy (Johnston & Zipursky 1980, Bussell et al 1988). IV IgG does cross the placenta and may provide protection for some fetuses (Davies et al 1986), although clearly not all of them (Mir et al 1988). The safety and efficacy of these alternative forms of therapy need to be tested in prospective studies. Currently, affected infants are usually delivered by elective caesarean section in order to facilitate the postnatal management of the infant (von dem Borne 1981, Blanchette 1988, Reznikoff-Etieant et al 1988, Editorial 1989). Whether caesarean section delivery will decrease the risk of ICH has not been proven.

(iv) Autoimmune thrombocytopenia

Neonatal thrombocytopenia secondary to maternal autoimmune disorders usually presents with a milder clinical course than for alloimmune thrombocytopenia. Typically the mother has ITP or, less frequently, other autoimmune disorders such as systemic lupus erythematosus (SLE), lymphoproliferative disorders or hyperthyroidism (Herman et al 1918, Nathan & Snapper 1958, Seip 1960, Karpatkin et al 1972, Kaden et al 1979, De Swiet 1985). The autoantibody is directed against antigens common both to the maternal and neonatal platelets.

Clinically, the affected infants are usually full-term healthy infants with either no clinical manifestations of thrombocytopenia or only mild manifestations (Kelton 1983). The platelet count is measured in the newborn either because the maternal diagnosis is known or suspected, or because the infant has mild manifestations such as petechiae. The diagnosis of maternal ITP should be differentiated if possible from mild thrombocytopenia associated with pregnancy (Burrows & Kelton 1988). The latter does not place either the mother or fetus at risk from haemorrhagic complications.

The management of the fetus and infant of the mother with ITP is controversial (Territo et al 1973, Karpatkin et al 1981, Cines et al 1982, Chirico et al 1983, Kelton 1983, Kryc & Corrigan 1983, Wenske et al 1983, 1984, Ciccimarra et al 1984, Karpatkin 1984, Newland et al 1984, Castaman et al 1985, Hanada et al 1985, Mazzucconi et al 1985, Le Gall et al 1986, Ronconi et al 1986, Barton et al 1987, Davidson et al 1987, Hara et al 1988, Daffos et al 1988, Blanchette et al 1989, Sacher & King 1989). Most infants affected by autoimmune thrombocytopenia in the mother are born with a platelet count greater than 50×10^9/litre (Burrows and Kelton 1991). ICH rarely, if ever, occurs prenatally nor is ICH clearly related to the birth process itself. Based on recent clinical studies the following recommendations can be made. The pregnant mother with autoimmune thrombocytopenia should be treated according to her own needs and not the very low risk needs of the fetus. The risk of cordiocentesis to determine the presence of thrombocytopenia is rarely indicated in ITP because of the inherent risk of the procedure itself and the low risk of maternal ITP for the fetus (Daffos et al 1988, Moise et al 1988). Fetal scalp sampling should be avoided because of the high technical failure rate in addition to the high false low platelet count results. There are no reliable predictors of severe thromboctyopenia in the infant (Kelton et al 1982, Barbui et al 1985). However as few as 3% of consecutive infants born to mothers with ITP have a platelet count less than 50×10^9/litre (Burrows & Kelton 1991). Following delivery the infant's platelet count usually falls over early postnatal life and the infant may require therapy at that time. A platelet count less than 50×10^9/litre is a useful guide for institution of therapy. The therapeutic interventions used in the past have included random platelet transfusions, exchange transfusion followed by platelet transfusion and corticosteroids (Territo et al 1973, Karpatkin et al 1981, Cines et al 1982, Kelton 1983, Mazzucconi et al 1985). More recently, IV IgG has been used and appears to be highly effective and safe in approximately 80% of infants (Cines et al 1982, Chirico et al 1983, Wenske et al 1983, Ciccimarra et al 1984, Castaman et al 1985, Hanada et al 1985, Le Gall et al 1986, Ronconi et al 1986, Stabile et al 1986, Barton et al 1987, Davidson et al 1987, Ballin et al 1988, Hara et al 1988, Blanchette et al 1989, Sacher & King 1989). It is not clear whether the addition of steroids to IV IgG offers added benefit. Prospective studies are required to confirm the high rate of response to IV IgG and the beneficial effects of IV IgG over other forms of therapy. Until these studies are completed, the currently available information would favour the use of IV IgG at a dose of 1 g/kg over several hours on two consecutive days or, as a second choice, the use of corticosteroids (Ballin et al 1988, Blanchette et al 1989).

3. Thrombocytopathy

The physiological differences in newborn platelet function compared to adults do not appear to result in an enhanced risk of bleeding in the absence

Table 8.2 Pathological disorders adversely affecting platelet function in newborns

1. Maternal
drugs (ex. aspirin)
dietary composition of essential fatty acids
diabetes
smoking
ethanol
2. Newborn
drugs (ex. Indomethacin)
dietary composition of essential fatty acids
vitamin E deficiency
perinatal aspiration syndrome
hyperbilirubinaemia
phototherapy
renal failure
liver failure

of secondary insults. However, the addition of impaired platelet function secondary to drugs or pathological states in mothers or infants may contribute to abnormal bleeding in newborns (Suvansri et al 1969, Bleyer & Breckenridge 1970, Corby & Schulman 1971, Stuart 1972, Levy & Garrettson 1974, Khurshid et al 1975, Maurer et al 1976, Ts'ao 1977, Friedman et al 1978, Stuart et al 1979, 1982, 1987, Cox et al 1980, Hicsomnez & Prozorova-Zamani 1980, Whaun et al 1980, Setzer et al 1982, Gersony et al 1983, Corrazza et al 1984, Ahlsten et al 1986, Kaapa et al 1986, Ostermann & van de Loo 1986, Murphy et al 1987). The perinatal events which may affect the infant's platelet function are listed in Table 8.2. The presence of a platelet function defect can be best demonstrated in newborns by the presence of a prolonged bleeding time. Platelet aggregation studies using the infants' platelets are difficult to perform because of the amount of blood required.

Abnormal platelet function will resolve when the underlying problem is corrected. If platelet dysfunction is contributing to bleeding then certain therapeutic modalities may be helpful. Cryoprecipitate has been used in adults and children to enhance platelet function, presumably by enhancing platelet vessel wall interaction by increasing the concentration of vWF. The latter is reflected by a shortening of the bleeding time as well as decreased clinical bleeding. The same approach can be used in infants with the bleeding time providing a test by which to assess the effect of a particular therapeutic intervention.

FLUID PHASE OF COAGULATION

1. Physiological process

(i) General

The presence and biochemical functions of components of the fluid phase of coagulation are similar for newborns and adults (Lammle & Griffin 1985, Colman et al 1987). However, there are some differences for coagulation proteins between newborns and adults necessitating reference ranges specifically for newborns. Complete reference ranges are available for healthy full-term and premature infants throughout the first 6 months of life (Andrew et al 1987a, 1988, 1990b). Tables 8.3 to 8.6 give mean values and upper and lower boundaries that encompass 95% of the population for the fluid phase components of haemostasis. These values are similar to smaller studies of infants at the time of birth (Cade et al 1969, Bleyer et al 1971, Jensen et al 1973, Holmberg et al 1974, Barnard et al 1979, Beverley et al 1984b, Forestier et al 1985, 1986).

The PT and APTT are both prolonged physiologically in many infants compared to adults (Tables 8.3 and 8.4). The long values for the PT and APTT reflect the slow rate and the decreased amount of thrombin generated in newborns compared to adults (Schmidt et al 1989b, Andrew et al 1990c). The latter are due to low levels of the four contact and four vitamin K-dependent proteins. However, the values for the PT and APTT in newborns are also affected by the sensitivity of the laboratory reagents used (Hirsh et al 1985, Koepke 1986). Within the last two decades, the widely varying sensitivities of differing PT reagents to low levels of the vitamin K-dependent proteins (usually secondary to coumarin therapy) have been described (Hirsh et al 1985). Indeed, the different reagents can result in several second discrepancies for the PT and thereby adversely affect patient management. The international normalized ratio (INR) provides a mechanism for correcting for differing sensitivities of PT reagents (see Chapter 9). The INR is calculated as

$$\left(\frac{\text{Patient PT (s)}}{\text{Control PT (s)}}\right)^{\text{ISI}}.$$

The international sensitivity index (ISI) corrects for the differing sensitivities of various reagents to low levels of the vitamin K-dependent factors. The variability in published values for the PT in newborns reflects in part the use of differing reagents. An insensitive rabbit thromboplastin reagent with an ISI of 2.5 was used to measure the PT values in Tables 8.3 and 8.4. The INR values are also given in Tables 8.3 and 8.4.

The APTT values are also affected by the sensitivity of the commercial reagents to low levels of certain coagulation factors or differing sensitivities to heparin (Koepke 1986). The APTT values in Tables 8.3 and 8.4 were measured with Dade Actin FS. Laboratories involved in the evaluation of newborns need to be aware of the effects of differing reagents on the PT and APTT.

The third screening test frequently used in newborns is the thrombin clotting time (TCT). The TCT can be prolonged by: (a) low levels of fibrinogen, (b) the presence of dysfibrinogenaemia, (c) heparin and (d) fibrin degradation products (Ockelford & Carter 1982). The amount of

Table 8.3 Reference values for coagulation tests in the healthy full-term infant during the first 6 months of life

	Day 1	Day 5	Day 30	Day 90	Day 180	Adult
PT (s)	13.0 (10.1–15.9)[a]	12.4 (10.0–15.3)[a]	11.8 (10.0–14.3)[a]	11.9 (10.0–14.2)[a]	12.3 (10.7–13.9)[a]	12.4 (10.8–13.9)
INR (s)	1.00 (0.53–1.62)	0.89 (0.53–1.48)	0.79 (0.53–1.26)	0.81 (0.53–1.26)	0.88 (0.61–1.17)	0.89 (0.64–1.17)
APTT (s)	42.9 (31.3–54.5)	42.6 (25.4–59.8)	40.4 (32.0–55.2)	37.1 (29.0–50.1)[a]	35.5 (28.1–42.9)[a]	33.5 (26.6–40.3)
TCT (s)	23.5 (19.0–28.3)[a]	23.1 (18.0–29.2)	24.3 (19.4–29.2)[a]	25.1 (20.5–29.7)[a]	25.5 (19.8–31.2)[a]	25.0 (19.7–30.3)
Fibrinogen (g/L)	2.83 (1.67–3.99)[a]	3.12 (1.62–4.62)[a]	2.70 (1.62–3.78)[a]	2.43 (1.50–3.79)[a]	2.51 (1.50–3.87)[a]	2.78 (1.56–4.00)
II (U/ml)	0.48 (0.26–0.70)	0.63 (0.33–0.93)	0.68 (0.34–1.02)	0.75 (0.45–1.05)	0.88 (0.60–1.16)	1.08 (0.70–1.46)
V (U/ml)	0.72 (0.34–1.08)	0.95 (0.45–1.45)	0.98 (0.62–1.34)	0.90 (0.48–1.32)	0.91 (0.55–1.27)	1.06 (0.62–1.50)
VII (U/ml)	0.66 (0.28–1.04)	0.89 (0.35–1.43)	0.90 (0.42–1.38)	0.91 (0.39–1.43)	0.87 (0.47–1.27)	1.05 (0.67–1.43)
VIII (U/ml)	1.00 (0.50–1.78)[a]	0.88 (0.50–1.54)[a]	0.91 (0.50–1.57)[a]	0.79 (0.50–1.25)[a]	0.73 (0.50–1.09)	0.99 (0.50–1.49)
vWF (U/ml)	1.53 (0.50–2.87)	1.40 (0.50–2.54)	1.28 (0.50–2.46)	1.18 (0.50–2.06)	1.07 (0.50–1.97)	0.92 (0.50–1.58)
IX (U/ml)	0.53 (0.15–0.91)	0.53 (0.15–0.91)	0.51 (0.21–0.81)	0.67 (0.21–1.13)	0.86 (0.36–1.36)	1.09 (0.55–1.63)
X (U/ml)	0.40 (0.12–0.68)	0.49 (0.19–0.79)	0.59 (0.31–0.87)	0.71 (0.35–1.07)	0.78 (0.38–1.18)	1.06 (0.70–1.52)
XI (U/ml)	0.38 (0.10–0.66)	0.55 (0.23–0.87)	0.53 (0.27–0.79)	0.69 (0.41–0.97)	0.86 (0.49–1.34)	0.97 (0.67–1.27)
XII (U/ml)	0.53 (0.13–0.93)	0.47 (0.11–0.83)	0.49 (0.17–0.81)	0.67 (0.25–1.09)	0.77 (0.39–1.15)	1.08 (0.52–1.64)
PK (U/ml)	0.37 (0.18–0.69)	0.48 (0.20–0.76)	0.57 (0.23–0.91)	0.73 (0.41–1.05)	0.86 (0.56–1.16)	1.12 (0.62–1.62)
HMWK (U/ml)	0.54 (0.06–1.02)	0.74 (0.16–1.32)	0.77 (0.33–1.21)	0.82 (0.30–1.46)[a]	0.82 (0.36–1.28)[a]	0.92 (0.50–1.36)
XIII:a (U/ml)	0.79 (0.27–1.31)	0.94 (0.44–1.44)[a]	0.93 (0.39–1.47)[a]	1.04 (0.36–1.72)[a]	1.04 (0.46–1.62)[a]	1.05 (0.55–1.55)
XIII:b (U/ml)	0.76 (0.30–1.22)	1.06 (0.32–1.80)[a]	1.11 (0.39–1.73)[a]	1.16 (0.48–1.84)[a]	1.10 (0.50–1.70)[a]	0.97 (0.57–1.37)

PT, prothrombin time; APTT, activated partial thromboplastin time: TCT thrombin clotting time; VIII, factor VIII procoagulant; vWF, von Willebrand factor; PK, prekallikrein; HMWK, high-molecular-weight kininogen; INR, international normalized ratio.

All factors except fibrinogen are expressed as units per millilitre (U/ml) where pooled plasma contains 1.0 U/ml. All values are expressed as mean followed in parentheses by the lower and upper boundaries encompassing 95% of the population. Between 40–77 samples were assayed for each value for the newborn. Some measurements were skewed due to a disproportionate number of high values. The lower limit which excludes the lower 2.5% of the population has been given (Andrew et al 1990b).

[a] Values that are indistinguishable from those of the adult.

Table 8.4 Reference values for coagulation tests in the healthy premature infant (30–36 weeks gestation) during the first 6 months of life

	Day 1	Day 5	Day 30	Day 90	Day 180	Adult
PT (s)	13.0 (10.6–16.2)[a]	12.5 (10.0–15.3)[a]	11.8 (10.0–13.6)[a]	12.3 (10.0–14.6)[a]	12.5 (10.0–15.0)[a]	12.4 (10.8–13.9)
INR	1.0 (0.61–1.7)	0.91 (0.53–1.48)	0.79 (0.53–1.11)	0.88 (0.53–1.32)	0.91 (0.53–1.48)	0.89 (0.64–1.17)
APTT (s)	53.6 (27.5–79.4)[b]	50.5 (26.9–74.1)[b]	44.7 (26.9–62.5)	39.5 (28.3–50.7)	37.5 (27.1–53.3)[a]	33.5 (26.6–40.3)
TCT (s)	24.8 (19.2–30.4)[a]	24.1 (18.8–29.4)[a]	24.4 (18.8–29.9)[a]	25.1 (19.4–30.8)[a]	25.2 (18.9–31.5)[a]	25.0 (19.7–30.3)
Fibrinogen (g/l)	2.43 (1.50–3.73)[a,b]	2.80 (1.60–4.18)[a,b]	2.54 (1.50–4.14)[a]	2.46 (1.50–3.52)[a]	2.28 (1.50–3.60)	2.78 (1.56–4.00)
II (U/ml)	0.45 (0.20–0.77)	0.57 (0.29–0.85)[b]	0.57 (0.36–0.95)[b]	0.68 (0.30–1.06)	0.87 (0.51–1.23)	1.08 (0.70–1.46)
V (U/ml)	0.88 (0.41–1.44)[a,b]	1.00 (0.46–1.54)[a]	1.02 (0.48–1.56)[a]	0.99 (0.59–1.39)[a]	1.02 (0.58–1.46)[a]	1.06 (0.62–1.50)
VII (U/ml)	0.67 (0.21–1.13)	0.84 (0.30–1.38)	0.83 (0.21–1.45)	0.87 (0.31–1.43)	0.99 (0.47–1.51)[a]	1.05 (0.67–1.43)
VIII (U/ml)	1.11 (0.50–2.13)[a]	1.15 (0.53–2.05)[a,b]	1.11 (0.50–1.99)[a,b]	1.06 (0.58–1.88)[a,b]	0.99 (0.50–1.87)[a,b]	0.99 (0.50–1.49)
vWF (U/ml)	1.36 (0.78–2.10)	1.33 (0.72–2.19)	1.36 (0.66–2.16)	1.12 (0.75–1.84)[a]	0.98 (0.54–1.58)[a]	0.92 (0.50–1.58)
IX (U/ml)	0.35 (0.19–0.65)[b]	0.42 (0.14–0.74)[b]	0.44 (0.13–0.80)	0.59 (0.25–0.93)	0.81 (0.50–1.20)	1.09 (0.55–1.63)
X (U/ml)	0.41 (0.11–0.71)	0.51 (0.19–0.83)	0.56 (0.20–0.92)	0.67 (0.35–0.99)	0.77 (0.35–1.19)	1.06 (0.70–1.52)
XI (U/ml)	0.30 (0.08–0.52)[b]	0.41 (0.13–0.69)[b]	0.43 (0.15–0.71)[b]	0.59 (0.25–0.93)[b]	0.78 (0.46–1.10)	0.97 (0.67–1.27)
XII (U/ml)	0.38 (0.10–0.66)[b]	0.39 (0.09–0.69)[b]	0.43 (0.11–0.75)	0.61 (0.15–1.07)	0.82 (0.22–1.42)	1.08 (0.52–1.64)
PK (U/ml)	0.33 (0.09–0.57)	0.45 (0.25–0.75)	0.59 (0.31–0.87)	0.79 (0.37–1.21)	0.78 (0.40–1.16)	1.12 (0.62–1.62)
HMWK (U/ml)	0.49 (0.09–0.89)	0.62 (0.24–1.00)[b]	0.64 (0.16–1.12)[b]	0.78 (0.32–1.24)	0.83 (0.41–1.25)[a]	0.92 (0.50–1.36)
XIII:a (U/ml)	0.70 (0.32–1.08)	1.01 (0.57–1.45)[a]	0.99 (0.51–1.47)[a]	1.13 (0.71–1.55)[a]	1.13 (0.65–1.61)[a]	1.05 (0.55–1.55)
XIII:b (U/ml)	0.81 (0.35–1.27)	1.10 (0.68–1.58)[a]	1.07 (0.57–1.57)[a]	1.21 (0.75–1.67)	1.15 (0.67–1.63)	0.97 (0.57–1.37)

PT, Prothrombin time; APTT, activated partial thromboplastin time; TCT, thrombin clotting time; VIII, Factor VIII procoagulant; vWF, von Willebrand factor; PK, prekallikrein; HMWK, high-molecular-weight kininogen; INR, international normalized ratio.

All factors except fibrinogen are expressed as units per millilitre (U/ml) where pooled plasma contains 1.0 U/ml. All values are given as a mean followed in parentheses by the lower and upper boundaries encompassing 95% of the population. Between 40–96 samples were assayed for each value for the newborn. Some measurements were skewed due to a disproportionate number of high values. The lower limits which excludes the lower 2.5% of the population has been given (Andrew et al 1990b).

[a]Values that are indistinguishable from the adult.

[b]Values different from those of the full-term infants.

Table 8.5 a Reference values for the inhibitors of coagulation in the healthy full-term infant during the first 6 months of life

	Day 1	Day 5	Day 30	Day 90	Day 180	Adult
ATIII (U/ml)	0.63 (0.39–0.87)	0.67 (0.41–0.93)	0.78 (0.48–1.08)	0.97 (0.73–1.21)[a]	1.04 (0.84–1.24)[a]	1.05 (0.79–1.31)
α_2M (U/ml)	1.39 (0.95–1.83)	1.48 (0.98–1.98)	1.50 (1.06–1.94)	1.76 (1.26–2.26)	1.91 (1.49–2.33)	0.86 (0.52–1.20)
C1-INH (U/ml)	0.72 (0.36–1.08)	0.90 (0.60–1.20)[a]	0.89 (0.47–1.31)	1.15 (0.71–1.59)	1.41 (0.89–1.93)	1.01 (0.71–1.31)
α_1AT (U/ml)	0.93 (0.49–1.37)[a]	0.89 (0.49–1.29)[a]	0.62 (0.36–0.88)	0.72 (0.42–1.02)	0.77 (0.47–1.07)	0.93 (0.55–1.31)
HCII (U/ml)	0.43 (0.10–0.93)	0.48 (0.10–0.96)	0.47 (0.10–0.87)	0.72 (0.10–1.46)	1.20 (0.50–1.90)	0.96 (0.66–1.26)
Protein C (U/ml)	0.35 (0.17–0.53)	0.42 (0.20–0.64)	0.43 (0.21–0.65)	0.54 (0.28–0.80)	0.59 (0.37–0.81)	0.96 (0.64–1.28)
Protein S (U/ml)	0.36 (0.12–0.60)	0.50 (0.22–0.78)	0.63 (0.33–0.93)	0.86 (0.54–1.18)[a]	0.87 (0.55–1.19)[a]	0.92 (0.60–1.24)

Table 8.5 b Reference values for the inhibitors of coagulation in the healthy premature infant (30–36 weeks gestation) during the first 6 months of life

	Day 1	Day 5	Day 30	Day 90	Day 180	Adult
ATIII (U/ml)	0.38 (0.14–0.62)[b]	0.56 (0.30–0.82)	0.59 (0.37–0.81)[b]	0.83 (0.45–1.21)[b]	0.90 (0.52–1.28)[b]	1.05 (0.79–1.31)
α_2M (U/ml)	1.10 (0.56–1.82)[b]	1.25 (0.71–1.77)	1.38 (0.72–2.04)	1.80 (1.20–2.66)	2.09 (1.10–3.21)	0.86 (0.52–1.20)
C1-INH (U/ml)	0.65 (0.31–0.99)	0.83 (0.45–1.21)	0.74 (0.40–1.24)[b]	1.14 (0.60–1.68)[a]	1.40 (0.96–2.04)	1.01 (0.71–1.31)
α_1AT (U/ml)	0.90 (0.36–1.44)[a]	0.94 (0.42–1.46)[a]	0.76 (0.38–1.12)[b]	0.81 (0.49–1.13)[a,b]	0.82 (0.48–1.16)[a]	0.93 (0.55–1.31)
HCII (U/ml)	0.32 (0.10–0.60)[b]	0.34 (0.10–0.69)	0.43 (0.15–0.71)	0.61 (0.20–1.11)	0.89 (0.45–1.40)[a,b]	0.96 (0.66–1.26)
Protein C (U/ml)	0.28 (0.12–0.44)[b]	0.31 (0.11–0.51)	0.37 (0.15–0.59)[b]	0.45 (0.23–0.67)[b]	0.57 (0.31–0.83)	0.96 (0.64–1.28)
Protein S (U/ml)	0.26 (0.14–0.38)[b]	0.37 (0.13–0.61)	0.56 (0.22–0.90)	0.76 (0.40–1.12)[b]	0.82 (0.44–1.20)	0.92 (0.60–1.24)

ATIII, antithrombin III; α_2M, α_2–macroglobulin; C1–INH, C1–esterase inhibitor; α_1AT, α_1-antitrypsin; HCII, heparin cofactor II.

All values are expressed in units per millilitre (U/ml) where pooled plasma contains 1.0 U/ml. All values are given as a mean followed in parentheses by the lower and upper boundaries encompassing 95% of the population. Between 40–75 samples were assayed for each value for the newborn. Some measurements were skewed due to a disproportionate number of high values. The lower limits which excludes the lower 2.5% of the populaton has been given (Andrew et al 1990b).

[a] Values that are indistinguishable from those of the adult.

[b] Values different from those of the full-term infant.

Table 8.6 **b** Reference values for the components of the fibrinolytic system in the healthy premature infant during the first 6 months of life

	Day 1	Day 5	Day 30	Day 90	Day 180	Adult
Plasminogen (U/ml)	1.95 (1.25–2.65)	2.17 (1.41–2.93)	1.98 (1.26–2.70)	2.48 (1.74–3.22)	3.01 (2.21–3.81)	3.36 (2.48–4.24)
TPA (ng/ml)	9.6 (5.0–18.9)	5.6 (4.0–10.0)[a]	4.1 (1.0–6.0)[a]	2.1 (1.0–5.0)[a]	2.8 (1.0–6.0)[a]	4.9 (1.4–8.4)
α_2AP (U/ml)	0.85 (0.55–1.15)	1.00 (0.70–1.30)[a]	1.00 (0.76–1.24)[a]	1.08 (0.76–1.40)[a]	1.11 (0.83–1.39)[a]	1.02 (0.68–1.36)
PAI (U/ml)	6.4 (2.0–15.1)	2.3 (0.0–8.1)[a]	3.4 (0.0–8.8)[a]	7.2 (1.0–15.3)	8.1 (6.0–13.0)	3.6 (0.0–11.0)

Table 8.6 **b** References values for the components of the fibrinolytic system in the healthy premature infant during the first 6 months of life

	Day 1	Day 5	Day 30	Day 50	Day 180	Adult
Plasminogen (U/ml)	1.70 (1.12–2.48)[b]	1.91 (1.21–2.61)[b]	1.81 (1.09–2.53)	2.38 (1.58–3.18)	2.75 (1.91–3.59)[b]	3.36 (2.48–4.24)
TPA (ng/ml)	8.48 (3.00–16.70)	3.97 (2.00–6.93)[a]	4.13 (2.00–7.79)[a]	3.31 (2.00–5.07)[a]	3.48 (2.00–5.85)[a]	4.96 (1.46–8.46)
α_2AP (U/ml)	0.78 (0.40–1.16)	0.81 (0.49–1.13)[b]	0.89 (0.55–1.23)[b]	1.06 (0.64–1.48)[a]	1.15 (0.77–1.53)	1.02 (0.68–1.36)
PAI (U/ml)	5.4 (0.0–12.2)[a,b]	2.5 (0.0–7.1)[a]	4.3 (0.0–10.9)[a]	4.8 (1.0–11.8)[a,b]	4.9 (1.0–10.2)[a,b]	3.6 (0.0–11.0)

TPA, tissue plasminogen activator; α_2AP, α_2-antiplasmin; PAI, plasminogen activator inhibitor.

For α_2AP, values are expressed as units per millilitre (U/ml) where pooled plasma contains 1.0 U/ml. Plasminogen units are those recommended by the Committee on Thrombolytic Agents. Values for TPA are given as nanograms per millilitre. Values for PAI are given as units per ml where 1 unit of PAI_1 activity is defined as the amount of PAI that inhibits the 1 international unit of human single-chain TPA. All values are given as a mean followed in parentheses by the lower and upper boundaries encompassing 95% of the population (Andrew et al 1990b).

[a] Values that are indistinguishable from those of the adult.

[b] Values that are different from those of the full-term infant.

thrombin used and the presence or absence of calcium in the buffer influence the sensitivity of the TCT to each of these variables. In Tables 8.3 and 8.4, a two-unit TCT was performed in a buffer containing calcium. This form of TCT is sensitive to heparin and fibrinogen concentration but is not sensitive to fibrinogen/fibrin degradation products (FDP) or dysfibrinogenaemias. Fibrinogen circulates in newborns in a fetal form characterized by an increased sialic acid content (Witt et al 1969, Galankis & Mosesson 1976, Hamulyak et al 1983). The physiological significance of fetal fibrinogen is uncertain. The TCT used in Tables 8.3 and 8.4 is insensitive to the presence of fetal fibrinogen.

Physiologically, the levels of the four vitamin K-dependent factors (II, VII, IX and X), in addition to the four contact factors (XI, XII, high-molecular-weight kininogen and prekallikrein) are approximately half the adult values. In contrast, levels of fibrinogen, factor VIII, vWF and factor XIII are similar or increased over the adult values. The net result of this unique balance of coagulation factors is a decrease in the total amount and rate at which thrombin is generated (Schmidt et al 1989a, Andrew et al 1990b). Indeed, the amount of thrombin generated in plasma from healthy infants is approximately half the normal adult values and similar to adults fully anticoagulated with either heparin or warfarin.

2. Congenital factor deficiencies

(i) General

The clinical spectrum of bleeding in newborns differs from children or adults (McDonald & Hathaway 1983, Montgomery et al 1985, Gibson 1989). First, the sites of bleeding are related to perinatal events. They include oozing from the umbilicus, cephalohaematomas, bleeding post-circumcision, bleeding from peripheral sites used for blood sampling and bleeding into the skin. Newborns appear to be particularly at risk for ICH secondary to congenital and acquired disorders. For example, the immune thrombocytopenias in infancy are associated with a much higher risk of ICH than childhood ITP despite similarly low platelet counts. Essentially, all congenital factor deficiencies that can cause bleeding are linked through case reports to ICH in infancy (Silverstein 1960, Girolami et al 1985, Ragni et al 1986, Abbondanzo et al 1988, Yoffe & Buchanan 1988). Deficiency of factor VII provides a striking example of this phenomenon (Ragni et al 1986). Similarly, the acquired disorder, vitamin K deficiency, is characterized by ICH, particularly in the early and late presentations (Lane & Hathaway 1985). Finally, because the total blood volumes of infants are so small, what may appear to be insignificant blood loss may rapidly place newborns in hypovolaemic shock.

The most common coagulation factor deficiencies to present in newborns are severe haemophilia A (factor VIII), and severe haemophilia B (factor IX) (Girolami et al 1985). Less frequently, deficiencies of fibrinogen, factors II, V, VII X, XI and XIII, and, rarely, vWD present in newborns (Silverstein 1960, Rapaport et al 1961, Lorand et al 1980, Mammen 1983a,b,c,d, Mariani & Mazzucconi 1983, Girolami et al 1985, Lane & Hathaway 1985, Ragni et al 1986, Abbondanzo et al 1988, Yoffe & Buchanan 1988). Although vWD is the most common haemostatic abnormality in children or adults, most forms of vWD cannot be confidently diagnosed in newborns by assays reflecting vWF activity or concentration. The physiological concentration of vWF as well as the high-molecular-weight multimeric forms of vWF are elevated at birth and persist into early infancy masking the presence of vWD (Katz et al 1989, Weinstein et al 1989). The definitive diagnosis of congenital factor deficiencies remains a low functional coagulation factor assay.

With the exception of factor XIII and α_2-antiplasmin (α_2AP), the severe form of congenital factor deficiencies prolong either or both the PT and APTT. Depending upon the results of these two tests, as well as the clinical problem, further specific assays can be performed to confirm the diagnosis. Any male infant suspected of having a congenital deficiency should have factor VIII and IX levels measured. The severe (less than 0.01 U/ml), moderate (0.01–0.05 U/ml) and mild (greater than 0.06 U/ml) forms of haemophilia A can be diagnosed at the time of birth because the lower limit of the reference range is 0.50 U/ml for factor VIII. Although the severe and moderate forms of haemophilia B can be confidently diagnosed in newborns, mild forms may require repeat testing for confirmation at a later time in infancy because the lower limit of the reference range is 0.15 U/ml at birth.

The diagnosis of other coagulation protein deficiencies may be particularly difficult if the physiological levels are low, or if the infant has already decompensated and developed DIC secondary to significant blood loss (Schmidt & Zipursky 1986). In the homozygote state, factor V and VII deficiencies (less than 0.10 and 0.03 U/ml, respectively) are easily distinguished from the physiological values for newborns. In contrast, the homozygous state for factors II and X (levels less than 0.20 and 0.10 U/ml, respectively) do overlap with the physiological levels. Measurement of the specific coagulation factor of concern in the parents or the use of molecular biology may be very helpful in identifying the presence of a defect in newborns.

Hypo- and afibrinogenaemias as well as homozygous factor XIII deficiency frequently present in newborns with delayed umbilical bleeding (Lorand et al 1980, Mammen 1983a). The identification of infants with factor XIII deficiency is particularly important because of the high risk of ICH at sometime during their lives and the ease and benefits of prophylactic therapy. The half-life of factor XIII is long and only very low levels of factor XIII are required for haemostasis (greater than 0.01 U/ml).

The therapeutic modalities for congenital factor deficiencies include plasma products (i.e. fresh frozen plasma (FFP) cryoprecipitate), and factor concentrates. The choice of therapeutic products is given in Table

Table 8.7 Treatment of infants with congenital or acquired factor deficiencies

Disorder	Treatment of choice	Alternative treatment
1. Inherited		
factor VIII	VIII concentrate, Cryo	FFP
factor IX	PCC	Plasma
factor II, VII, X	Plasma	PCC
factor V	FFP	—
factor XI	Plasma	—
factor XIII	Cryo, XIII concentrate	Plasma
afibrinogenemia	Cryo	Plasma
vWD	Cryo	FFP
Protein C	FFP, Protein C concentrate	—
2. Acquired		
Vitamin K	Vitamin K, plasma	PCC
Liver disease	Plasma, Cryo	ET
DIC	FFP, Cryo	ET, rarely
	Platelet concentrates	Heparin, treat underlying disorder

vWD, von Willebrand's Disease; Cryo, cryoprecipitate; PCC, prothrombin complex concentrate; FFP, fresh frozen plasma; ET, exchange transfusion.

8.7. The minimal haemostatic level necessary is directly linked to the particular deficiency and clinical situation.

3. Disseminated intravascular coagulation

(i) Clinical features

DIC is a haemostatic disorder secondary to a variety of underlying disease states (Boyd 1966, 1969, Markarian et al 1967, Anderson et al 1974, Zipursky & Jaber 1978, Corrigan 1979, Watkins et al 1980). Common underlying pathological disorders in newborns include respiratory distress syndrome (RDS), asphyxia, trauma, both viral and bacterial infections, hypothermia and perinatal aspiration due to meconium or amniotic fluid. The clinical spectrum of DIC in newborns is evolving and reflects improvements in perinatal care of sick newborns. For some infants, DIC is characterized by haemorrhagic or thrombotic complications whereas in other infants there may be minimal clinical signs of the DIC.

The diagnosis of DIC is based on both clinical features as well as abnormal laboratory tests. Laboratory tests compatible with the diagnosis of DIC include thrombocytopenia, prolongation of the screening tests (PT, APTT), low levels of specific coagulation proteins (fibrinogen, factors V and VIII), low levels of inhibitors (ATIII, HCII, protein C), positive paracoagulation test including the presence of elevated fibrinogen/fibrin split products, D-dimer and fibrin monomer. The paracoagulation tests measure the subtle effects of very small amounts of thrombin and/or plasmin and thereby identify mild in addition to severe forms of DIC (Ockelford & Carter 1982).

Positive results for the paracoagulation tests do not necessarily indicate the presence of DIC. For example, D-dimer indicates that cross-linked fibrin is being degraded in infants. Many infants at risk for DIC will also have extravascular extravasation of blood (i.e. intraventricular haemorrhage, cephalohaematoma) that may result in positive tests for D-dimer. To further complicate the interpretation of paracoagulation tests, the relationship between positive results and fibrin deposition in the microvasculature that impairs organ function is unclear. Some paracoagulation tests are positive in cord plasma from healthy infants, probably reflecting activation of haemostasis during the birth process, but not pathological fibrin deposition. Clearly, a combination of clinical and laboratory abnormalities are necessary for the diagnosis of DIC.

(ii) Clinical management

The cornerstone of management of DIC remains the successful treatment of the underlying disease state. The therapeutic modalities for the management of the secondary haemostatic complications include coagulation factor replacement with a variety of blood products including plasma (usually FFP), cryoprecipitate, exchange transfusions, platelet transfusions and, rarely, anticoagulant drugs (Skyberg & Jacobsen 1969, Gross & Melhorn 1971, De Lemos et al 1973, Hambleton & Appleyard 1973, Waltt et al 1973, Straub 1975, Zipursky et al 1979, Turner et al 1981, Gross et al 1982, Johnson et al 1982, Blajchman et al 1984). The argument that replacement therapy may 'fuel the fire' is theoretical. Unfortunately, there are few controlled studies that have documented improvements in laboratory tests and/or clinical course when coagulation replacement factor is given. This area requires further clarification. The presence of DIC does not necessarily indicate a need to intervene with coagulation factor replacement. For example, the need for treatment is unclear in infants with a rapidly resolving underlying problem, minimal clinical manifestations of haemostatic impairment, positive paracoagulation tests but only mildly abnormal screening tests. In contrast, infants with obvious haemorrhagic manifestations should be treated with coagulation factor replacement therapy until the primary problem resolves. Reasonable goals of therapy are to sustain a platelet count over 50×10^9/litre, a fibrinogen level greater than 1.0 g/l and a PT within the normal range for the infant. The role of newer plasma products such as ATIII and protein C concentrates is unclear and are currently undergoing evaluation in clinical studies (Hanada et al 1985, Von Kries et al 1985).

4. Vitamin K deficiency

(i) General

Infants who develop vitamin K deficiency are at greater risk of haemorrhagic complications than similarly affected adults in part because the levels of the four vitamin K-dependent coagulation proteins (II, VII, IX, X) are already physiologically low in infants (approximately 50% adult values). Thus, there is little reserve capacity when these coagulation factors are further decreased in vitamin K deficiency and infants are rapidly placed at risk of serious haemorrhaging.

Clinically, vitamin K deficiency in infancy can be classified into three patterns of presentation depending upon the timing of the presentation and concurrent problems (Lane & Hathaway 1985, Hathaway 1986, Shapiro et al 1986, Fetus & Newborn Committee 1988, Kries et al 1988). The classic form of vitamin K deficiency, haemorrhagic disease of the newborn (HDN), presents on days 2–5 of life in breast-fed, full-term infants, with gastrointestinal bleeding, widespread ecchymosis or bleeding from peripheral puncture sites. Of some concern is the occurrence of ICH as an initial bleeding site in these infants (Hathaway 1987, Hanawa et al 1988, Kries et al 1988, Shapiro et al 1988b). The vitamin K stores in infants are decreased compared to adults which in combination with the low intake of vitamin K in breast milk, as well as a sterile gut, place infants at risk of developing symptomatic vitamin K deficiency (Haroon et al 1982, Shirahata et al 1982, Widdershoven et al 1986b, Allison et al 1987, Hamulyak et al 1987, Olson 1987, Greer et al 1988, Hiraike et al 1988a,b, Mandelbrot et al 1988, Shinzawa et al 1989). Formula-fed infants receive higher amounts of vitamin K (approximately 830 μg/l) compared to breast-fed infants (<20 μg/l) and are therefore at a lower risk of developing HDN (Haroon et al 1982, Von Kries et al 1987). In the absence of vitamin K prophylaxis at birth the occurrence of HDN varies greatly depending upon the population and source of milk at birth. The frequency is likely about 1 in 200–400 infants in the absence of prophylactic therapy (Aballi & de Lamerens 1962, Sutherland & Glueck 1967).

The second form of vitamin K deficiency presents early in the first 24 h of life usually with serious bleeding, including ICH. The mothers of these infants often have been taking drugs that interfere with vitamin K stores or function in newborns (i.e. warfarin, anticonvulsants, rifampin, isoniazid) (Srinivasan et al 1982, Mountain et al 1970, Behrmann et al 1985, Binder 1986, Laosombat 1988).

The third form of HDN occurs later, beyond the first weeks of life in infants with a variety of other underlying disease states including chronic diarrhoea, short-term diarrhoea in breast-fed infants, infants with cystic fibrosis, a_1-antitrypsin deficiency, hepatitis and celiac disease (Muntean et al 1979, Forbes 1983, Chaou et al 1984, Payne & Hasegawa 1984, Editorial 1985, Motohara et al 1986, 1987, Goldschmidt et al 1988, Matsuda et al 1989).

Readily available laboratory tests that reflect the pathologically low levels of factors II, VII, IX and X secondary to vitamin K deficiency include the screening tests (PT, APTT) and coagulation factor assays. Specific assays for the decarboxylated forms of vitamin K-dependent factors and direct measurement of vitamin K have also been used. However not all of these assays are suitable for clinical use (Bloch et al 1984, Fujimara et al 1984, Kotohara et al 1985, Motohara et al 1986, 1987, Widdershoven et al 1986, 1988). In a vitamin K-deficient state decarboxylated forms of the vitamin K-dependent factors (PIVKA) are produced and can be measured directly or as a discrepancy between coagulant activity and immunological concentration of a particular vitamin K-dependent protein (Fujimura et al 1982). The use of the snake venom *Echis carinatum* which cleaves thrombin from both the decarboxylated and carboxylated forms of prothrombin in the absence of calcium, provides a rapid method for measuring the total prothrombin concentration (Shirahata et al 1982, Garrow et al 1986).

(ii) Prophylactic and therapeutic use of vitamin K

The evidence supporting the benefits of vitamin K prophylactic therapy has been recently summarized (Nathan & Oski, 1991). The conclusion that vitamin K prophylaxis is indicated comes from two strong randomized controlled trials (Vietti et al 1960, Sutherland & Glueck 1967), at least 14 controlled trials using biochemical evidence of vitamin K deficiency as surrogate outcomes (Astrowe & Palmerton 1941, Lehmann 1944, Aballi & de Lamerens 1962, Wefring 1962, Keenan et al 1971, O'Connor & Addiego 1986, Widdershoven et al 1986a,b, Motohara et al 1987, Von Kries et al 1987b, Ogata et al 1988) and studies of weaker designs (population surveys, case reports) (Shearer et al 1982, Bloch et al 1984, Hall & Pairaudeau 1987, Motohara et al 1987, Greer et al 1988, Hiraike et al 1988a,b). Recommendations for vitamin K prophylaxis have been published by many countries and are similar (Committee on Nutrition 1961, Aballi & de Lamerens 1962, Dunn 1982, McNinch et al 1983, Hathaway 1986, 1987, Shapiro et al 1986, Tripp & McNinch 1987, Fetus & Newborn Committee 1988, Brown et al 1989, Motohara et al 1989). The daily requirement for vitamin K in newborns is estimated to be approximately 1–5 μg/kg body weight. A single dose of 0.5–1 mg intramuscularly or an oral dose of 2–4 mg at birth provide effective prophylaxis. Usually vitamin K_1 is the form of vitamin K administered although low doses of vitamin K_3 may also be used. Whether oral vitamin K provides equivalent prophylaxis to intramuscular vitamin K when used in large populations of infants has not been determined (McNinch et al 1985, Sann et al 1985, O'Connor & Addiego 1986, Von Kries et al 1987). In research studies with small numbers of infants, oral vitamin K is absorbed and provides protection. However with the general use of oral vitamin K it is inevitable that some infants will not swallow all of an orally administered dose of vitamin K. Whether this problem is of a significant magnitude to recommend only intramuscular vitamin K has not been determined. In addition to general prophylaxis at birth, certain risk groups require additional vitamin K prophylaxis (i.e α_1-antitrypsin deficiency, chronic diarrhoea, cystic fibrosis, celiac disease). When a pregnant woman is receiving oral anticonvulsant therapy, vitamin K_1 should be given in the third trimester in amounts of approximately 5 mg/d.

Infants with haemorrhagic complications that may be due to vitamin K deficiency should be treated immediately with vitamin K. Confirmation of the diagnosis follows from results of laboratory tests. An infant with HDN should receive vitamin K either subcutaneously or intravenously but not intramuscularly as the latter may result in large haematoma formation at the site of injection. Vitamin K given intravenously has caused anaphylactic reactions in adults. The risk to newborns is unclear. Nevertheless, it seems advisable to administer intravenous vitamin K slowly. The systemically administered vitamin K requires approximately 2 h to result in some beneficial effect on the activity of the vitamin K-dependent factors. Infants with significant haemorrhagic manifestations should be treated with plasma in addition to vitamin K. However, if the bleeding is in the form of ICH or life threatening, then factor IX concentrates may be used. These products will immediately increase the vitamin K-dependent factor levels to a safe haemostatic concentration. However, factor IX concentrates may transmit hepatitis and may also cause thrombotic complications. The infant receiving factor IX concentrates should also receive both hepatitis B immunoglobulin and hepatitis B vaccination.

5. Liver disease

Haemostatic impairment associated with liver disease in newborns is similar to adults and is due to a combination of failure of hepatic synthetic functions, activation of the haemostatic system, poor clearance of the products of haemostasis as well as loss of haemostatic proteins into ascitic fluid (Kelly & Summerfield 1987). The goal of management for these infants is to maintain haemostasis until the liver regains normal function or, in the more severe cases, a liver transplantation is performed if appropriate and feasible.

6. Miscellaneous

Certain haemorrhagic manifestations occur with some frequency in newborns, usually linked to other underlying problems or the birth process itself.

(i) Intracranial haemorrhage

ICH occurs in both full-term and premature infants and may cause long-term morbidity (Hayden et al 1985). The most frequent form of ICH is intraventricular haemorrhage (IVH), which occurs primarily in premature infants weighing less than 1500 g. The diagnosis of IVH is made by ultrasound examination through the anterior fontanelle and less frequently by computerized tomography and magnetic resonance imaging. IVH is a complex problem (Burstein et al 1977, Volpe 1981, 1983, Shinnar et al 1982, Goddard-Finegold 1984, Ment et al 1987). In brief, IVH is characterized by bleeding from the fragile microvasculature of the subependymal germinal matrix which may extend into the lateral ventricles or into the brain parenchyma. Most IVH occur in the first 24 h of birth with almost all occurring in the subsequent 72 h. Approximately 10–20% of IVH will extend following the initial bleed. The concurrent problems associated with IVH include perinatal asphyxia, assisted ventilation usually for RDS, hypercardia, acidosis, hypoxia, pneumothorax and prematurity. Whether the physiological immaturity of the newborn coagulation system contributes to the occurrence and extent of IVH is unknown. Pathological alterations of the newborn's haemostatic system are associated with IVH in many infants. Thrombocytopenia, decreased concentrations of many coagulation proteins and evidence for activation of the haemostatic system are observed in infants with IVH (Gray et al 1968, Waltt et al 1973, Beverley et al 1984, McDonald et al 1984, Andrew et al 1987b, Lupton et al 1988, Turner et al 1985). In the single randomized control trial of FFP replacement in premature infants less than 1500 g did show a benefit with a reduction in IVH (Beverley et al 1985). Whether therapeutic intervention with plasma products will truly have a positive impact on IVH requires further study. Many alternative forms of therapy have been tested and recently reviewed (Ment et al 1987).

(ii) Respiratory distress syndrome

RDS in newborns is an acute lung disorder characterized by diffuse atelectases, high pulmonary oedema, hyaline membrane formation and right-to-left shunting of pulmonary blood flow (Strang 1966). Pathologically, RDS is characterized by fibrin deposition both intra-alveolarly and intravascularly, thereby suggesting that haemostasis is involved in the pathogenesis (Avery & Mead 1959, Gajl-Paczalska 1964). Numerous haemostatic abnormalities have been described in RDS and include prolongation of the screening tests, low levels of coagulation factors and inhibitors of coagulation (ATIII, protein C and HCII) (Liebermann 1961, Ambrus et al 1963, Stark et al 1968, El-Bardeesy & Johnson 1971, Markarian et al 1971, Mahasandana & Hathaway 1973, Watkins et al 1980, Andrew et al 1983, 1985, Arnold et al 1985, Peters et al 1984). It is quite conceivable that infants with RDS do have low-grade DIC resulting in activation of the haemostatic system and fibrin deposition. The potential benefits of coagulation factor replacement in RDS are unclear. In the past, intervention studies have been performed to assess the effect of both antithrombotic and thrombolytic therapy in RDS (Ambrus et al 1966, 1977, Markarian et al 1971). However, these trials were performed in the 1960s and 1970s and the results cannot be extrapolated to the current management of infants with RDS. More recently, intervention studies with ATIII concentrates have been conducted (Muntean & Rosegger 1989). However, the role of ATIII concentrates as well as other coagulation factor replacement therapy in RDS remain to be clarified.

7. Congenital inhibitor deficiencies

(i) General

Physiological levels of the inhibitors are also altered in newborns compared to adults. Levels for ATIII, heparin cofactor II (HCII), protein C and protein S are 50% or less of adult values (Aballi & de Lamerens 1962, Bleyer et al 1971, Buchanan 1978, 1986, Hathaway & Bonnar 1978, Gobel et al 1979, McDonald & Hathaway 1983, Montgomery et al 1985, Andrew et al 1987b, 1988, 1990b, Anderson et al 1988, Gibson 1989). In contrast, levels for C_1-esterase inhibitor, α_1-antitrypsin, $\alpha_2$antiplasmin (α_2AP) and α_2-macroglobulin (α_2M) are at or above adult values (Aballi & de Lamerens 1962, Bleyer et al 1971, Strothers et al 1975, Buchanan 1978, 1986, Hathaway & Bonnar 1978, Gobel et al 1979, McDonald & Hathaway 1983, Montgomery et al 1985, Andrew et al 1987a, 1988, 1990b, Gibson 1989, Bahakim et al 1990). Overall, newborn plasma inhibits thrombin at a slower rate than adult plasma and α_2M assumes a more important role as an inhibitor of thrombin than for adults.

The heterozygous state for deficiencies of ATIII, protein C or HCII rarely contribute to thrombotic complications during infancy (Bjarke et al 1974, Barnard & Hathaway 1979, Shapiro et al 1981, Mannino & Travner 1983, De Stefano et al 1987, Israels & Seshia 1987). This statement is based on the lack of perinatal problems in the vast majority of adults with these inherited disorders. Typically, the heterozygote adult begins to have problems with thromboembolic complications in the late second and early third decade of life. The emergence of clinical problems matches the physiological decrease in α_2M levels. The close relationship between α_2M levels and thrombotic complications in adults who are at risk on an inherited basis suggests that α_2M may have an important protective role in childhood.

The homozygote form of protein C deficiency does present in the neonatal period with extensive life-threatening complications (Griffen et al 1981, Marciniak et al 1985, Marlar et al 1989). Clinically, these infants present with purpura fulminans, severe DIC, central nervous system thrombosis, blindness and, less often, large-vessel thrombi. The diagnosis of the homozygote infant with protein C deficiency is dependent upon the clinical picture, a protein C level below the reference range for the affected infant and confirmation of the heterozygote state in the parents. Because the physiological levels of homozygous protein C can be as low as 0.12 U/ml measured immunologically, the clinical picture and the confirmation of the heterozygote state in both parents is necessary for the diagnosis to be made. The initial treatment of affected infants is replacement therapy with plasma (10 ml/kg approximately every 12 h). The long-term therapeutic modalities include oral anticoagulant therapy, protein C replacement with plasma products, including protein C concentrates, and liver transplantation (Casella et al 1988).

8. Acquired thrombotic complications

(i) Clinical features

Thromboembolic complications are usually secondary to underlying events in children and occur more frequently in sick infants than at any other time in childhood (Barnard & Hathaway 1979, Schmidt & Zipursky 1984, Schmidt & Andrew 1988). These infants are very ill with a number of underlying problems. The risk factors for thromboembolic complications in newborns include abnormalities in the vessel wall, disturbances of blood flow and alterations in blood coagulability. The presence of a high haematocrit and poor deformability of physiologically large red cells probably enhance blood viscosity and likewise contribute to the formation of thrombotic complications in infancy (Mennuti et al 1974, Aarts et al 1983).

Thrombotic complications occur in both arterial and venous vessels, secondary to catheters in the affected vessel, or, less frequently, spontaneously. In contrast to the adult, vessels in a wide variety of locations are affected in infancy and include radial, pulmonary, temporal, femoral and the aorta or inferior vena cava. Most of these thrombotic complications remain clinically silent and probably do not require further therapy. The latter statement is based on the high rate of clinically silent catheter-related thrombi in the aorta or the inferior vena cava that are not detected nor treated in most nurseries (Barnard & Hathaway 1979, Turitto & Weiss 1980, O'Neill et al 1981, Schmidt & Zipursky 1984, Jackson et al 1987, Schmidt & Andrew 1988). The lack of reports of follow-up complications support the current practice of non-intervention. In contrast, if an infant presents with morbidity or imminent mortality secondary to impaired flow to an organ or limb, intervention in addition to supportive care is warranted. Prior to treatment it is important to confirm the presence of a clot by radiological evaluation. A number of modalities are available although contrast angiography remains the reference standard (Vailas et al 1986, Seibert et al 1987, Schmidt & Andrew 1988). Active intervention therapy includes the use of anticoagulant drugs, thrombolytic agents and, for some infants, surgical removal of the clot.

(ii) Management

The anticoagulant drug of choice in newborns is standard heparin. The protocols used in newborns are directly extrapolated from adults and have not been validated in clinical trials in infants. Based on in vitro tests, plasma from newborns displays an apparent sensitivity to heparin compared to adults. These assays are dependent upon the conversion of endogenous prothrombin to thrombin (i.e. the APTT, PT and thrombin generation assays) (Schmidt et al 1989a). In contrast, plasma from newborns displays an apparent resistance to heparin in assays in which excess amounts of exogenous enzyme (i.e. Xa or thrombin) are added (Schmidt et al 1988, 1989a). Thus, the sensitivity or resistance of newborn plasma to heparin compared to the adult is an in vitro phenomenon reflecting the differing ratios of ATIII to enzyme in the assay system utilized. Which of these in vitro systems will most closely reflect the in vivo antithrombotic effect of heparin in newborns is not known. Until further clinical information is available it seems prudent to carefully follow the clinical response to heparin in combination with non-invasive monitoring (i.e. doppler, duplex ultrasound) in an affected infant. The starting doses of heparin per kilogram (50 U/kg bolus followed by 20 U/kg per hour) are extrapolated from the lower end of the therapeutic amounts of standard heparin used in the adult. Laboratory monitoring in the form of an APTT or heparin assay may be helpful to ensure that the heparin level is not above the adult therapeutic range as this may place infants at risk of bleeding (McDonald & Hathaway 1983, Levine & Hirsh 1986, Andrew & Schmidt 1988). The duration of treatment will be in part dictated by the underlying disease process. There is no evidence that newborns affected with a thrombotic complication require long-term anticoagulant therapy with oral anticoagulant drugs. If infants remain clinically stable, with no evidence of progression, the heparin can be stopped after 7–10 d and infants followed both clinically and with the use of non-invasive testing.

Infants who develop serious thrombotic complications complicated by organ or limb impairment may benefit from the use of thrombolytic agents (Corrigan 1988). The protocols followed for thrombolytic agents have been directly extrapolated from adults and not proven to be of benefit in newborns. The low plasminogen level in newborns probably limits the effectiveness of the thrombolytic agent used (Andrew et al 1989a, Corrigan et al 1989). Therefore, consideration should be given to administering FFP at the same time as the thrombolytic agent. The FFP will provide a source of both plasminogen and α_2AP. The therapeutic agents used in newborns include streptokinase, urokinase and, more recently, tissue plasminogen activator. The clinical response and resolution as measured by ultrasound should be monitored.

8. Conclusions

In summary, the laboratory evaluation of an infant suspected of having a haemorrhagic or thrombotic complication should include a complete blood count and blood smear, the PT, APTT, TCT and fibrinogen level. Other laboratory investigations are dependent upon the clinical problem and the family history, as well as the results of the initial testing. The appropriate management of infants with haemorrhagic complications is dependent upon the identification of the haemostatic defect. Replacement therapy with either specific factor concentrates, FFP, platelet concentrates or other forms of plasma products, including cryoprecipitate or exchange transfusions, may be indicated depending upon the underlying problem.

APPENDIX

Laboratory tests

1. Evaluation of platelet number and function

Platelet count determinations and the mean platelet volume can be measured for the infant with an EDTA-anticoagulated specimen of 120 µl of blood using a Coulter S^+ counter or other similar automated device.

The bleeding time in newborns has been performed with adult automated devices, modified template devices or Ivy bleeding times (Feusner 1980, Andrew et al 1987b, 1989b, 1990b). More recently, a modified automated device, made specifically for infants, has been tested and provides good reproducibility (Andrew et al 1990). To perform a bleeding time in newborns, the blood pressure cuff is adjusted according to the baby's weight; 30 mmHg in infants greater than 2 kg, 25 mmHg in infants weighing 1–2 kg, and 20 mmHg in infants weighing less than 1 kg (Feusner 1980). A single vertical incision of 2.5 mm in length and 0.5 mm in depth is made on the cleansed skin of the forearm with either an automated device, or a template device modified for newborns (Andrew et al 1987b, 1990b). Vertical incisions are chosen because of the very small arms and superficial location of veins in premature infants. Blood is absorbed from the incision every 15 s with filter paper until the bleeding stops. The upper limit of normal for the modified template is 200 s (Andrew et al 1987b) and for a modified automated device is 135 s (Andrew et al 1990b).

2. Evaluation of thrombocytopenia

A platelet count less than 150×10^9/litre signifies the presence of an underlying disease state although infants are unlikely to have serious bleeding if the degree of thrombocytopenia is mild. Further investigation depends upon the infant's condition and subsequent platelet counts. The examination of the stained peripheral blood film is important both to confirm the thrombocytopenia and to provide information regarding the mechanism(s) involved. The presence of large platelets may be observed on blood films and by direct sizing (see previous section). A bone marrow aspiration can be performed from either the tibia or posterior iliac crest using standard techniques. Particularly in newborns, the lack of megakaryocytes on bone marrow aspirates may reflect sampling difficulties rather than a true reduction in megakaryocyte number. Bone marrow biopsies accurately reflect megakaryocyte mass but are rarely indicated in newborns.

To accurately classify the mechanism of thrombocytopenia, the reference test is a platelet survival using radiolabelled autologous platelets (Joist et al 1983). Due to the limited blood volume in newborns, autologous platelet survivals are not feasible. However ABO compatible platelets from an unrelated, appropriately screened donor may be used instead (Castle et al 1987). After centrifugation and washing with acid–citrate–dextrose (ACD), platelets are resuspended with 30–50 μCi of ^{111}In-labelled oxine and incubated at room temperature for 30 min. The labelled platelets are then recentrifuged with ACD and subsequently resuspended in platelets-poor plasma. Each infant receives 8–15 μCi/kg of ^{111}In-labelled platelets (2–4 ml), with the higher dose used for organ imaging. The labelled platelets are injected into a peripheral intravenous line and blood sampling performed at 1, 6, 8, 12, 24, 48, 72 and 96 h after injection. The blood samples are obtained by microtechniques and consist of 0.5 ml of whole blood collected into EDTA. The ^{111}In radioactivity in the samples is measured in a gamma scintillation well counter and platelet survival curves constructed. The survival curves are fitted to linear, exponential and gamma functions by using the least-squares method in a digital computer (Murphy & Francis 1971). The gamma function is constructed from a multiple hit programme, and should be used for calculations of platelet survival. Radioactivity in the liver and spleen are expressed as a function of the radioactivity in the whole body by using appropriate computer-generated regions of interest. One can calculate the percentage recovery of injected platelets in the 1 h sample (assuming a blood volume of 80 ml/kg) as follows: percentage recovery = (c.p.m./ml) × total blood volume/injected dose. Imaging is performed by using a gamma scintillation camera with a large field of view.

Platelet associated IgG can be measured on 2 ml of whole blood collected into ACD using a variety of techniques. We have used an immunoradiometric assay for newborn samples but the small volumes of blood available for study limits the usefulness of this test (Kelton et al 1983).

3. Coagulation screening tests

Coagulation assays on neonatal plasma samples require the development of microtechniques from existing macroassays (Johnston & Zipursky 1980). The assays to be described require 1–2 ml of whole blood. Plastic tubes containing the correct amount of anticoagulant (usually 9 parts of blood to 1 part of sodium citrate) are prepared in the laboratory and kept in the nursery. The tubes are dated and replaced weekly. Plasma is prepared by centrifugation of the blood sample at 1700 g for 15 min, the plasma removed, placed in a clean plastic tube and recentrifuged for a further

5 min at the same speed. This plasma is removed and aliquoted for immediate and future testing. Before testing, the sample is screened for heparin with a sensitive 2 unit TCT. If a prolonged TCT is found, protamine sulphate is added to the aliquot to be tested and the TCT repeated. If the TCT is now normal, appropriate concentrations of protamine are added to the remaining plasma before the PT and APTT are tested.

The methods used to measure the PT and APTT are dependent on the volume of plasma and the equipment available. Both manual and automated methods are described. The manual method is performed in a water bath with a transparent front panel (see Fig. 8.1).

PT and APTT Manual method

PT. Into a 6 × 50 mm glass tube add 20 μl of plasma and incubate at 37°C for 1 min. Add 40 μl of prewarmed thromboplastin/calcium and start timer. The endpoint is reached when the first strand of fibrin forms.

APTT. Into a 6 × 50 mm glass tube add 20 μl of plasma and 20 μl of APTT reagent. Mix and incubate at 37°C for the time interval recommended for the APTT reagent used. Add 20 μl of calcium chloride solution (0.02 M or 0.025 M). Start timer and record the time of fibrin formation.

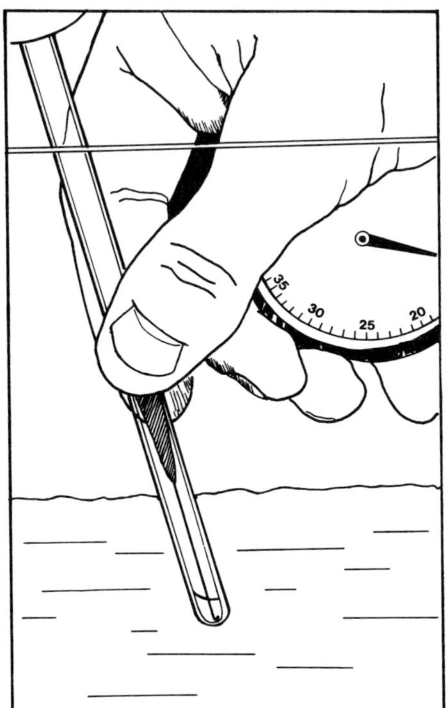

Fig. 8.1 The manual method for coagulation tests is performed in a water bath with a transparent front panel.

Automated method

The method described is for an ACL automated analyser (Instrumentation Laboratory).

For both the PT and APTT, 160 μl of plasma is placed in a micro sample cup (Kodak micro tube No. 1212115, Kodak, Canada).

For the PT, 50 μl of plasma is automatically pipetted into the rotor followed by 100 μl of thromboplastin. A fibrinogen value is calculated by the delta change in light scatter from the PT reaction (see p. 240).

For the APTT, 50 μl of plasma is pipetted from the micro plasma cup into the rotor. The instrument automatically adds the reagent and calcium chloride solution after the recommended incubation time.

Other automated instruments, capable of using reduced plasma volumes, can be used. The protocols for each particular instrument are followed.

TCT

The TCT functions as a screen for heparin contamination and the presence of low fibrinogen levels. The method described is a calcium thrombin clotting time, which makes it relatively insensitive to FDP and to fetal fibrinogen.

Reagents.

Bovine thrombin. Diluted to 100 U/ml in normal saline. The thrombin is aliquoted and frozen at −70°C and is diluted to 2 U/ml for use.

Seeger's buffer. 33.5 ml of 0.15 M sodium chloride, 6.6 ml of 1% calcium chloride solution, 13.3 ml of Acacia (15% solution in 0.15 M sodium chloride), 66.6 ml of imidazole (Glyoxaline buffer, pH 7.3).

Method. Into a 6 × 50 mm glass tube add 60 μl of Seeger's titration mixture, 20 μl of plasma and 20 μl of 2 U/ml thrombin. Start timer. The endpoint is the first appearance of fibrin.

The control plasma time for a 2 U/ml TCT must be 23–27 s. If the TCT is prolonged, 1 μl of protamine sulphate (1 U/ml) is added to 20 μl of plasma and the TCT repeated. If the test is now normal, an appropriate amount of protamine is added to the plasma for the PT and APTT.

Fibrinogen

The measurement of fibrinogen is a useful screening test for the newborn. Three different methods are described.

The first method is the thrombin clottable assay of Clauss (Clauss 1957).

Dilutions of a fibrinogen standard plasma are prepared in a test-tube or reaction cup depending on the instrumentation available:

Dilution	Plasma volume (μl)	Buffer volume (μl)
1:10	10	90
1:15	10	140
1:20	5	95

1:30	5	145
1:40	5	195.

100 μl of the diluted plasma is incubated at 37°C for 2–3 min. 50 μl of thrombin (100 U/ml) is added and the timer started. Each dilution is measured in duplicate and the results plotted on log–log paper as concentration against time (Fig. 8.2). Two dilutions are made for the control plasma and 1:10 and 1:20 dilutions are assayed as above.

For newborn samples the first dilution made is 1:10. The second dilution is dependent on the result obtained with the first dilution and either a 1:5 or 1:20 dilution is made and assayed.

The second method is a capillary fibrinogen method which is based on the Clauss assay. Micropipettes are prepared by diluting a standard preparation of heparin to 50 U/ml in water. A standard glass 100 μl micropipette is rinsed with the heparin solution, the residual liquid is blown out and the tubes dried.

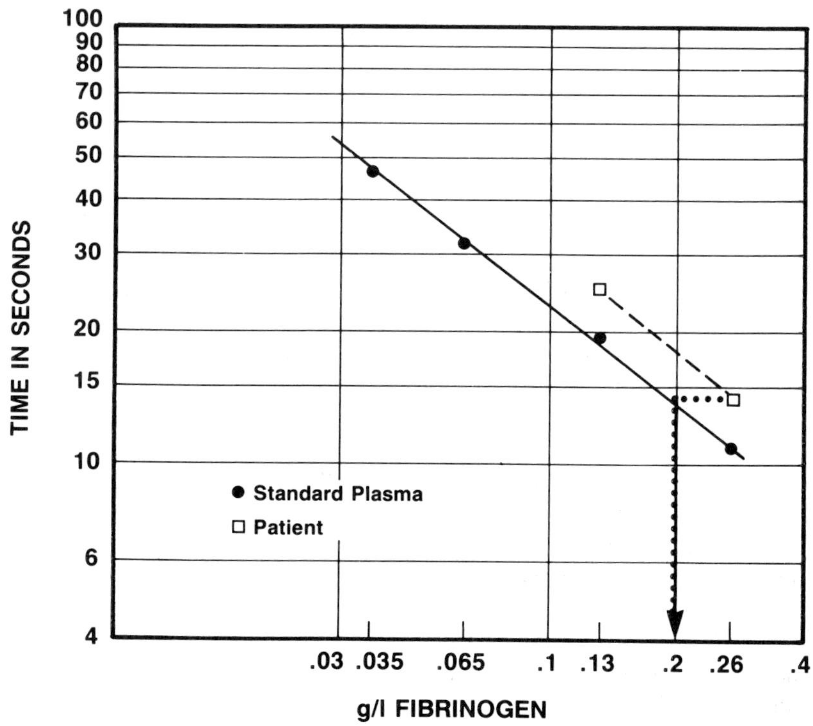

Fig. 8.2 Concentration of fibrinogen versus time for the thrombin clottable assay of Clauss (Clauss 1957). The solid line represents a standard line derived from the clotting time of the diluted fibrinogen standards 1:10 (0.26 g/l), 1:20 (13 g/l), 1:40 (0.65 g/l) and 1:80 (0.035 g/l). The dotted line joins the clotting times of 1:10 and 1:20 dilutions of patient plasma. In this case the 1:10 dilution has a clotting time of 14 s equivalent to a fibrinogen concentration of 0.20. The fibrinogen concentration is multiplied by 10 to convert to grams per litre.

To prepare the blood collecting tube, 400 μl of veronal buffer and 10 μl of buffered sodium citrate is pipetted into a 12 × 75 mm plastic tube.

The method for collection and assay is as follows. 100 μl of capillary blood is drawn into the heparinized tube and immediately rinsed into the citrate/buffer tube. The blood is centrifuged and the diluted plasma removed. 100 μl of the diluted plasma is pipetted into the reaction tube, followed by 50 μl of thrombin (100 U/ml) (Clauss method). The dilution of plasma used is calculated from the haematocrit:

$$\frac{\text{Plasma volume per 100 μl of blood}}{\text{Buffer/anticoagulant + Plasma volume}} = \text{Dilution.}$$

The third method is a fibrinogen value calculated by the ACL coagulometer, which is an accurate estimate of fibrinogen in normal plasmas. However, an over-estimation of fibrinogen is obtained in patients receiving thrombolytic therapy and in some cases of DIC. The level and type of fibrin/fibrinogen degradation product determines the degree of short polymer assembly and therefore false high values on the ACL analyser.

4. *Coagulation factor assays*

Factors VIII, IX, XI, and XIII

These factors are assayed in an identical manner with the variable being the particular factor-deficient plasma. The method, based on the one-stage assay of Biggs (Biggs 1972), is modified for use on semi-automated and automated instruments.

Method. Dilutions of standard plasma are made in either a 12 × 75 mm test-tube or reaction cuvette of the instrument (1:10 = 10 μl of plasma and 90 μl of veronal buffer; 1:20 = 5 μl of plasma and 95 of buffer, etc.).

Method for an automated instrument. Into the reaction cuvette pipette, 100 μl of each dilution of diluted plasma, 100 μl of a deficient plasma and 100 μl of APTT reagent. Mix and incubate for the recommended time. Add 20 μl of prewarmed calcium chloride solution (0.02 or 0.025 M).

Method for a manual microtechnique. Into a 6 × 50 mm glass tube, pipette 20 μl of diluted plasma, 20 μl of deficient plasma and 20 μl of APTT reagent. Mix and incubate for the recommended time. Add 20 μl of prewarmed calcium chloride solution.

The clotting times are determined and the results plotted against concentration (units per millilitre) on semi-log paper. The patient plasma is diluted 1:10 and 1:20 in buffer and the results are read off the standard curve. By making the plasma dilution directly into the reaction well or test-tube only 15 μl of patient plasma is required for each assay. If manual testing is done, the four assays will use only 15 μl of plasma.

Factors II, V, VII and X

These factors are assayed in an identical manner using plasma deficient in the factor of interest. Factor VII and factor X are prepared by immunodepletion of normal plasma. Factor II-deficient plasma is prepared from bovine plasma by adsorption with tricalcium phosphate (50 mg/ml of plasma). The preparation is stirred continually for 10 min and then centrifuged (Owren 1949). Factor V-deficient plasma is prepared by prolonged incubation of normal plasma collected into sodium oxalate. Dilutions of standard and patient plasma are prepared as described previously (Biggs 1972).

Method. Into a 12 × 75 mm test tube or reaction cup, pipette 25 μl of diluted plasma and 25 μl of deficient plasma. Mix and add 100 μl of prewarmed thromboplastin. The clotting times are plotted on semi-log paper against the concentration of the factor of interest. The four extrinsic assays can be measured using a total of 30 μl of plasma.

5. *Paracoagulation assays*

D-dimer and FDP assays utilize a latex agglutination technique and are both commercially available (Greenberg et al 1987).

D-dimer assay (see also Chapter 6)

25 μl of latex beads coated with monoclonal D-dimer antibody are pipetted onto a clear glass slide. 10 μl of plasma is added, mixed and the slide gently rocked for 3 min. The sample is observed for agglutination. Depending on the degree of agglutination, either a 1:2 or 1:8 dilution is made. If the sample is positive at a 1:8 dilution, further dilutions may be made or a result of >2000 ng/ml reported. Positive and negative controls are included.

Fibrinogen/fibrin degradation products

Preparation of serum samples. Into a 6 × 50 mm glass tube, pipette 25 μl of plasma, 25 μl of a mixture of 0.1 M ε-amino-n-caproic acid in 0.025 M calcium chloride solution. Add 1 μl of 5000 U/ml thrombin. Mix and leave for 30 min at room temperature (1 μl of 5000 U/ml thrombin). The tube is centrifuged to obtain serum.

Method. The starting serum sample is a 1:2 dilution and, if required, further dilutions are made in a saline glycine buffer. (Buffer: 7.5 g of glycine, 8.5 g of sodium chloride, made up to 980 ml with distilled water. The pH is adjusted to 8.2 with 2 N sodium hydroxide. The volume is brought up to 1000 ml with water.) Onto a ringed glass slide pipette, place 10 μl of latex particles coated with an antihuman fibrinogen or antihuman D- and E-fibrinogen fragments and then add 10 μl of each dilution of serum. Mix gently and rock for 2 min and observe for agglutination of the latex particles. The normal value in our laboratory is <0.025 g/l.

Thrombin–ATIII complexes

These complexes are assayed using a commercially available kit (e.g. Hoechst, Behring Diagnostics). The assay is an enzyme-linked immunological assay utilizing antihuman thrombin antibodies as the capture antibody and ATIII antibodies conjugated with horseradish peroxidase as the second antibody. Blood taking must be atraumatic to avoid false high values. The method used is as described by the manufacturer.

6. *Evaluation of vitamin K deficiency*

To distinguish between liver disease and vitamin K deficiency, two rapid assays of prothrombin are made (Corrigan & Kryc 1980). One is a standard calcium-dependent biological assay using thromboplastin as the activator. The second assay uses the snake venom *Echis carinatus* as the activator. This venom is specific for the activation of prothrombin and has no calcium requirements. It will therefore activate the decarboxylated forms of prothrombin (i.e. PIVKA).

Method. Dilutions of normal plasma are made in veronal buffer for the standard curve starting with 1:5 (1.0 U/ml), 1:10 (0.5 U/ml), etc. Into a glass tube or instrument reaction well, pipette 50 μl of each dilution of plasma, 50 μl factor II-deficient plasma and 50 μl of Ecarin[1]. Start timer.

A standard curve is constructed with concentration (in units per millilitre) versus time (in seconds) on log–log paper. Patient and control plasmas are diluted 1:5 and 1:10 and assayed as above. The values are read off the standard line. The biological assay for factor II is described under coagulation factor assays (see p. 241)

7. *Coagulation inhibitors*

The inhibitors ATIII, protein C, protein S and HCII are measured both immunologically and functionally. Immunological assays for the serine protease inhibitors can be measured using a Mancini radial immunodiffusion plate (Mancini et al 1965), Laurell rocket electrophoresis (Laurell 1965) or commercial enzyme-linked immunoabsorbent assay (ELISA) (Amiral et al 1984). We measure ATIII by radial immunodiffusion with commercially available antibodies (Atlantic Antibodies), and proteins C and S by ELISA assays (Diagnostica Stago). The plates are precoated and the method described by the manufacturer is used. HCII antibody is obtained from Diagnostica Stago and measured by Laurell rocket electrophoresis using 5 μl of plasma.

---

[1] Ecarin (Diagnostica Stago). A vial is diluted with 1 ml of water and 1 ml of 0.15 M saline. It can be used fresh or freeze–thawed.

Functional assays for the serine protease inhibitors are measured using commerically available chromogenic kits. Protein C and ATIII are assayed using Berichrom kits from Behring (Hoechst). A commercial kit from Diagnostica Stago is available for the HCII functional assay.

Protein C assay

The protein C kit contains protein C activator, a lyophilized extract from the venom of *Agkistrodon contortrix*, Hepes buffer (pH 8.25) and lyophilized substrate (3.3 mM). The reagents are prepared according to manufacturers' instructions.

Method. To a cuvette add 25 μl of plasma and 250 μl of venom. The sample is mixed and incubated for 5 min. 50 μl of substrate is added and the delta absorbence per minute is calculated.

ATIII assay

The ATIII kit contains α-thrombin with heparin and aprotinin, hydrochloric acid buffer (pH 8.2) and 2 mM substrate.

Method. Plasmas are diluted 1: 40 in saline (5 μl and 195 μl of buffer). 25 μl of the diluted plasma is pipetted into a cuvette followed by 500 μl of diluted thrombin. This is incubated for 3 min and 50 μl substrate added. The change in delta absorbance is measured.

HCII assay

The HCII assay uses the following reagents: thrombin (2.75 U/ml), substrate (0.9 μmol/ml) and buffer pH 8.4 containing 0.1 mg/ml dermatan sulphate.

Method. The assay has been adapted for use on an ACL 300 R analyser, which is programmed as follows:

Loading conditions:
Sample volume, 60 μl
Reagent volume (position 2), 60 μl
Reagent volume (position 3), 60 μl

Incubation and acquisition conditions:
Reaction time, 120 s
Inter-ramp interval, 3 s
Delay time, 0 s
Acquisition time, 90 s
Speed, 1200 r.p.m.

Dilutions of a standard plasma are made in assay buffer (1:40, 1:80, 1:160). Control and patient samples are diluted 1:80. The standards are placed in positions 1, 2 and 3 of the sample holder. Buffer is placed in position 4 followed by controls and patients. Thrombin is placed in reagent holder 2 and substrate in 3.

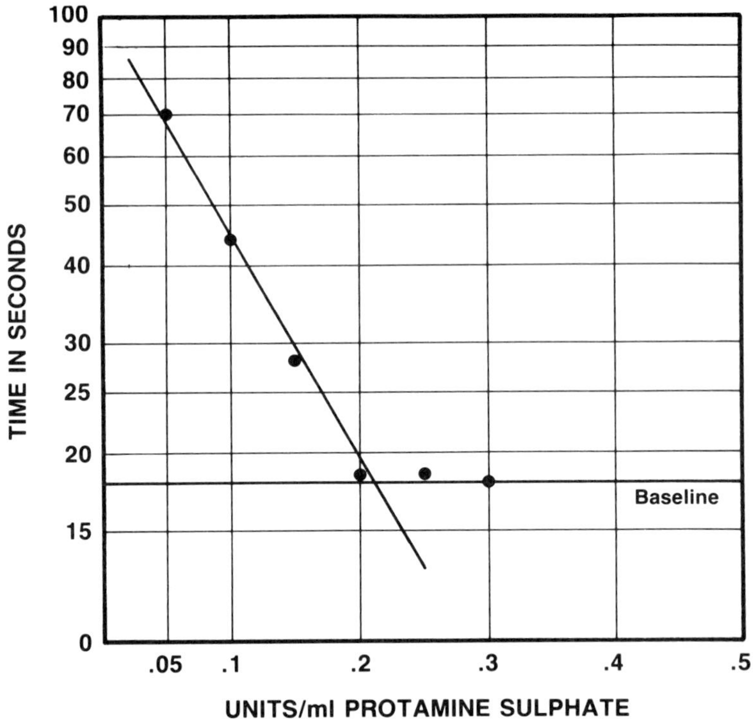

Fig. 8.3 Measurement of heparin activity by the protamine assay. The point at which the line crosses the normal baseline is equal to the heparin concentration.

The ACL analyser will automatically pick up plasma, thrombin and substrate, incubate and read for the appropriate times. The data is transmitted to a computer and delta absorbances determined using the ACL research program. The delta absorbances are plotted on linear graph paper.

The assay can also be done using microtitre plates and read as an endpoint method on a microtitre plate reader or in test-tubes and transferring to a cuvette for reading at 405 nm in a spectrophotometer.

8. Heparin assays

Two assays for heparin measurement are the protamine sulphate neutralization test (Refn & Vestergaard 1954) and the Xa inhibition assay (Teien & Lie 1977).

Protamine assay

This is a thrombin inhibition assay and considered to be the reference assay for determining therapeutic heparin ranges. Varying concentrations of protamine sulphate are added to plasma and thrombin times measured.

Method. Microsample into a 6 × 50 mm glass tube, add 20 µl of plasma, 1 µl of a protamine dilution and 20 µl of thrombin (~3 U/ml). Start timer and record the clotting time.

This first concentration of protamine will be dependent on the initial thrombin time of the sample. The longer the TCT, the greater the concentration of protamine added to the sample. The procedure is repeated 3–4 times with differing protamine dilutions and the clotting times are plotted on semi-log paper versus the protamine sulphate concentrations. A straight line should be obtained and the point at which the line crosses the normal baseline is equal to the heparin concentration (see Fig. 8.3).

Xa heparin assay

This is a chromogenic method and a number of commercial kits are available. The manufacturers' method is followed. The principle of the assay is as follows. Xa is added to plasma diluted in a buffer containing ATIII and the mixture is incubated for exactly 1 min. A Xa-specific substrate is added and the delta absorbance measured. The amount of Xa inhibited is inversely proportional to the concentration of heparin in plasma. This assay uses 10 µl of plasma compared to a protamine heparin assay which requires a minimum of 100 µl of plasma.

REFERENCES

Aarts P A M M, Bolhuis P A, Sakariassen K S, Heethaar R M, Sixma J J 1983 Red blood cell size is important for adherence of blood platelets to artery subendothelium. Blood 62: 214–217

Aballi A J, de Lamerens S 1962 Coagulation changes in the neonatal period and in early infancy. Pediatric Clinics of North America 9: 785–817

Abbondanzo S L, Gootenberg J E, Lofts R S, McPherson R A 1988 Intracranial haemorrhage in congenital deficiency of factor XIII. American Journal of Pediatric Haematology and Oncology 10: 65–68

Adner M M, Fisch G R, Starobin S G 1969 Use of 'compatible' platelet transfusions in treatment of congenital isoimmune thrombocytopenic purpura. New England Journal of Medicine 280: 244–247

Ahlsten G, Ewald U, Tuvemo T 1983 Cord blood platelet aggregation: Quality control by a two-sample technique. Upsala Journal of Medical Sciences 88: 9–15

Ahlsten G, Ewald U, Tuvemo T 1985 Arachidonic acid induced aggregation of platelets from human cord blood compared with platelets from adults. Biology of the Neonate 47: 199–204

Ahlsten G, Ewald U, Tuvemo T 1986 Maternal smoking reduces prostacyclin formation in human umbilical arteries. A study on strictly selected pregnancies. Acta Obstetrica Gynecologica Scandinavica 65: 645–649

Alebouyeh M, Lusher J M, Ameri M R, Evans R K, Robinson A 1978 The effect of 5-hydroxytryptamine and epinephrine on newborn platelets. European Journal of Pediatrics 128: 163–168

Alexander W A, Cooper B, Handin R I 1978 Characterization of the human platelet α-adrenergic receptor. Journal of Clinical Investigation 61: 1136–1144

Allison P M, Mummah-Schendel L L, Kindberg C G, Harms C S, Bang N U, Suttie J W 1987 Effects of a vitamin K-deficient diet and antibiotics in normal human volunteers. Journal of Laboratory and Clinical Medicine 110: 180–188

Ambrus C M, Weintraub D H, Dunphy D, Dowd J E, Pickren J W, Niswander K R, Ambrus J L 1963 Studies on hyaline membrane disease. I. The fibrinolysin system in pathogenesis and therapy. Pediatrics 32: 10–24
Ambrus C M, Weintraub D, Ambrus J L 1966 Studies on hyaline membrane disease. III. Therapeutic trial of urokinase-activated human plasmin. Pediatrics 38: 231–243
Ambrus C M, Choi T S, Cunnanan E et al 1977 Prevention of hyaline membrane disease with plasminogen. A cooperative study. Journal of the American Medical Association 237: 1837–1841
Amiral J, Adalbert B, Adam M 1984 Application of enzyme immunoassays to coagulation testing. Clinical Chemistry 30: 1512–1516
Anderson J M, Brown J K, Cockburn F 1974 On the role of disseminated intravascular coagulation on the pathology of birth asphyxia. Developmental Medicine and Child Neurology 16: 581–591
Andersson T R, Bangstad H, Larsen M L 1988 Heparin cofactor II and antithrombin and protein C in plasma from term and preterm infants. Acta Paediatrica Scandinavica 77: 485–488
Andrew M 1991 The hemostatic system in the infant. In: Nathan D, Oski F (eds) Haematology of infancy and childhood, 4th edn W B Saunders, Boston (in press)
Andrew M, Karpatkin M 1982 A simple screening test for evaluating prolonged partial thromboplastin times in newborn infants. Journal of Pediatrics 101: 610
Andrew M, Kelton J 1984 Neonatal thrombocytopenia. Clinical Perinatology 11: 359–391
Andrew M, Massicotte-Nolan P M, Karpatkin M 1983 Plasma protease inhibitors in premature infants: Influence of gestational age, postnatal age and health status. Proceedings of the Society for Experimental Biology and Medicine 173: 495–500
Andrew M, Massicotte-Nolan P, Mitchell L, Cassidy K 1985 Dysfunctional antithrombin III in sick premature infants. Pediatric Research 19: 237–239
Andrew M, Paes B, Milner R, Johnston M, Mitchell L, Tollefsen D M, Powers P 1987a The development of the human coagulation system in the fullterm infant. Blood 70: 165–172
Andrew M, Castle V, Saigal S, Carter C, Kelton J 1987b Clinical impact of neonatal thrombocytopenia. Journal of Pediatrics 110: 457–464
Andrew M, Mitchell L, Berry L, Schmidt B, Hatton M W 1988 Fibrinogen has a rapid turnover in the healthy newborn lamb. Pediatric Research 23: 249–252
Andrew M, Paes B, Milner R et al 1988 Development of the human coagulation system in the healthy premature infant. Blood 72: 1651–1657
Andrew M, Brooker L, Weitz J 1989a Fibrin clot lysis by thrombolytic agents is impaired in the newborn. Thrombosis and Haemostasis 62: 288 (abstract)
Andrew M, Castle V, Mitchell L, Paes B 1989b A modified bleeding time in the infant. American Journal of Haematology 30: 190–191
Andrew M, Mitchell L, Paes B, Berry L, Burrows R, Khambalia B, Ofosu F 1990a A circulating anticoagulant in the fetus and mother. Pediatric Research 27: 262a (abstract)
Andrew M, Paes B, Johnston M 1990b Development of the hemostatic system in the neonate and young infant. American Journal of Pediatric Haematology Oncology 12: 95–104
Andrew M, Schmidt B 1988 Seminars in Thrombosis and Haemostasis 14: 28–32.
Andrew M, Schmidt B, Mitchell L, Paes B, Ofosu F 1990c Thrombin generation in newborn plasma is critically dependent on the concentration of prothrombin. Thrombosis and Haemostasis 63: 27–30
Andrew M, Paes B, Bowker J, Vegh P 1990 Evaluation of an automated bleeding time device in the newborn. American Journal of Haematology 35: 275–277
Arad I D, Alpan G, Sznajderman S D, Eldor A 1986 The mean platelet volume (MPV) in the neonatal period. American Journal of Perinatology 3: 1–3
Arnold J, O'Brodovich H, Whyte R, Coates G 1985 Pulmonary thromboemboli after neonatal asphyxia. Journal of Pediatrics 106: 806–809
Astrowe P S, Palmerton E S 1941 Clinical studies with vitamin K in newborn infants. Journal of Pediatrics 18: 507–515
Avery M E, Mead J 1959 Surface properties in relation to atelectasis and hyaline membrane disease. American Journal of Disease of Children 97: 517–523
Bahakim H, Gader A, Galil A, Babbar F A-A, Gaafar T H, Edrees Y B 1990 Coagulation parameters in maternal and cord blood at delivery. Annals of Saudi Medicine 10: 149–155
Ballin A, Koren G, Kohelet D, Burger R, Greenwald M, Bryan C A, Zipursky A 1987 Reduction of platelet counts induced by mechanical ventilation in newborn infants. Journal of Pediataric 111: 445–449

Ballin A, Andrew M, Ling E, Perlman M, Blanchette 1988 High-dose intravenous gammaglobulin therapy for neonatal autoimmune thrombocytopenia. Journal of Pediatrics 112: 789–792
Barbui T, Cortelazzo S, Viero P, Buelli M, Casarotto C 1985 Idiopathic thrombocytopenic purpura and pregnancy. Maternal platelet count and antiplatelet antibodies do not predict the risk of neonatal thrombocytopenia. Ricerca in Clinica e in Laboratorio 15: 139–144.
Barnard D R, Hathaway W E 1979 Neonatal thrombosis. American Journal of Pediatric Haematology/Oncology 1: 235–244
Barnard D R, Simmons M A, Hathaway W E 1979 Coagulation studies in extremely premature infants. Pediatric Research 13: 1330–1335
Barradas M A, Mikhailidis D P 1986 An investigation of maternal and neonatal platelet function. Biological Research in Pregnancy and Perinatology 7: 60-65
Barton J C, Saleh M N, Stedman C M, Lobuglio A T 1987 Case report: Immune thrombocytopenia: effects of maternal gammaglobulin infusion on maternal and fetal serum, platelet, and monocyte IgG. American Journal of Medical Science 293: 112–118
Behrmann B A, Chan W K, Finer N N 1985 Resurgence of hemorrhagic disease of the newborn, a report of 3 cases. Canadian Medical Association Journal 133: 884–885
Beverley D W, Chance G W, Inwood M J, Schaus M, O'Keefe B 1984a Intraventricular haemorrhage and haemostasis defects. Archives of Disease in Childhood 59: 444–448
Beverley D W, Inwood M J, Chance G W, Schaus M, O'Keefe B 1984b 'Normal' haemostasis parameters: a study in a well-defined inborn population of preterm infants. Early Human Development 9: 249–257
Beverley D W, Pitts-Tucker T J, Congdon J, Arthur R J, Tate I G 1985 Prevention of intraventricular haemorrhage by fresh frozen plasma. Archives of Disease in Childhood 60: 710–713
Biggs R 1972 Human blood coagulation. In: Biggs R (ed) Haemostasis and thrombosis. Blackwell Scientific, Oxford p 614
Binder L 1986 Hemorrhagic disease of the newborn: an unusual etiology of neonatal bleeding. Annals of Emergency Medicine 15: 935–938
Bjarke B, Herin P, Blomback M 1974 Neonatal aortic thrombosis. A possible clinical manifestation of congenital antithrombin III deficiency. Acta Paediatrica Scandinavica 63: 297–301
Blajchman M A, Sheridan D, Rawls W E 1984 Risks associated with blood transfusion in newborn infants. Clinics in Perinatology 11: 403–413
Blanchette V S 1988 Neonatal alloimmune thrombocytopenia: a clinical perspective. Current Studies in Haematology and Blood Transfusion 54: 112–126
Blanchette V S, Sacher R A, Ballem P J, Bussel J B, Imbash P 1989 Commentary on the management of autoimmune thrombocytopenia during pregnancy and in the neonatal period. Blut 59: 121–123
Bleyer W A, Breckenridge R T 1970 Studies on the detection of adverse drug reactions in the newborn. II. The effects of prenatal aspirin on newborn hemostasis. Journal of the American Medical Association 213: 2049–2053
Bleyer W A, Hakami N, Shepard T H 1971 The development of hemostasis in the human fetus and newborn infant. Journal of Pediatrics 79: 838–853
Bloch C A, Rothberg A D, Bradlow B A 1984 Mother–infant prothrombin precursor status at birth. Journal of Pediatric Gastroenterology and Nutrition 3: 101–103
Boyd J F 1966 Disseminated fibrin thromboembolism in stillbirths; a histological picture similar to one form of maternal hypofibrinogenemia. Journal of Obstetrics and Gynaecology in the British Commonwealth 73: 629–639
Boyd J F 1969 Disseminated fibrin thromboembolism among neonates dying more than 48 hours after birth. Journal of Clinical Pathology 22: 663–671
Brockmeier F K, Nordhagen R, Finne P H 1983 Neonatal alloimmune thrombocytopenia. Acta Paediatrica Scandinavica 72: 583–587
Brown S G, McHugh G M, Shapleski J, Wotherspoon P A, Taylor B J, Gillett W R 1989 Should intramuscular vitamin K prophylaxis for haemorrhagic disease of the newborn be continued? A decision analysis. New Zealand Medical Journal 102: 3–5
Buchanan G R 1978 Neonatal coagulation: normal physiology and pathophysiology. Clinical Haematology 1: 85–109
Buchanan G 1986 Coagulation disorders in the neonate. Pediatric Clinics of North America 33: 203–220

Burrows R F, Kelton J G 1988 Incidentally detected thrombocytopenia in healthy mothers and their infants. New England Journal of Medicine 319: 142–145
Burrows R F, Kelton J G 1990 Low fetal risks in pregnancies associated with idiopathic thrombocytopenic purpura do not justify obstetrical interventions. American Journal of Obstetrics and Gynecology 163: 147–150
Burrows R F, Caco C C, Kelton J G 1988 Neonatal alloimmune thrombocytopenia: Spontaneous in utero intracranial haemorrhage. American Journal of Haematology 28: 98–102
Bussell J P, Berkowitz R L, McFarland J G, Lynch L, Chitkara U 1988 Antenatal treatment of neonatal alloimmune thrombocytopenia. New England Journal of Medicine 319: 1374–1378
Cade J F, Hirsh J, Martin M 1969 Placental barrier to coagulation factors: Its relevance to the coagulation defect at birth and to haemorrhage in the newborn. British Medical Journal 2: 281–283
Casella J F, Bontempo F A, Markel H, Lewis J H, Zitell B J, Starzl T E 1988 Successful treatment of homozygous protein C deficiency by hepatic transplantation. Lancet 1: 435–437
Castaman G, Rodeghiero F, Ronconi G F, Dini E 1985 Successful treatment of neonatal autoimmune thrombocytopenia with high-dose intravenous immunoglobulins. Haematologica (Pavia) 70: 276–277 (letter)
Castle V, Andrew M, Kelton J, Carter C, Giron D, Johnston M 1986 Frequency and mechanism of neonatal thrombocytopenia. Journal of Pediatrics 108: 749–755
Castle V, Coates G, Kelton J, Andrew M 1987 ^{111}Indium oxine platelet survivals in the thrombocytopenic infant. Blood 70: 652–656
Chaou W-T, Chou M-L, Eitzman D V 1984 Intracranial haemorrhage and vitamin K deficiency in early infancy. Journal of Pediatrics 105: 880–884
Chirico G, Duse M, Ugazio A, Rondini G 1983 High-dose intravenous gamma-globulin therapy for passive immune thrombocytopenia in the neonate. Journal of Pediatrics 103: 654–655
Ciccimarra F, De Curtis M, Paludetta R, Romano G, Troncone R 1984 Treatment of neonatal passive immune thrombocytopenia. Journal of Pediatrics 105: 677–678 (letter)
Cines D B, Dusak B, Tomaski A, Mennutti M, Schreiber A D 1982 Immune thrombocytopenic purpura and pregnancy. New England Journal of Medicine 306: 826–831
Clauss A 1957 Gerinnungsphysiologische Schnellmethod zur Bestimmung des Fibrinogens Acta Haematologica 17: 237–246
Colman R W, Marder V J, Salzman E W, Hirsh J 1987 Overview of hemostasis. In: Colman R W, Hirsh J, Marder V J, Salzman E W (eds) Hemostasis and thrombosis principles and clinical practice. J B Lippincott, Philadelphia p 3–8
Corby D G, Barr T P 1981 Decreased alpha-adrenergic receptors in newborn platelets. Cause of abnormal response to epinephrine. Developmental Pharmacology and Therapeutics 2: 215–225
Corby D G, O'Barr T P 1981 Neonatal platelet function: a membrane-related phenomenon? Haemostasis 10: 177–185
Corby D G, Schulman I 1971 The effects of antenatal drug administration on aggregation of platelets of newborn infants. Journal of Pediatrics 79: 307–313
Corby D G, Zuck T F 1976 Newborn platelet dysfunction: a storage pool and release defect. Thrombosis and Haemostasis 36: 200–207
Corrazza M S, Davis R F, Merritt A, Bejar R, Cvetnic W 1984 Prolonged bleeding time in preterm infants receiving indomethacin for patent ductus arteriosus. Journal of Pediatrics 105: 292–296
Corrigan J 1988 Neonatal thrombosis and the thrombolytic system. Pathophysiology and therapy. American Journal of Pediatric Haematology/Oncology 10: 83–91
Corrigan J J 1979 Activation of coagulation and disseminated intravascular coagulation in the newborn. American Journal of Pediatric Haematology/Oncology 1: 245–249
Corrigan J J, Kryc J J 1980 Factor II (prothrombin) levels in cord blood. Correlation of coagulant activity with immunoreactive protein. Journal of Pediatrics 97: 979–983
Corrigan J J, Sluth J J, Jeter M, Lox C D 1989 Newborn's fibrinolytic mechanism: components and plasmin generation. American Journal of Haematology 32: 273–278

Cox A C, Rao G H R, Gerrard J M, White J G 1980 The influence of vitamin E quinone on platelet structure, function and biochemistry. Blood 55: 907–914
Daffos F, Forestier F, Muller J Y, Reznikoff-Etievant M, Habibi B, Capella-Pavlovski M, Maigret P, Kaplan C 1984 Prenatal treatment of alloimmune thrombocytopenia. Lancet ii: 632 (letter)
Daffos F, Capella-Pavlovsky M, Forestier F 1985 Fetal blood sampling during pregnancy with use of a needle guided by ultrasound: a study of 606 consecutive cases. American Journal of Obstetrics and Gynecology 153: 655–660
Daffos F, Forestier F, Kaplan C, Cox W 1988 Prenatal diagnosis and management of bleeding disorders with fetal blood sampling. American Journal of Obstetrics and Gynecology 158: 939–946
Daiguji M, Meltzer H Y, U'Prichard D C 1981 Human platelet α_2 adrenergic receptors: Labelling with ^{3}H yohimbine, a selective antagonist ligand. Life Sciences 28: 2705–2715
Davidson B N, Rayburn W F, Bishop R C, Fleming W P, Beer A E 1987 Immunoglobulin therapy for autoimmune thrombocytopenic purpura during pregnancy. A report of two cases. Journal of Reproductive Medicine 32: 107–109
Davies S V, Murray J A, Gee H, Giles H McC 1986 Transplacental effect of high-dose immunoglobulin in idiopathic thrombocytopenia purpura (ITP). Lancet i: 1098–1099
De Stefano V, Leone G, De Carolis M P et al 1987 Antithrombin III in fullterm and preterm newborn infants: three cases of neonatal diagnosis of AT III congenital defect. Thrombosis and Haemostasis 57: 329–331
De Swiet M 1985 Maternal autoimmune disease and the fetus. Archives of Disease in Childhood 60: 794–797
De Lemos R A, McLaughlin G W, Koch H F, Diserens H W 1973 Abnormal partial thromboplastin time and survival in respiratory distress syndrome. Effect of exchange transfusion. Pediatric Research 7: 396 (abstract)
Derycke M, Dreyfus M, Ropert J C, Tchernia G 1985 Intravenous immunoglobulin for neonatal isoimmune thrombocytopenia. Archives of Disease in Childhood 60: 667–669
Dunn P M 1982 Vitamin K for all newborn babies (C). Lancet ii: 770 (letter)
Editorial 1985 Late onset of hemorrhagic disease of the newborn. Nutrition Reviews 43: 303
Editorial 1989 Management of alloimmune neonatal thrombocytopenia. Lancet i: 137
El-Bardeesy M W, Johnson A M 1971 Serum proteinase inhibitors in infants with hyaline membrane disease. Journal of Pediatrics 81: 579–587
Fetus and Newborn Committee 1988 Canadian Pediatric Society: the use of vitamin K in the perinatal period. Canadian Association Medical Journal 139: 127–130
Feusner J H 1980 Normal and abnormal bleeding time in neonates and young children utilizing a fully standardized template technique. American Journal of Pathology 74: 73–77
Feusner J H, Slichter S J, Harker L A 1983 Acquired haemostatic defects in the ill newborn. British Journal of Haematology 53: 73–84
Forbes D 1983 Delayed presentation of haemorrhagic disease of the newborn. Medical Journal of Australia 2: 136–138
Forestier F, Daffos F, Rainaut M, Sole Y, Amiral J 1985 Vitamin K dependent proteins in fetal hemostasis at mid trimester pregnancy. Thrombosis and Haemostasis 53: 401–403
Forestier F, Daffos F, Galacteros F, Bardakjian J, Rainaut M, Berezard Y 1986 Hematological values of 163 normal fetuses between 18 and 30 weeks of gestation. Pediatric Research 20: 342–346
Friedman J M, Aster R H 1985 Neonatal alloimmune thrombocytopenic purpura and congenital porencephaly in two siblings associated with 'new' maternal antiplatelet antibody. Blood 65: 1412–1415
Friedman Z, Whitman V, Maisels M J, Berman W, Marks K H, Vesell E S 1978 Indomethacin disposition and indomethacin induced platelet dysfunction in premature infants. Journal of Clinical Pharmacology 18: 272–279
Fujimura Y, Mimura Y, Kinoshita S, Yoshioka A, Kitawaki T, Yoshioka K 1982 Studies on vitamin K-dependent factor deficiency during early childhood with special reference to prothrombin activity and antigen level. Haemostasis 11: 90–95
Fujimura Y, Okubo Y, Sakai T, Sugimoto M, Takase T, Yoshioka A, Fukui H 1984 Studies on precursor proteins PIVKA-II, -IX, and -X in the plasma of patients with 'hemorrhagic disease of the newborn'. Haemostasis 14: 211–217

Gader A M A, Bahakim H, Jabber F A, Lambourne A L, Gaafar T H 1988 Dose–response aggregometry in maternal/neonatal platelets. Thrombosis and Haemostasis 60: 314–318
Gajl-Paczalska K 1964 Plasma protein composition of hyaline membrane in the newborn as studied by immunofluorescence. Archives of Disease in Childhood 39: 226–231
Galankis D K, Mosesson M W 1976 Evaluation of the role of in vivo proteolysis (fibrinogenolysis) in prolonging the thrombin time of human umbilical cord fibrinogen. Blood 48: 109–118
Garrow D, Chisholm M, Radford M 1986 Vitamin K and thrombotest values in full term infants. Archives of Disease in Childhood 61: 349–351
Gersony W M, Peckham G J, Ellison R C, Miettinen O S, Nadas A S 1983 Effects of indomethacin in premature infants with patent ductus arteriosus: results of a national collaborative study. Journal of Pediatrics 102: 895–906
Gibson B 1989 Neonatal haemostasis. Archives of Disease in Childhood 64: 503–506
Gill F M 1983 Thrombocytopenia in the newborn. Seminars in Perinatology 7: 201–212
Girolami A, De Marco L, Dal Bo Zanon R, Patrassi R, Cappellato M G 1985 Rarer quantitative and qualitative abnormalities of coagulation. Clinics in Haematology 14: 385–411
Gobel U, Voss H C Petrich C, Jurgens H, Oliver A 1979 Etiopathology and classification of acquired coagulation disorders in the newborn infant. Klinische Wochenschrift 57: 81–86
Goddard-Finegold J 1984 Periventricular, intraventricular haemorrhages in the premature newborn. Update on pathologic features, pathogenesis and possible means of prevention. Archives of Neurology 41: 766–771
Gogstad G O, Brostad F, Krutnes M-B, Hagen I, Solum N O 1982 Fibrinogen-binding properties of the human platelet glycoprotein IIb–IIIa complex: a study using crossed-radioimmunoelectrophoresis. Blood 60: 663–671
Goldschmidt B, Bors S, Szabo A 1988 Vitamin K-dependent clotting factors during longterm parenteral nutrition in fullterm and preterm infants. Journal of Pediatrics 112: 108–111
Grant J A, Scrutton M C 1980 Interaction of selective α-adrenoceptor agonists and antiagonists with human and rabbit blood platelets. British Journal of Pharmacology 71: 121–134
Gray O P, Ackerman A, Fraser A J 1968 Intracranial haemorrhage and clotting defects in low birth weight infants. Lancet i: 545–581
Greenberg C S, Devine D V, McCrae K M 1987 Measurement of plasma fibrin D-dimer levels with the use of a monoclonal antibody coupled to latex beads. American Journal of Clinical Pathology 87: 94–100
Greer F R, Mummah-Schendel L L, Marshall S, Suttie J W 1988 Vitamin K_1 (phylloquinone) and Vitamin K_2 (menaquinone) status in newborns during the first week of life. Pediatrics 81: 137–140
Griffen J H, Evatt B, Zimmerman T S, Kleiss A J, Wideman C 1981 Deficiency of protein C in congenital thrombotic disease. Journal of Clinical Investigation 68: 1370–1373
Gross S, Melhorn D K 1971 Exchange transfusion with citrated whole blood for disseminated intravascular coagulation. Journal of Pediatrics 78: 415–419
Gross S J, Filston H C, Anderson J C 1982 Controlled study of treatment for disseminated intravascular coagulation in the neonate. Journal of Pediatrics 100: 445–448
Gruel Y, Boizard B, Daffos F, Forestier F, Caen J, Wautier J L 1986 Determinations of platelet antigens and glycoproteins in the human fetus. Blood 68: 488–492
Hall J G, Levin J, Kuhn J P, Ottenheimer E J, van Berkum K A P, McKusick K A 1969 Thrombocytopenia with absent radius. Medicine 48: 411–439
Hambleton G, Appleyard W J 1973 Controlled trial of fresh frozen plasma in asphyxiated low birthweight infants. Archives of Disease in Childhood 48: 31–35
Hamulyak K, de Boer-van den Berg M A G 1987 The placental transport of [^{3}H]vitamin K_1 in rats. British Journal of Haematology 65: 335–338
Hamulyak K, Nieuwenhuizen W, Devillee P P, Hemker H C 1983 Re-evaluation of some properties of fibrinogen purified from cord blood of normal newborns. Thrombosis Research 32: 301–320
Hanada H, Ono I 1985 A neonate with passive ITP effectively treated with high-dose intravenous gammaglobulin. Rinsho Ketsueki 27: 808
Hanada T, Abe T, Takita H 1985 Antithrombin III concentrates for treatment of disseminated intravascular coagulation in children. American Journal of Pediatrics 7: 3–8

Hanawa Y, Maki M, Murata B et al 1988 The second nation-wide survey in Japan of vitamin K deficiency in infants. European Journal of Pediatrics 147: 472–477
Hara T, Kukita J, Yamashita H et al 1988 Intravenous gammaglobulin for prolonged passive immune thrombocytopenia. Acta Paediatrica Japan 30: 627–631
Harker L A, Slichter S J 1972 The bleeding time as a screening test for evaluation of platelet function. New England Journal of Medicine 287: 155–159
Haroon Y, Shearer M J, Rahim S, Gunn W G, McEnery G, Barkhan P 1982 The content of phylloquinone (vitamin K_1) in human milk, cow's milk and infant formula foods determined by high-performance liquid chromatography. Journal of Nutrition 112: 1105–1117
Hathaway W E 1986 ICTH Subcommittee on neonatal hemostasis. Thrombosis and Haemostasis 55: 145
Hathaway W E 1987 New insights on vitamin K. Haematology/Oncology Clinics of North America 1: 367–379
Hathaway W, Bonnar J 1978. Perinatal coagulation. Grune & Stratton, New York
Hayden C K, Shattuck K E, Richardson C J, Ahrendt D K, House R, Swischu K 1985 Subependymal germinal matrix haemorrhage in fullterm neonates. Pediatrics 75: 714–718
Hedberg V A, Lipton J M 1988 Thrombocytopenia with absent radii. A review of 100 cases. American Journal of Pediatric Haematology/Oncology 10: 51–64
Hegde U M 1985 Immune thrombocytopenia in pregnancy and the newborn. British Journal of Obstetrics and Gynaecology 92: 657–659
Herman J, Resnitzky P, Fink A 1918 Association between thyrotoxicosis and thrombocytopenia. A case report and review of the literature. Israel Journal of Medical Sciences 14: 469–475
Herman J H, Jumbelic M I, Anconer R J, Kickler T S 1986 In utero cerebral haemorrhage in alloimmune thrombocytopenia. American Journal of Pediatric Haematology/Oncology 8: 312–317
Hicsomnez G, Prozorova-Zamani V 1980 Platelet aggregation in neonates with hyperbilirubinemia. Scandinavian Journal of Haematology 24: 67–70
Hiraike H, Kimura M, Itokawa Y 1988a Determination of K vitamins (phylloquinone and menaquinones) in umbilical cord plasma by a platinum-reduction column. Journal of Chromatography 430: 143–148
Hiraike H, Kimura M, Itokawa Y 1988b Distribution of K vitamins (phylloquinone and menaquinones) in human placenta and maternal and umbilical cord plasma. American Journal of Obstetrics and Gynecology 158: 564–569
Hirsh J, Ofosu F, Cairns J 1985 Advances in antithrombotic therapy. In: Hoffbrand A V (ed) Recent advances in haematology. Churchill Livingstone, Edinburgh, vol 4, p 333–367
Holmberg L, Henriksson P, Ekelund H, Astedt B 1974 Coagulation in the human fetus, comparison with term newborn infants. Journal of Pediatrics 85: 860–864
Imbach P, Barandun S, d'Apuzzo V et al 1981 High-dose intravenous gammaglobulin for idiopathic thrombocytopenic purpura in childhood. Lancet i: 1228–1231
Israels S J, Seshia S S 1978 Childhood stroke associated with protein C or S deficiency. Journal of Pediatrics 111: 562–564
Israels S J, Gowen B, Gerrard J M 1978 Contractile activity of neonatal platelets. Pediatric Research 21: 293–295
Jackson J C, Truog W E, Watchko J F, Mack L A, Cyr D R, van Belle G 1987 Efficacy of thromboresistant umbilical artery cathertes in reducing aortic thrombosis and related complications. Journal of Pediatrics 110: 102–105
Jacqz E M, Barrow S E, Dollery C T 1985 Prostacyclin concentrations in cord blood and in the newborn. Pediatrics 76: 954–957
Jenkins C S, Phillips D R, Clemetson K J, Meyer D, Larrieu M-J, Luscher E F 1976 Platelet membrane glycoproteins implicated in ristocetin-induced aggregation. Journal of Clinical Investigation 57: 112–124
Jensen A H, Josso S, Zamet P, Monset-Couchard M, Minkowski A 1973 Evolution of blood clotting factors in premature infants during the first 10 days of life: a study of 96 cases with comparison between clinical status and blood clotting factor levels. Pediatric Research 7: 638–644
Johnson C A, Snyder M S, Weaver R L 1982 Effects of fresh frozen plasma infusions on coagulation screening tests in neonates. Archives of Disease in Childhood 57: 950–952
Johnston M, Zipursky A 1980 Microtechnology for the study of the blood coagulation system in newborn infants. Canadian Journal of Medical Technology 42: 159–164

Joist H J, Baker K R, Welch M J 1983 Methodologic and basic aspects of Indium^{111} labelled platelets. Seminars in Thrombosis and Haemostasis 9: 86–99
Jones C R, McCabe R, Hamilton C A, Reid J L 1985 Maternal and fetal platelet responses and adrenoreceptor binding characteristics. Thrombosis and Haemostasis 53: 95–98
Kaapa P, Knip M, Viinikka L, Ylikorkala O 1986a Increased platelet thromboxane B_2 production in newborn infants of diabetic mothers. Prostaglandins Leukoktrienes, Medicine 21: 299–304
Kaapa P, Uhari M, Nikkari J, Viinikka L, Ylikorkala O 1986b Dietary fatty acid and platelet thromboxane production in puerperal women and their offspring. American Journal of Obstetrics and Gynecology 155: 146–149
Kaden B R, Rosse W, Hauch T W 1979 Immune thrombocytopenia in lymphoproliferative diseases. Blood 53: 545–551
Kaplan C, Daffos F, Forestier F, Cox W L, Lyon-Caen M C, Dupuy-Montean M C, Salmon C 1988 Management of alloimmune thrombocytopenia: antenatal diagnosis and in utero transfusion of maternal platelets. Blood 72: 340–343
Karpatkin M 1984 Corticosteroid therapy in thrombocytopenic infants of women with autoimmune thrombocytopenia. Journal of Pediatrics 105: 623–625
Karpatkin M, Porges R F, Karpatkin S 1981 Platelet counts in infants of women with autoimmune thrombocytopenia: Effects of steroid administration to the mother. New England Journal of Medicine 305: 936–939
Karpatkin M, Mannucci P M, Mannuccio Manniuci P, Bhogal M, Vigano S, Nardi M 1986 Low protein C in the neonatal period. British Journal of Haematology 62: 137–142
Karpatkin S, Strick N, Karpatkin M G, Siskind A W 1972 Cumulative experience in the detection of antiplatelet antibody in 234 patients with idiopathic thrombocytopenic purpura, systemic lupus erythematosus and other clinical disorders. American Journal of Medicine 52: 776–785
Katz J, Hodder F S, Aster R S, Bennetts G A, Cairo M S 1984 Neonatal isoimmune thrombocytopenia. The natural course and management and the detection of maternal antibody. Clinical Pediatrics 23: 159–162
Katz J A, Moake J L, McPherson P D, Weinstein M J, Moise K J 1989 Relationship between human development and disappearance of unusually large von Willebrand factor multimers from plasma. Blood 73: 1851–1858
Keenan W J, Jewett T, Glueck H I 1971 Role of feeding and vitamin K in hypoprothrombinemia of the newborn. American Journal of Disease in Children 121: 271–277
Kelly D A, Summerfield J A 1987 Hemostasis in liver disease. Seminars in Liver Disease 7: 182
Kelton J G 1983 Management of the pregnant patient with idiopathic thrombocytopenic purpura. Annals of Internal Medicine 99: 796–800
Kelton J G, Blanchette V S, Wilson W E, Powers P, Pai K R, Effer S B, Barr R D 1980 Neonatal thrombocytopenia due to passive immunization. Prenatal diagnosis and distinction between maternal platelet alloantibodies and autoantibodies. New England Journal of Medicine 302: 1401–1403
Kelton J G, Inwood M J, Barr R M et al 1982 The prenatal prediction of thrombocytopenia in infants of mothers with clinically diagnosed immune thrombocytopenia. American Journal of Obstetrics and Gynecology 144: 449–454
Kelton J G, Denome G, Walker C, Horsewood P, Gauldie K 1983 Measurement of platelet-associated IgG using an immunoradiometric assay. Journal of Immunoassay 4: 65–82
Khurshid M, Lee T J, Pealre I R, Bloom A L 1975 Vitamin E deficiency and platelet functional defect in a jaundiced infant. British Medical Journal 4: 19–21
Kiefel V, Santoso S, Glockner W M, Katzman B, Mayr W R, Mueller-Eckhardt C 1989 Post-transfusion purpura associated with an anti-Bak. Vox Sanguinis 56: 93–97
Kieffer N, Biozard B, Didry, Wauthier J-L, Nurden A T 1984 Immunochemical characterization of the platelet-specific alloantigen Lek^a: a comparative study with the PL^{A1} alloantigen. Blood 64: 1212–1219
Kipper S, Sieger L 1982 Whole blood platelet volumes in newborn infants. Journal of Pediatrics 101: 763–766
Kisker C T, Perlman, Bohlken D, Wicklund B 1988 Measurement of prothrombin mRNA

during gestation and early neonatal development. Journal of Laboratory and Clinical Medicine 112: 407–412
Koepke J A 1986 Partial thromboplastin time — proposed performance guidelines. ICSH Panel on the APTT. Thrombosis and Haemostasis 55: 143–144
Koztalanyi G, Jobst K, Kellermayer M, Ludany A 1980 ADP-induced surface changes of adult and newborn platelets. British Journal of Hematology 46: 257–262
Kries R B, Shearer M J, Gobel U 1988 Vitamin K in infancy. European Journal of Pediatrics 147: 106–112
Kryc J J, Corrigan J J 1983 Idiopathic thrombocytopenic purpura during pregnancy. A pediatric viewpoint. American Journal of Pediatric Haematology/Oncology 5: 21–25
Lam A H, Shulman L A 1985 Ultrasound in congenital intracranial haemorrhage secondary to isoimmune thrombocytopenia. Pediatric Radiology 15: 8–11
Lammle B, Griffin J H 1985 Formation of the fibrin clot: the balance of procoagulant and inhibitory factors. Clinics in Haematology 14: 281–343
Landolfi R, De Cristofaro R, Ciabattoni G, De Carolis S, Durazzis S, Mancini S, Bizzi B 1988 Placental-derived PGI_2 inhibits cord blood platelet function. Haematologica (Pavia) 73: 207–218
Lane P A, Hathaway W E 1985 Medical progress: vitamin K in infancy. Journal of Pediatrics 106: 351–359
Laosombat V 1988 Hemorrhagic disease of the newborn after maternal anticonvulsant therapy: a case report and literature review. Journal of the Medical Association of Thailand 71: 643–648
Laurell C B 1965 Antigen-antibody crossed electrophoresis. Analytical Biochemistry 10: 358–361
Le Gall E, Picaud J C, Treguier C, Fiant M, Oger M O, Jezequel C 1986 High-dose intravenous gammaglobulin therapy for autoimmune thrombocytopenia in two neonates. Archives Francaises de Pediatrie 43: 191–193
Lecompte T 1988 Hereditary thrombocytopenias. Current Studies in Haematology and Blood Transfusion 55: 162–173
Lehmann J 1944. Vitamin K as a prophylactic in 13 000 infants. Lancet i: 493–494
Levine M N, Hirsh J 1986 Hemorrhagic complications of anticoagulant therapy. Seminars in Thrombosis and Hemostasis 12: 39–57
Levy G, Garrettson L K 1974 Kinetics of salicylate elimination by newborn infants of mothers who ingested aspirin before delivery. Pediatrics 53: 201–209
Liebermann J 1961 The nature of the fibrinolytic enzyme defect in hyaline membrane disease. New England Journal of Medicine 265: 363–369
Lorand L, Losowsky M S, Miloszewski K J M 1980 Human factor XIII: fibrin stabilizing factor. Progress in Hemostasis and Thrombosis 5: 245–290
Lupton B A, Hill A, Whitfield M F, Carter C J, Wadsworth L D, Roland E H 1988 Reduced platelet count as a risk factor for intraventricular haemorrhage. American Journal of Diseases of Children 142: 1222–1224
McDonald M M, Hathaway W E 1983 Neonatal haemorrhage and thrombosis. Seminars in Perinatology 7: 213–225
McDonald M M, Johnson M L, Rumack C M, Koops B L, Babb C, Guggenheim M A, Hathaway W E 1984 Role of coagulopathy in newborn intracranial haemorrhage. Pediatrics 74: 26–31
McFarland J G, Frenzke M, Aster R H 1989 Testing of maternal sera in pregnancies at risk for neonatal alloimmune thrombocytopenia. Transfusion 29: 128–133
McGill M, Mayhaus C, Hoff R, Carey P 1987 Frozen maternal platelets for neonatal thrombocytopenia. Transfusion 27: 347–349
McGrath K, Minchinton R, Cunningham I, Ayberk H 1989 Platelet anti-Bak^b, antibody associated with neonatal alloimmune thrombocytopenia. Vox Sanguinis, 57: 182–184
McIntosh S, O'Brien R T, Schwarz S O, Pearson H 1973 Neonatal isoimmune purpura: response to platelet infusions. Journal of Pediatrics 82: 1020–1027
McNinch A W, Orme R L, Tripp J W 1983 Haemorrhagic disease of the newborn returns. Lancet i: 1089–1093
McNinch A W, Upton C, Samuels M, Shearer M J, McCarthy P, Tripp J H, Orme R L 1985 Plasma concentrations after oral or intramuscular vitamin K_1 in neonates. Archives of Disease in Childhood 60: 814–818

Mahasandana C, Hathaway W E 1973 Circulating anticoagulants in the newborn: Relation to hypercoagulability and the idiopathic respiratory distress syndrome. Pediatric Research 7: 670–673
Mammen E F 1983a Fibrinogen abnormalities. Seminars in Thrombosis and Haemostasis 9: 1–9
Mammen E F 1983b Factor V deficiency. Seminars in Thrombosis and Hemostasis 9: 17–18
Mammen E F 1983c Factor II abnormalities. Seminars in Thrombosis and Hemostasis 9: 13–16
Mammen E F 1983d Factor X abnormalities. Seminars in Thrombosis and Hemostasis 9: 31–33
Mancini G, Carbonara O, Heremans J F 1965 Immunochemical quantitation of antigens by single radial immunodiffusion. Journal of Immunochemistry 2: 235–254
Mandelbrot L, Guillaumont M, Forestier F, Lefrere J J, Daffos F, Crozin D, Leclerq M 1988 Placental transfer of vitamin K_1 and its implications in fetal hemostasis. Thrombosis and Haemostasis 60: 39–43
Mannino F L, Travner D A 1983 Stroke in neonates. Journal of Pediatrics 102: 605–610
Marciniak E, Wilson H D, Marlar R A 1985 Neonatal purpura fulminans: a genetic disorder related to the absence of protein C in blood. Blood 65: 15–20
Mariani G, Mazzucconi M G 1983 Factor VII congenital deficiency. Hemostasis 13: 169–177
Markarian M, Lindley A, Jackson J J, Bannon A 1967 Coagulation factors in pregnant women and premature infants with and without the respiratory distress syndrome. Thrombosis Diathesis Haemorrhagica 17: 585–594
Markarian M, Githens J H, Fernandez F, Jackson J J, Bannon A E, Lindley A, Lubchenco L O 1971 Hypercoagulability in premature infants with special reference to the respiratory distress syndrome and haemorrhage. 1. Coagulation studies. Biology of the Neonate 17: 84–97
Marlar R A, Montgomery R R, Broekmans A W, Working Party 1989 Diagnosis and treatment of homozygous protein C deficiency. Journal of Pediatrics 114: 528–534
Martin B, Robin H, Williams R, Ornelas W 1983 Neonatal graft vs. host disease following transfusion of maternal platelets. Transfusion 23: 417 (abstract)
Martin-Bouyer G, Khanh N B, Linh P D et al 1983 Epidemic of haemorrhagic disease in Vietnamese infants caused by warfarin-contaminated talcs. Lancet i: 230–233
Massey G V, McWilliams N B, Mueller D G, Napolitano A, Maurer H M 1987 Intravenous immunoglobulin in treatment of neonatal alloimmune thrombocytopenia. Journal of Pediatrics 111: 133–135
Matsuda I, Nishiyama S, Motohara K, Endo F, Ogata T, Futagoishi Y 1989 Late neonatal vitamin K deficiency associated with subclinical liver dysfunction in human milk-fed infants. Journal of Pediatrics 114: 602–605
Maurer H M, Haggins J C, Still W J S 1976 Platelet injury during phototherapy. American Journal of Hematology 1: 89–96
Mazzucconi M G, Francesconi M, Fidani P et al 1985 Pregnancy, delivery and detection of antiplatelet antibodies in women with idiopathic thrombocytopenic purpura. Haematologica (Pavia) 70: 506–509
Mehta P, Vasa R, Newman L, Karpatkin M 1980 Thrombocytopenia in the high-risk infant. Journal of Pediatrics 97: 791–794
Mennuti M, Schwartz R H, Gill F 1974 Obstetric management of isoimmune thrombocytopenia. American Journal of Obstetrics and Gynecology 118: 565–568
Ment L R, Duncan C C, Ehrenkranz R A 1987 Intraventricular haemorrhage of the preterm neonate. Seminars in Perinatology 11: 132–141
Mir N, Samson D, House M J, Kavan I Z 1988 Failure of antenatal high-dose immunoglobulin to improve fetal platelet count in neonatal alloimmune thrombocytopenia. Vox Sanguinis 55: 188
Moise K J, Carpenter R J, Cotton D B, Wasserstrom N, Kirshon B, Cano L 1988 Percutaneous umbilical cord blood sampling in the evaluation of fetal platelet counts in pregnant patients with autoimmune thrombocytopenia purpura. Obstetrics and Gynecology 72: 346–350
Montgomery R R, Marlar R A, Gill J C 1985 Newborn haemostasis. Clinical Haematology 14: 443–460
Morell A, Skvaril F, Van Loghem E, Kleemola M 1971 Human IgG subclasses in maternal and fetal serum. Vox Sanguinis 21: 481–492

Motohara K, Endo F, Matsuda I 1985 Effect of vitamin K administration of acarboxy prothrombin (PIVKA-II) levels in newborns. Lancet ii: 242–246
Motohara K, Endo F, Matsuda I 1986 Vitamin K deficiency in breast-fed infants at one month of age. Journal of Pediatric Gastroenterological Nutrition 5: 931–933
Motohara K, Endo F, Matsuda I 1987 Screening for late neonatal vitamin K deficiency by acarboxyprothrombin in dried blood spots. Archives of Disease in Childhood 62: 370–375
Motohara K, Matsukane I, Endo F, Kiyota Y, Matsuda I 1989 Relationship of milk intake and vitamin K supplementation to vitamin K status in newborns. Pediatrics 84: 90–93
Mountain K R, Hirsh J, Gallius A S 1970 Neonatal coagulation defect due to anticonvulsant drug treatment in pregnancy. Lancet i: 265–268
Mueller-Eckhardt C, Becker T, Weishert M, Witz C, Santosa S 1986 Neonatal alloimmune thrombocytopenia due to fetomaternal Zw^b incompatibility. Vox Sanguinis 50: 94–96
Mueller-Eckhardt C, Kiefel V, Grubert A et al 1989 348 cases of suspected neonatal alloimmune thrombocytopenia. Lancet i: 363–366
Mull M M, Hathaway W E 1970 Altered platelet function in newborns. Pediatric Research 4: 229–237
Muntean W, Rosegger H 1989 Antithrombin III concentrate in preterm infants with IRDS: an open, controlled, randomized clinical trial. Thrombosis and Haemostasis 62: 288 (abstract)
Muntean W, Petck W, Rosanelli K, Mutz I D 1979 Immunologic studies of prothrombin in newborns. Pediatric Research 13: 1262–1265
Murphy E A, Francis M E 1971 The estimation of blood platelet survival. II. The multiple hit model. Thrombosis Diathesis Haemorrhagica 25: 53–80
Murphy W G, Moore J C, Kelton J G 1987 Calcium dependent cysteine protease activity in the sera of patients with thrombotic thrombocytopenic purpura. Blood 70: 1683–1687
Nachman R L, Jaffe E A Weksler B B 1971 Immuno-inhibition of ristocetin induced aggregation. Journal of Clinical Investigation 59: 143–158
Nathan D J, Snapper I 1958 Simultaneous placental transfer of factors responsible for LE cell formation and thrombocytopenia. American Journal of Medicine 25: 647–653
Newland A C, Boots M A, Patterson K G 1984 Intravenous IgG for autoimmune thrombocytopenia in pregnancy. New England Journal of Medicine 310: 261–262
Nicolini U, Rodeck C H, Kochenour N K, Greco P, Fisk N M, Letsky E 1988 In utero platelet transfusion for alloimmune thrombocytopenia. Lancet ii: 506 (letter)
O'Connor M E, Addiego J E 1986 Use of oral vitamin K_1 to prevent hemorrhagic disease of the newborn infant. Journal of Pediatrics 108: 616–619
O'Neill J A, Neblett W W III, Born M L 1981 Management of major thromboembolic complications of umbilical artery catheters. Journal of Pediatric Surgery 16: 972–978
Ockelford P A, Carter C J 1982 Disseminated intravascular coagulation: The application and utility of diagnostic tests. Seminars in Thrombosis and Hemostasis 8: 198–216
Ogata T, Motohara K, Endo F et al 1988 Vitamin K effect in low birth weight infants. Pediatrics 81: 423–427
Okomura T, Jamieson T A 1976 Platelet glycocalicin: a single receptor for platelet aggregation induced by thrombin ristocetin. Thrombosis Research 8: 701–706
Olson J A 1987 Recommended dietary intakes (RDI) of vitamin K in humans. American Journal of Clinical Nutrition 45: 687–692
Ostermann H, van de Loo J 1986 Factors of the hemostatic system in diabetic patients. A survey of controlled studies. Haemostasis 16: 386–416
Owren P A 1949 A quantitative one stage method for the assay of prothrombin. Scandinavian Journal of Clinical and Laboratory Investigation 1: 81–83
Payne N R, Hasegawa D K 1984 Vitamin K deficiency in newborns: a case report in α-1-antitrypsin deficiency and a review of factors predisposing to hemorrhage. Pediatrics 73: 712–716
Pearson H A, McIntosh S 1978 Neonatal thrombocytopenia. Clinical Haematology 7: 111–122
Pearson H A , Shulman N R, Marder V J, Cone T E 1964 Isoimmune neonatal thrombocytopenic purpura. Clinical and therapeutic considerations. Blood 23: 154–177
Peters M, Jansen E, ten Cate J W, Kahle L H, Ockelford P, Breederveld C 1984a Neonatal antithrombin III. British Journal of Haematology 58: 579–587
Peters M, ten Cate J W, Breederveld C, De Leeuw R, Emeis J, Koppe J 1984b Low antithrombin III levels in neonates with idiopathic respiratory distress syndrome: poor prognosis. Pediatric Research 18: 273–276

Podolsak B 1973 Thrombopoiesis in newborn infants after exchange blood transfusion. Zeitschrift fur Kinderheilkd 114: 13–26
Ragni M V, Lewis J J, Spero J A, Hasiba U 1986 Factor VII deficiency. American Journal of Haematology 10: 79–88
Rapaport S I, Proctor R R, Patch J J, Yettra M 1961 The mode of inheritance of PTA deficiency: evidence for the existence of major PTA deficiency and minor PTA deficiency. Blood 18: 149–165
Refn I, Vestergaard L 1954 The titration of heparin with protamine. Scandinavian Journal of Clinical and Laboratory Investigation 6: 284–287
Reznikoff-Etieant M F, Kaplan C, Durieux I, Huchet J, Salmon C, Netter A 1988 Alloimmune thrombocytopenias, definition of a group at risk; a prospective study. Current Studies in Haematology and Blood Transfusion 55: 119–124
Ronconi G F, Castaman G, Fantuz E, Rodeghiero F 1986 Treatment of passive-acquired immune thromboctyopenia of the newborn with high-dose intravenous gammaglobulin infusion. Pediatria Medica E Chirurgica (Vincenz) 7: 567–568
Sacher R A, King J C 1989 Intravenous gammaglobulin in pregnancy: a review. Obstetrical and Gynecological Survey 44: 25–34
Samuels P, Main E K, Tomaski A, Mennuti M T, Gabbe S A, Cines D B 1987 Abnormalities in platelet antiglobulin tests in preeclamptic mothers and their neonates. American Journal of Obstetrics and Gynecology 157: 109–113
Sann L, Leclercq M, Guillaumont M, Trouyez R, Bethenod M, Bourgeay-Causse M 1985 Serum vitamin K_1 concentrations after oral administration of vitamin K_1 in low birth weight infants. Journal of Pediatrics 107: 608–611
Schmidt B, Andrew M 1988 Neonatal thrombotic disease: prevention, diagnosis and therapy. Journal of Pediatrics, 113: 407–410
Schmidt B, Zipursky A 1984 Thrombotic disease in newborn infants. Clinics in Perinatology 11: 461–488
Schmidt B, Zipursky A 1986 Disseminated intravascular coagulation masking neonatal hemophilia. Journal of Pediatrics 109: 886–888
Schmidt B, Mitchell L, Ofosu F, Andrew M 1988 Standard assays underestimate the concentration of heparin in neonatal plasma. Journal of Laboratory and Clinical Medicine 112: 641–643
Schmidt B, Ofosu F A, Mitchell L, Brooker L A, Andrew M 1989a Anticoagulant effects of heparin in neonatal plasma. Pediatric Research 25: 405–408
Schmidt B, Mitchell L, Ofosu F, Andrew M 1989b Alpha-2-macroglobulin is an important progressive inhibitor of thrombin in neonatal and infant plasma. Thrombosis and Haemostasis 62: 1074–1077
Seibert J J, Taylor B J, Williamson S L, Williams B T, Szabo J S, Corbitt S L 1987 Sonographic detection of neonatal umbilical-artery thrombosis. American Journal of Roentgenology 148: 965–968
Seip M 1960 Systemic lupus erythematosus in pregnancy with haemolytic anaemia, leukopenia, and thrombocytopenia in the mother and her newborn infant. Archives of Disease in Childhood 35: 364–366
Setzer E S, Webb I B, Wassenaar J W, Reeder J D, Mehta P S, Eitzman D V 1982 Platelet dysfunction and coagulopathy in intraventricular hemorrhage in the premature infant. Journal of Pediatrics 100: 599–605
Shapiro M E, Riodvien R, Bauer K A, Salzman E W 1981 Acute aortic thrombosis in antithrombin III deficiency. Journal of the American Medical Association 245: 1759–1781
Shapiro A D, Jacobson L J, Aramon M E, Manco-Johnson M J, Hulac P, Lane P, Hathaway W E 1986 Vitamin K deficiency in the newborn infant: prevalence and perinatal risk factors. Journal of Pediatrics 109: 675–680
Shearer M J, Barkhan P, Rahhim S, Stimmler L 1982 Plasma vitamin K_1 in mothers and their newborn babies. Lancet ii: 460–463
Shibata Y, Miyaji T, Ichikawa Y, Matsuda I 1986a A new platelet antigen system, Yuk^a/Yuk^b. Vox Sanguinis 51: 334–336
Shibata Y, Matsuda I, Miyaji T, Ichikawa Y 1986b Yuk^a, a new platelet antigen involved in two cases of neonatal alloimmune thrombocytopenia. Vox Sanguinis 50: 177–180
Shinnar S, Molteni A, Gammon K, D'Souza B J, Altman J, Freeman J M, 1982 Intraventricular hemorrhage in the premature infant: a changing outlook. New England Journal of Medicine 306: 1464–1468

Shinzawa T, Mura T, Tsunei M, Shiraki Z 1989 Vitamin K absorption capacity and its association with vitamin K deficiency. American Journal of Disease in Childhood 143: 686–689
Shirahata A, Nojiri T, Takaragi S, Horiuchi T, Yamada K 1982 Normotest screenings and prophylactic oral administration for idiopathic vitamin K deficiency in infancy. Acta Haematologica (Japan) 45: 867–875
Shulman N R, Aster R H, Pearson H A, Hiller M C 1962 Immunoreactions involving platelets. VI. Reactions of maternal isoantibodies responsible for neonatal purpura. Differentiation of a second platelet antigen system. Journal of Clinical Investigation 41: 1059–1069
Shulman N R, Marder V J, Hiller M C, Collier E M 1964 Platelet and leukocyte isoantigens and their antibodies: serologic, physiologic and clinical studies. Progress in Haematology 4: 222–304
Sidiropoulos D, Straume B 1984 The treatment of neonatal isoimmune thrombocytopenia with intravenous immunoglobulin (IgG i.v.). Blut 48: 383–386
Silverstein A 1960 Intracranial bleeding in hemophilia. Archives of Neurology 3: 141–157
Skyberg D, Jacobsen C D 1969 Defibrination syndrome in a newborn, and its treatment with exchange transfusion. Acta Paediatrica Scandinavica 58: 83–86
Srinivasan G, Seeler R A, Tiruvury A, Pildes R S 1982 Maternal anticonvulsant therapy and hemorrhagic disease of the newborn. Obstetrics and Gynecology 59: 250–252
Stabile A, Pesaresi M A, Sopo S M, Segni G 1986 Effective high-dose intravenous gammaglobulin therapy for passive immune thrombocytopenia in the neonate. European Journal of Pediatrics 146: 90–91
Stark C R, Abramson D, Erkan V 1968 Intravascular coagulation and hyaline-membrane disease of the newborn. Lancet i: 1180–1181
Strang L B 1966 The pulmonary circulation in the respiratory distress syndrome. Pediatric Clinics of North America 13: 693–730
Straub P W 1975 A case against heparin therapy of intravascular coagulation. Thrombosis Diathesis Haemorrhagica 33: 107–112
Strothers J, Boulton F, Wild R, Ibbotson R, Mila P, Lloyd M, Snodgrass H 1975 Neonatal coagulation. Lancet i: 408–409 (letter)
Stuart M J 1972 Vitamin E deficiency: its effect on platelet-vascular interaction in various pathologic states. Annals of the New York Academy of Sciences 277.
Stuart M J 1977 Storage pool deficiency in neonatal platelets. Thrombosis and Haemostasis 38: 4 (abstract)
Stuart M J 1978 The neonatal platelet: evaluation of platelet malonyl dialdehyde formation as an indicator of prostaglandin synthesis. British Journal of Haematology 39: 83–90
Stuart M J 1979 Platelet function in the neonate. American Journal of Pediatric Hematology/ Oncology 1: 227–234
Stuart M J, Allen J B 1982 Arachidonic acid metabolism in the neonatal platelet. Pediatrics 69: 714–718
Stuart M J, Dusse J 1985 In vitro comparison of the efficacy of cyclooxygenase inhibitors on the adult versus neonatal platelet. Biology of the Neonate 47: 265–269
Stuart J, Breeze E G, Picken A M, Wood B S 1973 Capillary blood coagulation profile in the newborn. Lancet ii: 1467–1471
Stuart M J, Elrad H, Graeber J E, Hakanson D O, Sunderji S G, Barvirchak M N 1979 Increased synthesis of prostaglandin endoperoxides and platelet hyperfunction in infants of mothers with diabetes mellitus. Journal of Laboratory and Clinical Medicine 94: 12–26
Stuart M J, Gross S J, Elrad H, Graeber J E 1982 Effects of acetylsalicylic acid ingestion on maternal and neonatal hemostasis. New England Journal of Medicine 307: 909–912
Stuart M J, Dusse J, Clark D A, Walenga R W 1984 Differences in thromboxane production between neonatal and adult platelets in response to arachidonic acid and epinephrine. Pediatric Research 18: 823–826
Stuart M, Wu J, Sunderji S, Cranley C 1987 Effect of amniotic fluid on platelet thromboxane production. Journal of Pediatrics 11: 289–292
Suarez C R, Menendez C E, Walenga J M, Fareed J 1984 Neonatal and maternal hemostasis. Value of molecular markers in the assessment of hemostatic status. Seminars in Thrombosis and Haemostasis 10: 280–284
Suarez C R, Gonzalez J, Menendez C, Fareed J, Fresco R, Walenga J 1988 Neonatal and maternal platelets: activation at time of birth. American Journal of Haematology 29: 18–21

Sutherland J M, Glueck H I 1967 Hemorrhagic disease of the newborn; breast feeding as a necessary factor in the pathogenesis. American Journal of Disease in Children 113: 524–533
Suvansri U, Cheung W H, Sawitsky A 1969 The effect of bilirubin on the human platelet. Journal of Pediatrics 74: 240–246
Tate D Y, Carlton G T, Johnson D et al 1981 Immune thrombocytopenia in severe neonatal infections. Journal of Pediatrics 98: 449–453
Tchernia G, Dreyfus M, Laulrian Y, Derycke M, Mirica C, Kerbrat G 1984 Management of immune thrombocytopenia in pregnancy: response to infusions of immunoglobulins. American Journal of Obstetrics and Gynecology 148: 225–226
Teien A N, Lie M 1977 Evaluation of amidolytic heparin assay method. Increased sensitivity by adding purified antithrombin III. Thrombosis Research 10: 399–410
Territo M, Finklestein J, Oh W, Hobel C, Kattlove H 1973 Management of autoimmune thrombocytopenia in pregnancy and in the neonate. Obstetrics and Gynecology 41: 579–584
Ts'ao C 1977 Comparable inhibition of PRP of neonates and adults by aspirin. Haemostasis 6: 118–126
Ts'ao C H, Green D, Schultz K 1976 Function and ultrastructure of platelets of neonates; enhanced ristocetin aggregation of neonatal platelets. British Journal of Haematology 32: 225–233
Turitto V T, Weiss H J 1980 Red blood cells: their dual role in thrombus formation. Science 207: 541–543
Turner T, Prouse C V, Prescott R J, Cash J D 1981 A clinical trial on the early detection and correction of haemostatic defects in selected high-risk neonates. British Journal of Haematology 47: 65–75
Vailas G N, Brouillette R T, Scott J P, Shkolnik A, Conway J, Wiringa K 1986 Neonatal aortic thrombosis: recent experience. Journal of Pediatrics 109: 101–108
Vietti T J, Murphy T P, James J A, Pritchard J A 1960 Observation on the prophylactic use of vitamin K in the newborn. Journal of Pediatrics 56: 343–346
Volpe J J 1981 Neonatal intraventricular hemorrhage. New England Journal of Medicine 304: 886–891
Volpe J J 1983 Intraventricular hemorrhage: incidence, neuropathology, and pathogenesis. Neonatology Letter 1:1
von dem Borne A E G K, Von Riesz E, 1980 Bak^a, a new platelet-specific antigen involved in neonatal alloimmune thrombocytopenia . Vox Sanguinis 9: 113–120
von dem Borne A E G K, van Leeuwen E F, von Reisz L E, van Boxtel C J, Engelfriet C P 1981 Neonatal alloimmune thrombocytopenia: detection and characterization of the responsible antibodies by the platelet immunofluorescent test. Blood 57: 649–656
Von Kries R, Stannigel H, Gobel U 1985 Anticoagulant therapy by continuous heparin–antithrombin III infusion in newborns with disseminated intravascular coagulation. European Journal of Pediatrics 114: 191–194
Von Kries R, Kreppel S, Becker A, Gobel U, Tangermann R 1987a Acarboxyprothrombin activity after oral prophylactic vitamin K. Archives of Disease in Childhood 62: 938–940
Von Kries R, Shearer M J, McCarthy P T, Haug M, Hanzer G, Gobel U 1987b Vitamin K_1 content of maternal milk: influence of the stage of lactation, lipid composition, and vitamin K_1 supplements given to the mother. Pediatric Research 22: 513–517
Von Kries R, Becker A, Gobel U 1987c Vitamin K in the newborn: influence of nutritional factors on acarboxy-prothrombin detectability and factor II and VII clotting activity. European Journal of Pediatrics 146: 123–127
Walenga R W, Sunderji S G, Stuart M J 1988 Formation of hydroxyeicosatetraenoic acids (HETE) in blood form adults versus neonates: reduced production of 12-HETE in cord blood. Pediatric Research 24: 563–567
Waltt H, Kurz R, Mitterstieler G, Fodisch J H, Hohenauer L, Rossler H 1973 Intracranial haemorrhage in low birth weight infants and prophylactic administration of coagulation factor concentrates. Lancet i: 1284–1288
Watkins M N, Swan S, Caprini J A, Gardner T H, Zuckerman L, Vagher J P 1980 Coagulation changes in the newborn with respiratory failure. Thrombosis Research 17: 153–175

Wefring K W 1962 Hemorrhage in the newborn and vitamin K prophylaxis. Journal of Pediatrics 61: 686–692

Weinstein M J, Blanchard R, Moake J L, Vosburgh E, Moise K 1989 Fetal and neonatal von Willebrand factor (vWF) is unusually large and similar to the vWF in patients with thrombotic thrombocytopenia purpura. British Journal of Haematology 72: 68–72

Weiss J H, Aledort M K, Kochwa S 1968 The effect of salicylate on the haemostatic properties of platelets in man. Journal of Clinical Investigation 47: 2169–2180

Wenske C, Gaedicke G, Kuenzlen E, Heyes C H, Mueller-Eckhardt C, Kleihauer F, Lauritzen C 1983 Treatment of idiopathic thrombocytopenic purpura in pregnancy by high-dose intravenous immunoglobulin. Blut 46: 347–353

Wenske C, Gaedicke G, Heyes H 1984 Idiopathic thrombocytopenic purpura in pregnancy and neonatal period. Blut 48, 377–382

Whaun J M, Smith G R, Sochor V A 1980 Effect of prenatal drug administration on maternal and neonatal platelet aggregation and PF4 release. Haemostasis 9: 226–237

Whaun J, 1973 The platelet of the newborn infant: 5-hydroxythryptamine uptake and release. Thrombosis Diathesis Haemorrhagica 30: 327–333

Whaun J H 1980 The platelet of the newborn infant: adenine nucleotide metabolism and release. Thrombosis Haemostasis 43: 99–103

Widdershoven J, Kollee L, van Munster P, Bosman A M, Monnens L 1986a Biochemical vitamin K deficiency in early infancy: diagnostic limitation of conventional coagulation tests. Helvetica Pediatrica Acta 41: 195–201

Widdershoven J, Motohara K, Endo F, Matsuda I, Monnens L 1986b Influence of the type of feeding on the presence of PIVKA-II in infants. Helvetica Paediatrica Acta 41: 25–29

Widdershoven J, Lambert W, Motohara K, Monnens L, de Leenheer A, Matsuda I, Endo F 1988 Plasma concentrations of vitamin K_1 and PIVKA-II in bottle-fed and breast-fed infants with and without vitamin K prophylaxis at birth. European Journal of Pediatrics 148: 139–142

Witt I, Muller H, Kunter L J 1969 Evidence for the existence of fetal fibrinogen. Thrombosis Diathesis Haemmorrhagica 22: 101–109

Yoffe G, Buchanan G R 1988 Intracranial haemorrhage in newborn and young infants with hemophilia. Journal of Pediatrics 113: 333–336

Zipursky A, Jaber H M 1978 The haematology of bacterial infections in newborn infants. Clinics in Haematology 7: 175–193

Zipursky A, Johnston M, deSa D, Hsu E, Milner R 1979 Clinical and laboratory diagnosis of hemostatic disorders in newborn infants. American Journal of Pediatric Hematology/Oncology 1: 217–226

9. The implementation of international normalized ratios for standardization of the prothrombin time in oral anticoagulant control

Jean M. Thomson

The need for standardization of the prothrombin time has arisen from a continued worldwide use of many different prothrombin time (PT) systems for oral anticoagulant control incorporating a variety of thromboplastin reagents, techniques, instruments and methods of expressing results. Many reports have been published, over several decades, highlighting the effects of these variables on the PT test. In particular, the wide differences in sensitivity of various thromboplastins to the coumarin-induced defect can have a profound effect on anticoagulant dosage and subsequent intensity of anticoagulation (ICTH & ICSH 1979, Loeliger 1979, Loeliger et al 1985a). These can be of such magnitude that a several-fold variation in warfarin dosage ensues (Lam Po Tang & Poller 1975, Poller & Taberner 1982).

THE WORLD HEALTH ORGANIZATION SCHEME

Over the years, many attempts have been made to remedy the situation by the introduction of schemes to standardize the PT. The ultimate aim of all of them has been to achieve uniformity in oral anticoagulant dosage.

In 1983 the World Health Organization (WHO) introduced a new approach towards international standardization of the PT in oral anticoagulant control (WHO Expert Committee on Biological Standardization 1983). Recommendations for the scheme, based on thromboplastin calibration (Loeliger and Lewis 1982), emerged from a collaborative study performed under the auspices of the European Community Bureau Commun de Référence (BCR) (Loeliger et al 1981, Hermans et al 1983). The various steps leading towards this achievement had extended over many previous years and included proposals from distinguished teams of scientists from several countries who were actively engaged in seeking progress towards a reliable system of standardization of the PT. These have been summarized in a previous edition of this book (Tomenson & Thomson 1985) and are therefore not included in the present chapter.

In summary, the WHO scheme is based on the establishment of primary and secondary international reference preparations (IRP) for thromboplastin and the adoption of a statistical model for the calibration of working thromboplastins against these reference materials. It was found that when logarithms of PT performed with an IRP were plotted against logarithms of PT measured with a test preparation under calibration, on the same set of plasmas obtained from normal controls and stabilized, anticoagulated patients, the relationship was linear or very close to linear (Kirkwood 1983). The slope of the calibration line thus obtained has been defined as the International Sensitivity Index (ISI) which quantifies the responsiveness of the thromboplastin in terms of the primary IRP.

IRP for thromboplastin

The first primary IRP for thromboplastin was designated 67/40. Its ISI was defined arbitrarily as 1.0. This was a combined preparation containing adsorbed plasma together with tissue extract from human brain, to be used with its own specified technique. Henceforth, the reagent was described as 'human combined'. Because of limited supplies and the possibility of loss of stability, 67/40 was replaced in 1984 by a Quick test thromboplastin (BCT/253 human plain), i.e. Quick test reagent (Thomson et al 1984), which was designated as the second WHO primary IRP. The WHO Expert Committee on Biological Standardization (1984) decreed that future IRP should be calibrated against BCT/253.

Other IRP for thromboplastin have been recognized by the WHO and BCR. Those from the WHO are available in limited supply, free of charge, to national control laboratories from this organization, whereas IRP from the BCR must be purchased. The latter are mainly used by manufacturers of thromboplastin. These additional preparations were provided because supplies of the primary material were necessarily restricted. They are coded respectively as BCT/099 (human plain), OBT/79 (bovine combined) and RBT/79 (rabbit plain); each with an independent BCR community reference material (CRM) number. In 1985 an additional IRP, under the auspices of the International Committee for Standards in Haematology (ICSH) was prepared (Thomson et al 1986). The material was designated BCT/441 (human plain) and was intended for use by national control laboratories in developing and Eastern bloc countries where, for currency or other problems, IRP are unable to be purchased from the BCR. Calibrations of all of these preparations are related in a step-wise manner from the primary IRP. In consequence, a hierarchical scheme has emerged. The current, established structure of available IRP is illustrated in Fig. 9.1. The establishment of IRP from different animal sources arose principally from the belief that 'like versus like' calibration, i.e. species specificity, was of importance in thromboplastin calibration (Hermans et al 1983), although evidence on which this was based was equivocal.

The calibration of routine working reagents begins with the calibration of manufacturers' house standards against an IRP. The exercises are carried

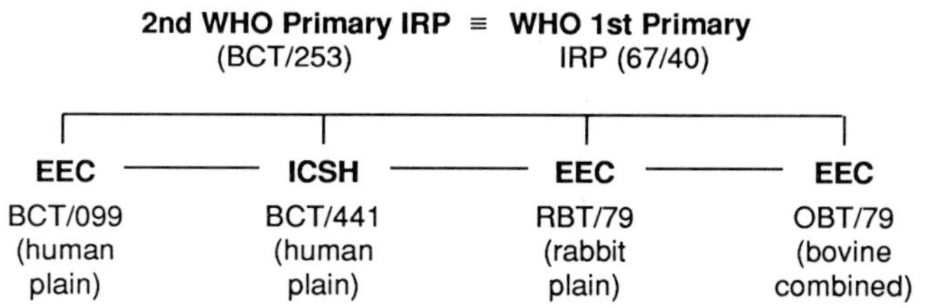

Fig. 9.1 The current established hierarchical structure of international reference preparations (IRP) for thromboplastin.

out by these manufacturers who then proceed to assign ISI to subsequent production batches, using their house standards as the calibrant.

International Normalized Ratios

The ISI of a thromboplastin quantifies its responsiveness to the coumarin defect in patients' plasma, in terms of the primary IRP. According to the WHO system, once a thromboplastin reagent has been calibrated, PT results obtained with it can be expressed on a common scale as International Normalized Ratios (INR). The use of IRP for thromboplastin and the adoption of INR should greatly facilitate the application of common and well-defined therapeutic ranges for oral anticoagulant control, independent of the thromboplastin employed (Loeliger & Lewis 1982).

The INR is the PT ratio (patient PT/normal PT) which it is estimated would have been obtained if the primary IRP 67/40 had been used in the PT. A patient's prothrombin ratio can be converted into an INR by the formula

$$\text{INR} = (\text{Prothrombin ratio})^{\text{ISI}},$$

i.e. raising the prothrombin ratio obtained with the local reagent to the power of its ISI. Alternatively, it can be derived from a nomogram (p. 283).

In 1985 the ICSH and the International Committee on Thrombosis and Haemostasis (ICTH) formally proposed the adoption of the WHO scheme (ICSH & ICTH 1985). To achieve uniformity in PT testing in oral anticoagulant control, manufacturers of thromboplastins were requested to indicate the relationship of each production batch to the WHO IRP by assigning an ISI to each lot of their material. The international committees recommended the provision of package inserts comprising tables or graphs giving equivalent INR which correspond to PT in seconds, ratios, etc. The committees also advised clinicians to employ INR when prescribing dosage of oral anticoagulants and the scientific press were urged to encourage the use of the new terminology in their publications.

Technical requirements for the INR system have been detailed by the WHO (WHO Expert Committee on Biological Standardization 1983,

1984) and its validation has been confirmed in several international, collaborative calibrations (e.g. Hermans et al 1983, Thomson et al 1984, 1986). It is gratifying that most of the major manufacturers of thromboplastin have accepted the system and are complying with ICSH/ICTH recommendations concerning the calibration of their production batches and the assigning of ISI. An increasing number of national committees and professional bodies have supported the adoption of the WHO scheme. As a result it is now becoming widespread, customary practice to report PT as INR in oral anticoagulant control in western Europe, Canada, Australasia, South Africa, Japan and some developing countries. The USA has been slow to adopt the system but the major manufacturers of thromboplastin and warfarin are now giving their support to the use of INR.

The precision of the calibration procedure

Undoubtedly, the INR system has had a considerable impact, but questions still remain on the reliability of its implementation. It cannot be disputed that its introduction represents considerable progress in providing improved standards of safety and effectiveness of oral anticoagulant dose administration. Nevertheless, its application has revealed some inaccuracies and limitations.

In the first place the precision of the ISI is influenced by both within- and between-laboratory variation in the calibration procedure. There is, therefore, an inherent imprecision in the estimation of the ISI (Loeliger et al 1985b). When the system was first introduced there were no reliable guidelines as to the requirements to achieve an accurate ISI. The impression was that a single, full calibration exercise, i.e. 20 normal plasmas and 60 coumarins would suffice in order to assign an accurate ISI to the product. Subsequent experience has shown that multicentre calibration is essential for a reliable ISI because of the many variables which affect the reliability of a single centre's ISI result. Should a systematic error arise at one centre, it could remain undetected if reliance is placed only on the ISI value of this single calibration. It is not surprising, therefore, that when the exercise is conducted by more than one laboratory it becomes more accurate. This has been demonstrated in calibrations of IRP which, by necessity, have been performed on a multicentre, international, collaborative basis. A high standard of precision, measured by the standard error of the mean (SEM) of the ISI has been achieved in these exercises. For example, a coefficient of variation (CV) of as low as 1.2% was obtained in the calibration of the WHO IRP BCT/253 (Thomson et al 1984).

In view of the cumulative evidence, and in order to achieve accuracy and good precision in PT testing, it is now recommended that calibration of manufacturers' house standards should be performed by at least three experienced, independent laboratories. The aim should be to maintain the precision (CV) of the ISI to $\leq 5\%$. When successive batches of working thromboplastin are calibrated, it should be possible to achieve the CV of the slope in the region of $\leq 3\%$.

A second variable affecting the accuracy of the ISI calibration is the response of the manufacturers' production batches of thromboplastin to the coumarin-induced defect in an individual patient's plasma, i.e. the sensitivity of the reagent. Using high sensitivity thromboplastins, with ISI close to 1.0, interlaboratory error in PT testing has been shown in the United Kingdom and the Netherlands to amount to 7–8% (CV) (Van Dijk-Wierda et al 1977, Poller et al 1979). Under well-controlled conditions, taking all of the preceding factors into account, it is estimated that the overall CV of the INR is likely to be between 11 and 13.5% if the thromboplastin employed is a high sensitivity reagent (Loeliger 1984, Loeliger et al 1985b). With low sensitivity thromboplastins (high ISIs) the total error will be higher, amounting to 20% or more due to a greater between-laboratory variation. Further, more recent evidence on the advantages of high ISI thromboplastins is given in subsequent sections of this chapter.

The stability of manufacturers' production batches is another important consideration. ISI values may be assigned to a product some considerable time before the thromboplastin is marketed. Constant surveillance by the producer is necessary, during the shelf life of the reagent, to monitor its stability. The derivation of the ISI of a reagent, in accordance with the WHO protocol (1983), needs to be undertaken with each production batch of individual manufacturer's reagents. Stringent requirements are stipulated, particularly in regard to the source of plasma samples necessary for this exercise. These must be obtained from patients who have been receiving oral anticoagulants for at least 6 weeks, i.e. stabilized on treatment. They should also exhibit a wide range of prothrombin times, spanning the therapeutic interval.

THE APPLICATION OF THE INR SYSTEM

The relatively complex mathematics of the INR system has to some extent retarded its widespread introduction and caused some difficulties and errors (Poller 1988). However, the facility to read INR values directly from manufacturers' package inserts has simplified one aspect for the user. Values provided are usually equivalent to observed prothrombin times or ratios according to the ISI of the reagent. With some thromboplastins more than one set of INR are available, based on different mean normal control values. However, this policy has not been validated in clinical practice and can lead to inaccuracy and confusion.

In theory, by using reagents with assigned ISI, INR results from patients receiving oral anticoagulant therapy should be the same irrespective of the thromboplastin employed. In practice, this has not always proved to be the case. Some of the most reliable data illustrating this point has emerged from multicentre surveys. One example comes from the National External

Table 9.1 Mean INR values obtained in serial UK NEQAS surveys with two commonly used thromboplastins

Survey No.	Thromboplastin A	Thromboplastin B
60	5.26	6.14
	2.31	2.53
	2.99	3.41
	2.85	2.87
61	3.0	3.0
	2.7	2.5
	3.2	3.7
62	2.93	3.08
	3.62	4.34
	1.85	1.95
63	1.81	1.81
	2.41	2.47
	2.29	2.32
64	2.34	2.76
	3.33	3.91
65	3.65	4.05
	2.95	2.35
66	2.20	2.35
	2.47	2.78

19 test samples from long-term, coumarinized patients.
$t = 2.83$, $P < 0.02$.

Quality Assessment Scheme (NEQAS) in the UK which has revealed that INR obtained on the same lyophilized test samples with different thromboplastin reagents may disagree (Poller 1987a). A consistent trend has been observed in serial surveys; some commercial brands of thromboplastin tending to give higher or lower mean INR values than others on the same plasmas (Table 9.1). There are several possible reasons. The most immediate explanation is that there could be a calibration error in the manufacturers' ISI, which would not be surprising given the relative complexity of the calibration procedure. There was in fact evidence of some inaccuracy in some manufacturers' ISI values when the system was first adopted. One published report found that the ISI were too low according to an independent assessment by two hospital laboratories, both of which had considerable experience in thromboplastin calibration (Poller 1987b). For instance, for an INR of 4.0 obtained using an IRP, the equivalent INR using two different commercial thromboplastins would have been 4.9; a difference of clinical significance. It is gratifying, however, that manufacturers have in general become more aware of the inherent pitfalls which can arise during calibration of their reagents. Consequently, some adjustments of ISI have been made by some manufacturers.

A second possible source of error in ISI calibration relates to the source of IRP. It is conceivable, given that different manufacturers are using alternative routes of calibration, e.g. via human brain (plain) or rabbit brain (plain) IRP, that this may be introducing some error in calibration. For instance, it was shown in the BCR exercise (Hermans et al 1983) that the precision of the calibration of the human brain (plain) IRP, BCT/099, was considerably greater than that with the rabbit brain (plain) IRP, RBT/79. Any inherent error in this calibration is necessarily transposed to subsequent calibrations with these IRP.

A third explanation may arise from a problem which was previously thought to be due to a species effect. The coumarin-induced coagulation defect is complex, affecting clotting factors II, VII, IX and X and the anticoagulants protein C and S. Commercial tissue thromboplastins vary considerably in their responsiveness to these clotting factors, the most sensitive approximating to an ISI of 1.0 and the least to an ISI of approximately 2.8. Efforts are made in calibration to minimize these differences by only incorporating plasmas in the calibration from long-term stabilized patients. Nevertheless, if the test reagent and the IRP differ considerably in response to the coumarin clotting factors, it is likely that the calibration will be less accurate. The previous concept of the need to use 'like-to-like' calibration, i.e. human versus human, rabbit versus rabbit, may therefore have been confused with the above.

In all events, the present multiplicity of reference preparations and complexity of the hierarchical relationship is undesirable for biological standards. It is possible that the anomalies in INR values with the manufacturers' reagents would be reduced if a single spine calibration scheme could be developed.

WHO recommendations specify that plasma samples from patients in the early induction phase of oral anticoagulation are excluded from calibration exercises. This may have some bearing on subsequent anticoagulant dosage in these patients. ISI values are rarely derived from plasmas obtained from hospitalized cases. It is not inconceivable, therefore, that different calibration results may be achieved from plasmas derived from patients during the induction of therapy (Tomenson 1984). Likewise, it cannot be assumed that INR are as dependable during the early stages of coumarin treatment when the vitamin K-dependent clotting factors are depressed at different levels (Poller 1987a). During this same period, the varying response of different thromboplastins to the coumarin-induced defect is likely to be more evident than when patients are stabilized on treatment.

In the light of these speculations, a study was performed to assess the reliability of the INR system during the induction phase of coumarin administration (McKernan et al 1988). PT were measured daily with a variety of commercial thromboplastin reagents, in addition to the WHO IRP BCT/253, in patients following commencement of oral anticoagulation. As expected, INR obtained with different reagents on consecutive days of testing showed a wide divergence. The explanation for the differences in response can only be attributed to varying sensitivity of the thromboplastins to the coumarin-induced defect. Specific assays of factors II, VII and X with the different reagents confirmed this view. Some consistent trends with the thromboplastins were also noted; demonstrated by a tendency to overestimate or underestimate the INR. Again, one reason may have been that the respective ISI of the reagents required slight adjustment since INR values were invariably 'out of line' with those derived directly from the IRP. The greatest differences were, however, believed to arise from variations in sensitivity between the different thromboplastins which might be expected during the induction phase when the vitamin K-dependent clotting factors are depressed at varying rates. INR values in the induction phase and in non-stabilized patients may not be sufficiently precise. This problem can only be rectified by the routine use of sensitive (low ISI) thromboplastins (p. 281).

As previously indicated, in the new system for standardization of the PT, the responsiveness of a thromboplastin reagent to the coumarin defect is quantified by the ISI. From this value it should in theory be possible to derive the equivalent INR across the range of different thromboplastin reagents. The data from external quality assessment surveys of the PT has demonstrated that there are limitations in the reliability of INR achieved in this way with the present generation of thromboplastin reagents. UK NEQAS studies have shown that improved performance and better precision in INR between centres have been obtained the closer the ISI is to 1.0 (Poller et al 1988). In theory, the higher the ISI rises above 1.0, i.e. the less responsive the reagent, the larger the error in transposing the patient's observed prothrombin ratio (PR) into the INR. In other words, the error of the INR is quantitatively dependent on the ISI; the higher the ISI the greater the increase in variability.

An additional factor influencing the reliability of INR is the precision of the observed PR with different thromboplastin reagents. Any imprecision in determining the local PR will be carried over into the conversion to the INR. Figure 9.2 shows the relationship between INR and PR for two reagents with ISI of 1.0 and 2.0, respectively. An increase in the PR gives a much larger increase in the INR with the less sensitive reagent (ISI of 2.0). It follows that the variance of the INR is greater the higher the ISI, i.e. the variance of the INR when transforming a PR to an INR is dependent on the slope (the ISI). If the variance is expressed as a CV then, in theory, the CV of the INR should approximate to the CV of the PR multiplied by the ISI.

To test the theory, Taberner et al (1989) conducted a study to assess the influence of the ISI on the precision of the INR. Data was obtained from over 400 centres participating in the UK NEQAS. The interlaboratory SD for the PR was determined from cumulative results from 20 coumarin test samples tested with three different thromboplastins. Two were rabbit brain reagents (ISI of 1.1 and 1.4) and the third originated from human brain material (ISI of 1.0). The mean PR and its SD were linear when plotted on

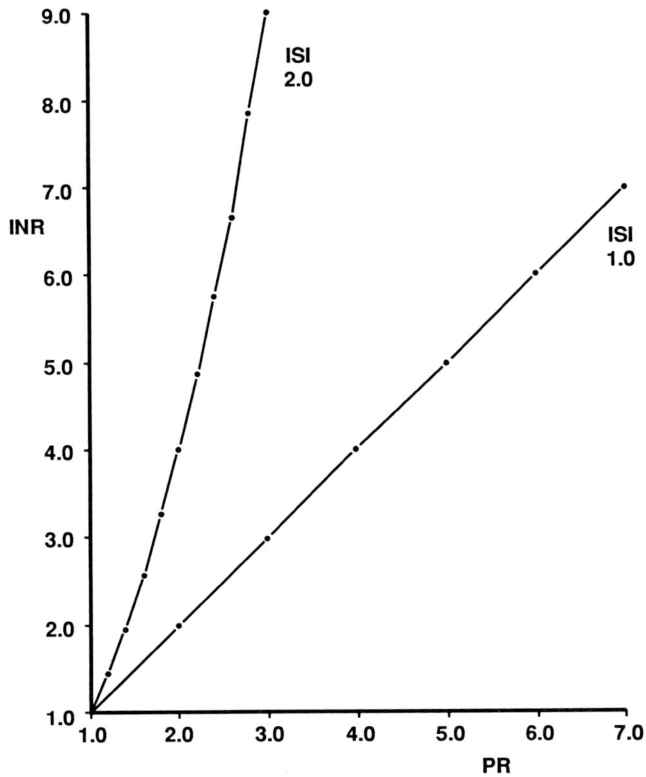

Fig. 9.2 The differing relationships between INR and PR for two thromboplastins (ISI values of 1.0 and 2.0).

a logarithmic scale (Fig. 9.3a), as had previously been shown (Poller et al 1988). However, the slope and intercepts of the two rabbit brain thromboplastins differed. When these relationships were expressed as CV versus PR they became curves (Fig. 9.3b). The actual mean CV achieved in the cumulative external quality assessment surveys, from which the data for the two rabbit brain thromboplastins had been derived, were compared with those predicted. It was found that they were in close agreement (Fig. 9.4). From these observations it was concluded that the ISI of a thromboplastin has a major influence on the interlaboratory variability of the INR. Manufacturers should be encouraged to produce reagents with ISI values as close to 1.0 as possible to avoid loss of precision when PR are expressed as INR. The study also revealed that any comparisons of precision of different thromboplastin reagents should always be made following transformation to INR so that the results will be on the same scale.

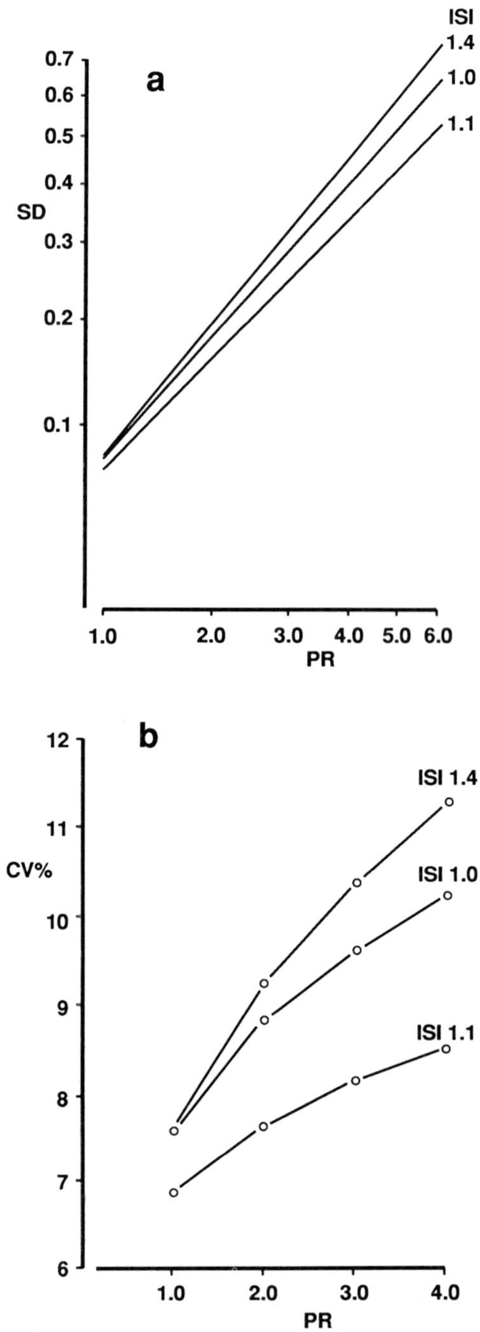

Fig. 9.3 **a** Relationship between SD and PR for three thromboplastins (ISI values of 1.0, 1.1 and 1.4) in serial NEQAS in blood coagulation surveys. Reproduced by permission of the Organizer. **b** Theoretical relationship between CV and PR.

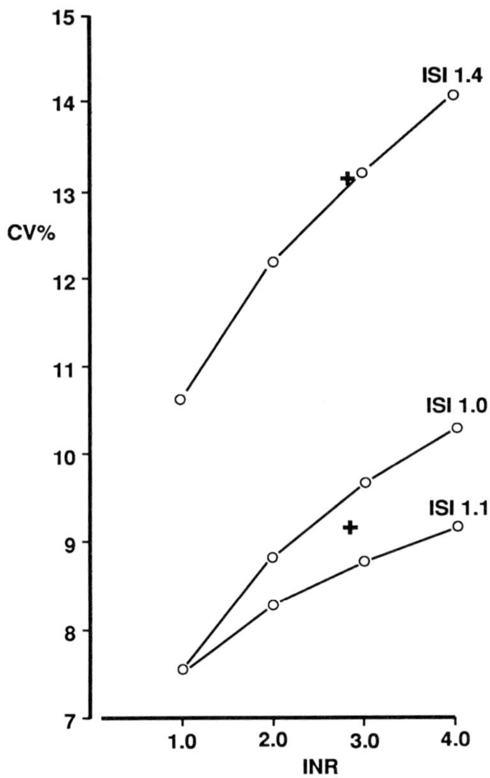

Fig. 9.4 Theoretical relationship between CV and INR. Upper cross represents mean CV and INR obtained in serial NEQAS surveys for thromboplastin with an ISI of 1.4. Lower cross represents similar results for a thromboplastin with an ISI of 1.1

The effects of different methods of endpoint detection

A major consideration in the assessment of the reliability of the INR system is the effect of different methods of endpoint detection on the INR. A manual method normally employs a tilt tube technique, where the timing of clot formation is determined by visual assessment. Although it is commonly considered as the reference method for PT testing and the recommended procedure for calibration exercises, variations in INR still occur from differences in technique of individual operators. For instance, the speed and angle of tilting of the tube in which the test is performed require special attention (Thomson 1980). Deviations may also arise from the use of test-tubes of varying diameter and/or different surfaces.

Since the introduction of standardization of the PT, the need for uniformity of technique has become more apparent. External quality assessment surveys have greatly assisted in improvement of standards of performance of the test. In the UK, where a manual technique is used by almost half of the hospitals, results from the NEQAS have maintained a low overall CV in serial PT exercises (Poller et al 1988, Poller 1989). The thromboplastin reagent with the lowest ISI (1.1), however, gave the lowest overall CV (9.2%), indicating the superiority of a low ISI reagent as well as demonstrating the good precision (CV 8.6%) obtainable with a manual technique. The overall figure for the percentage deviation at all UK hospitals participating in the four UK NEQAS surveys conducted in 1989, using different thromboplastin reagents and the manual method, was 11.4%.

The effect of automation

There is a universal trend in many countries towards automation of the PT. In North America, coagulometers are now employed almost exclusively and in the majority of centres. Their use is also widespread in Western Europe and most other developed countries. Numerous publications have shown that PT results derived by an automated method vary between different models and makes of instruments. Not only, therefore, may the reagent component influence the INR but also the significant and sometimes appreciable coagulometer effect must be considered.

The most meaningful analyses of reagent/instrument combinations (systems) have again been derived from large databases such as those obtained from external quality assessment surveys, e.g. the American College of Pathologists (CAP) (Evatt et al 1981a,b) and the UK NEQAS. These have demonstrated discrepant findings and mean differences in PT results with different automated and semi-automated systems. Hitherto, PT results in North America have mainly been expressed as simple clotting times or observed PR. The effects of instrumentation on INR from the CAP surveys could therefore not be evaluated.

It has, however, been possible to assess the impact of automation on INR in the UK where the ISI system has been universally adopted since 1984. In the UK the manual technique has always been regarded as the reference method and the yardstick of performance. Figure 9.5 provides a comparison of coagulometer and manual results, expressed as CV (%) of INR. The data was obtained from serial NEQAS surveys (Poller 1989) and indicates that, overall, coagulometer results are less precise than the manual technique and that they have an effect on the INR.

PT results from serial NEQAS surveys were examined in a study which was specifically conducted to assess the effect of coagulometers (Poller et al 1989). Mean coagulometer PT values were plotted for each of 20 coumarin test plasmas issued in serial surveys conducted between April 1986 and October 1987 against the mean manual result for the same plasmas. This analysis was based on a logarithmic scale and orthogonal regression analysis. It was thus possible to determine the slope parameter and CV for each system, i.e. each reagent/instrument combination. Although there were dif-

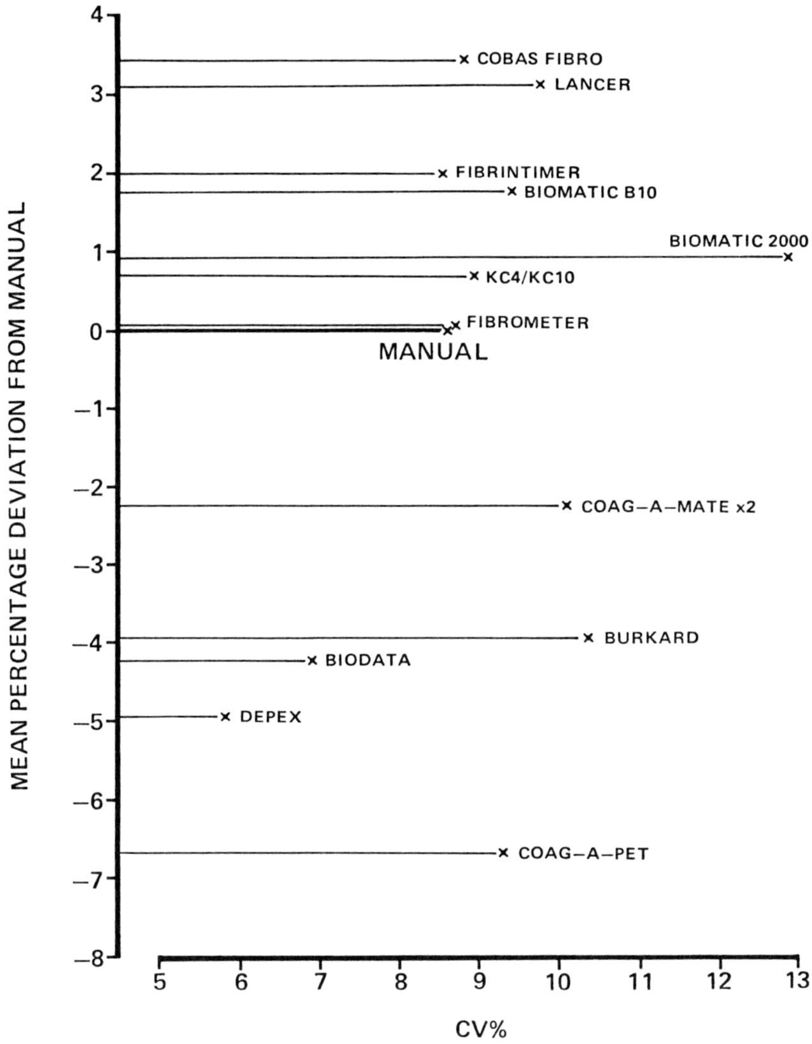

Fig. 9.5 Accuracy (percentage deviation from manual INR) and precision (CV% of INR) with coagulometers in UK NEQAS surveys. (From Poller (1989), reproduced by permission of the author and the publishers, British Medical Journal.)

ferences across the range of instruments the regression slopes were similar irrespective of whether results were expressed as direct PT (s) or transformed to INR. The CV of the slope of the INR was, however, greater with the majority of instrument/reagent systems indicating that there was an additional error arising from the conversion of the PT, to INR and that the use of the ISI system did not compensate for the coagulometer effect. Seven of the eight types of coagulometer examined tended to overestimate

Table 9.2 Overall mean regression slopes and CV

Instrument	Estimated slope parameter PT (CV)	INR (CV)	Average No. of users
Reagent A			
Coag-a-Mate ×2	0.97 (1.98)	0.97 (1.89)	17
Fibrintimer	0.93 (1.27)	0.92 (1.62)	15
Biodata	0.95 (1.69)	0.94 (1.94)	7
Lancer	0.91 (2.38)	0.89 (2.93)	6
Coag-a-Pet	0.95 (2.58)	0.95 (2.57)	6
Burkard	1.02 (1.63)	1.01 (2.43)	16
Biomatic 2000	0.94 (1.92)	0.92 (2.49)	8
KC4/KC10	0.93 (1.42)	0.92 (1.60)	24
Reagent B			
KC4/KC10	0.86 (2.0)	0.86 (1.67)	9

the INR, i.e. the slope was <1.0 (Table 9.2). The CV of the slopes was valuable as a guide to the precision of the different systems although those with the best precision did not always provide INR which most closely approximated to the manual results. A common finding was that of good agreement between manual and automated INR values, with plasma samples which gave INR of approximately 3.0 (approximately 42.0 s with Manchester Reagent). However, coagulometer INR tended to be lower at less intense (INR <3.0) and higher at more intense degrees of anticoagulation (INR >3.0).

In the same study, within-instrument variability with one type of coagulometer, the KC4/KC10, with one type of thromboplastin, Manchester Reagent (i.e. one system), was evaluated. This system was analysed because it is currently employed by a larger number of centres than other instrument/reagent combinations in the UK. It was disconcerting to find that individual regression slopes varied widely, between 0.80 and 0.96, indicating that within-instrument differences were similar to and as great as those produced by the different systems. As a first step to remedy the situation, local adjustment of instruments may be required. The availability of a range of INR calibrated coumarin plasmas could well be an asset in bringing instruments of the same model and manufacturer into closer agreement with each other. Until better within-instrument performance is achieved, the use of a correction factor to make allowance for instrument variables or an adjustment of the ISI for all models of one instrument type would not seem feasible or appropriate.

In the Netherlands the majority of oral anticoagulant clinics employ Thrombotest for PT testing. Almost all of these centres perform the tests by a micromethod with a Lode coagulometer. A study was conducted to investigate whether the ISI for Thrombotest, which in accordance with the WHO calibration method is based on a manual techniquc, is appropriate for a micromethod using a Lode coagulometer (Peters et al 1989). As in the British evaluation, ISI values were calculated by orthogonal regression from the PT of normal controls and patient samples from six experienced laboratories. Although the precision (CV) of the micromethod was shown to be the same as that of the manual method there were significant differences between the PT of both normal subjects and anticoagulated patients with manual and automated methods. Overall, PT measured by Lode coagulometers were longer and the ISI values ranged from 1.00 to 1.07, amounting on average to be 3% higher than that of the manual method. The investigation provides a further example of within-instrument variation sufficient to give rise to differences in INR.

A single-centre evaluation aiming to examine the instrument effect on the ISI has been reported in Australia (Ray & Smith 1989). Calibrations were performed on five different types of instruments with Thromborel S (Behring) reagent against the Australian Reference Thromboplastin tested manually. Significant instrument effects on the ISI were noted. The authors concluded that individual laboratories may need to calculate the ISI value of their own test systems. This recommendation, although well intended, may not provide the solution to the problem because, as discussed earlier, the possible inherent error of an ISI determined in a single-centre calibration is considerable.

Poggio et al (1989) found significant variations in ISI with two thromboplastins calibrated against an IRP, using four different coagulometers. Some inaccuracy in INR values resulted.

In the United Kingdom the most commonly used PT systems are currently the KC4/KC10 and Coag-a-Mate ×2/×C and Manchester Reagent. These two systems have been evaluated, in detail, in a prospective field study designed to compare their effect on PT and INR (Thomson et al 1991). Centres employing these systems were issued 20 test plasmas with a wide scatter of INR values spanning the therapeutic interval. Results were compared by linear and logarithmic orthogonal regression with the calibrated manual PT values of the test plasmas. With the majority, considerable within-instrument variability was again apparent, sufficient to be meaningful in clinical terms. However, a substantial minority of participants obtained good agreement with the manual reference values (Fig. 9.6a). This shows that close approximation to the manual result is attainable with an automated method of endpoint detection.

An overall pattern of results, characteristic for each instrument, emerged. The KC results agreed well with the manual results when the PT were between 25 and 30 s (INR between 1.6 and 2.0) but values tended to be shorter than for the manual method with lower values (<25.0 s) and longer with higher values (>30.0 s), i.e. a cross-over effect (Figs 9.6b & 9.7). The same pattern was also observed in serial NEQAS surveys with two other instruments, the Fibrintimer and Lancer (Poller et al 1989). With the Coag-a-Mate, however, PT were consistently slightly shorter than the manual re-

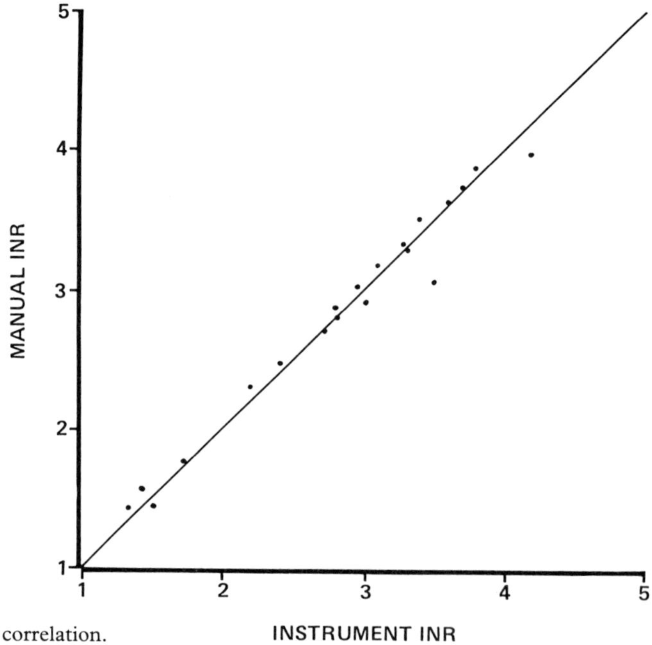

a A linear correlation.

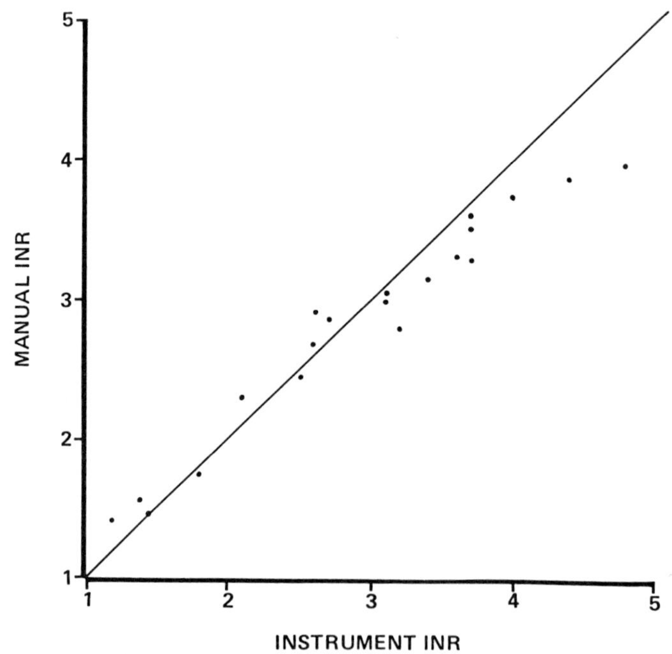

b A non-linear relationship. (cross-over)

Fig. 9.6 INR obtained by two centres using KC/10 (Amelung) instruments, correlated with respective overall reagent manual mean INR.

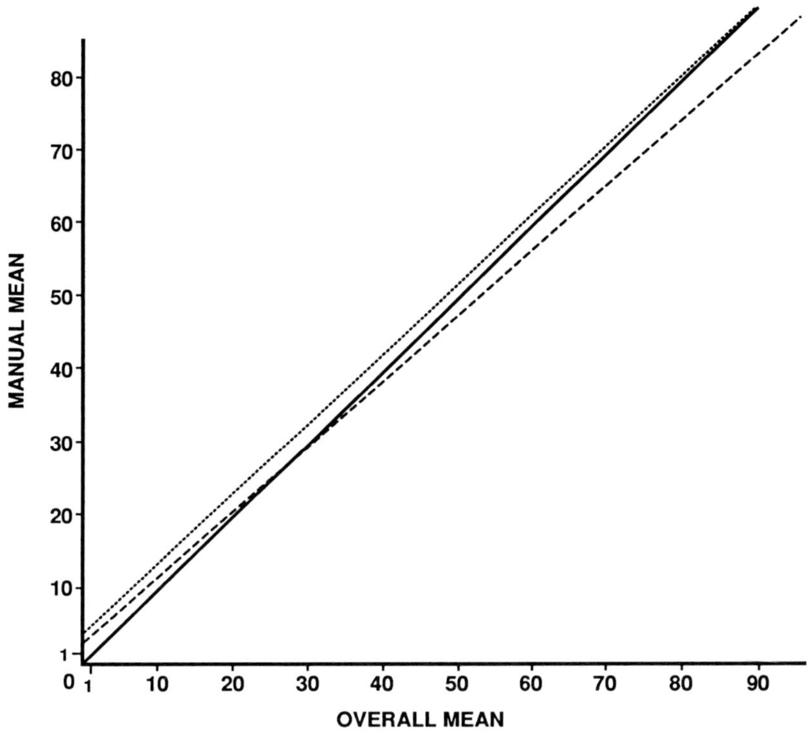

Fig. 9.7 Mean orthogonal regression lines of the KC (-----) Coag-a-Mate (.......) and the line of coincidence (▬).

sults over the whole range of test plasmas spanning the therapeutic interval (Fig. 9.7). In clinical terms this would mean that a slightly larger dose of warfarin would be prescribed to achieve INR values >3.0 with the Coag-a-Mate than with the manual technique whereas with KC instruments, to achieve the same INR, the dose would be likely to be less. The mean deviation from a manual INR of 4.0 was –0.1 with the Coag-a-Mate whereas it was +0.3 overall with the KC instruments. These observations were based on the mean results of the two systems. Some individual instruments of both types, however, showed much more discrepant values from the manual method. Effects on dosage with these may therefore be much more marked.

The effect of the mean normal control value

Since the INR system is based upon PR the normal control time used to derive the latter is obviously of fundamental importance. In general, normal PT measured by automated and semi-automated techniques are shorter than when tested manually. However, contrary to the general assumption, it does not follow that when the normal value is shorter the PT of coumarin plasmas will also be shortened in proportion, i.e. the instrument PR is altered from the manual ratio.

The relationship between normal and coumarin PT was investigated in the Coag-a-mate/KC study. (Thomson et al 1991). The mean instrument normal PT (MNPTs) with both coagulometers were, not unexpectedly, found to be shorter than the manual value. There was, however, an undesirable lack of agreement on normal values between laboratories using the same model of instrument. Individual centres using to same system gave a wide scatter of normal control results ranging from less than 13.0 s to more than 16.0 s. Moreover, the degree of shortening of the MNPT did not parallel that of the abnormal samples and there was, in fact, a total lack of correlation between these values. Results with the Coag-a-Mate are given as an example (Fig. 9.8). Another important observation arising from this

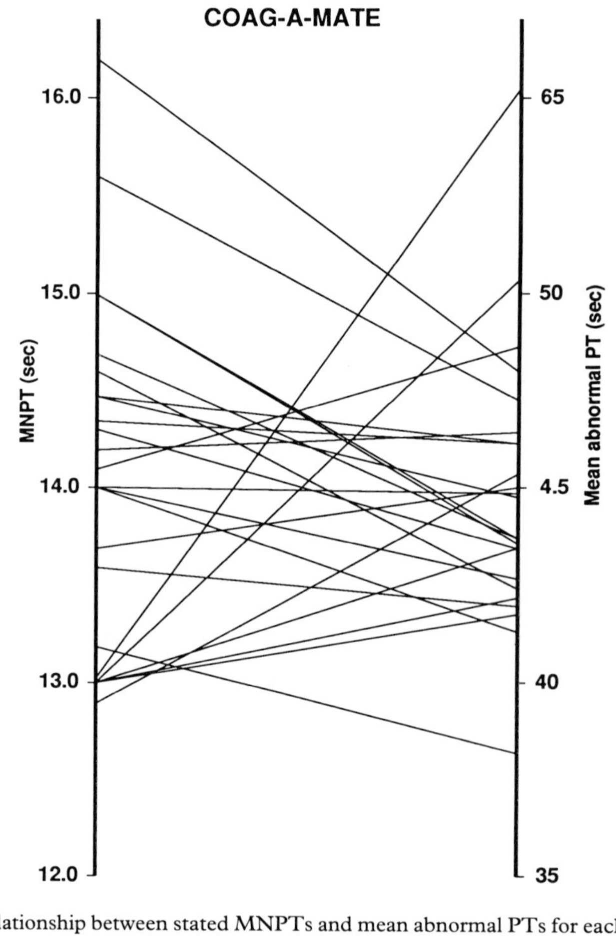

Fig. 9.8 Relationship between stated MNPTs and mean abnormal PTs for each centre using a Coag-a-Mate.

study was that the degree of disagreement between instrument and manual INR was related to the normal control values. The greater the difference between them, the greater the instrument deviation from the manual INR. This negative correlation was significant at the 1% level for the two systems (Fig. 9.9). Correction of the instrument effect on the PT would therefore not be feasible using the local MNPT to derive INR. With the KC system the mean percentage deviation of the instrument INR from the manual INR was significantly reduced, however, when the instrument value was calculated from the MNPT supplied in the chart provided by the manufacturer of the Manchester Reagent thromboplastin.

Instrument effects appear to undermine the reliability of a system of standardization based on a simple PT ratio and of an INR derived from it. ISI values are by definition derived from calibration exercises employing the manual PT technique. From the above evidence it is apparent that ISI obtained in this way may not always be applicable when a Coagulometer is used. Unfortunately, the extent of interinstrument variability does not at present allow the correction of coagulometer effects by the assignment of a system-specific ISI to all instruments or systems of one type. A system-related ISI could otherwise have provided an answer to this problem (British Society for Haematology 1990). As an initial step some local adjustment of instruments seems necessary to bring models of the same type

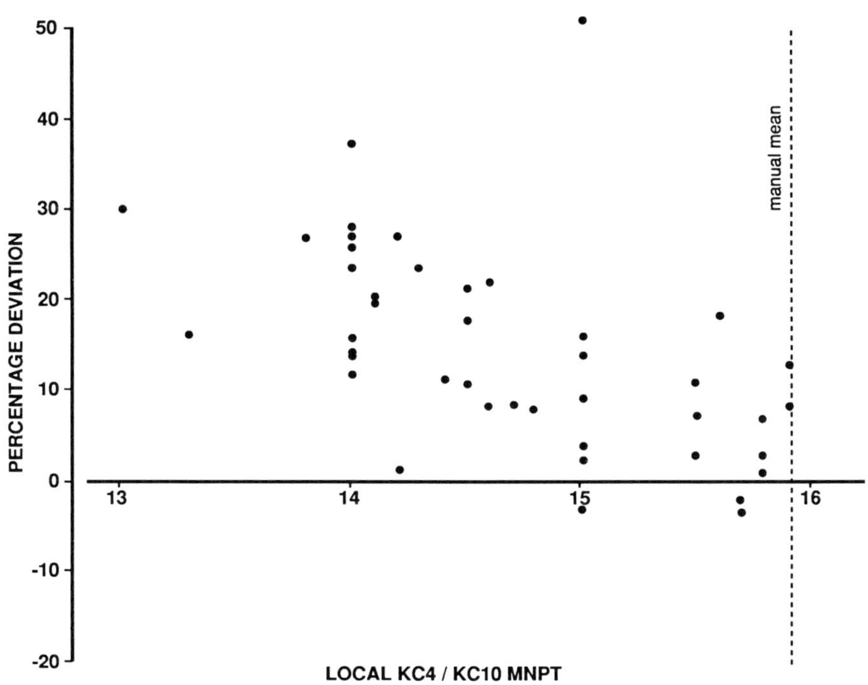

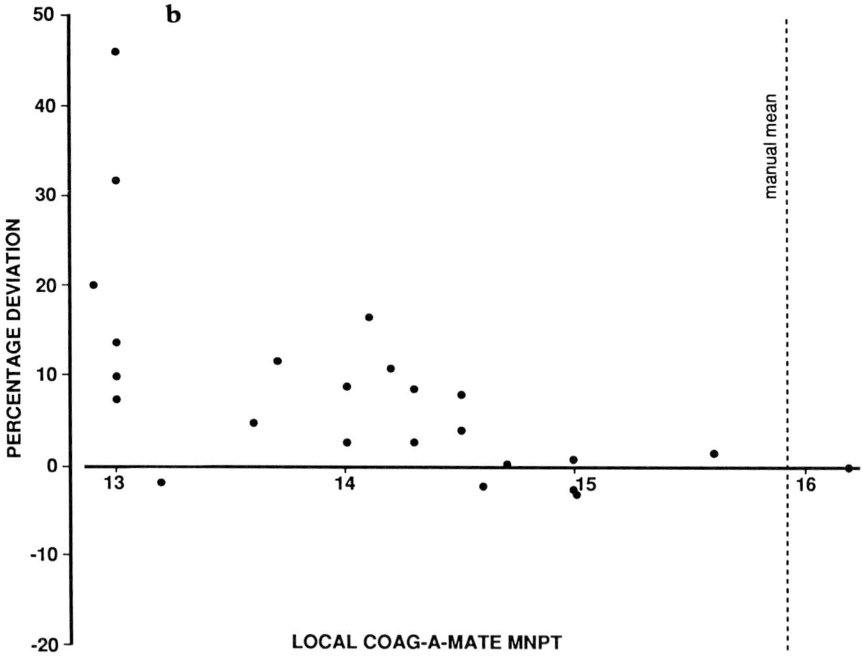

Fig. 9.9 Mean percentage deviation of coagulometer INR from manual results for each centre, plotted against the stated local MNPT. **b** When local MNPT are used to derive INR for Coag-a-Mate.

more in line with each other and with the manual technique. The wider application of reference plasmas calibrated in PT or INR may help to resolve this difficulty.

A variety of opinions is expressed on the correct source of the MNPT used to obtain an INR and the issue remains controversial and unresolved. In practice, it has been shown that the use of the manual ISI and the MNPT from a manufacturer's chart, if reliably derived, gives INR which are closer to the manual result than the use of a coagulometer-derived MNPT and the manual ISI (Thomson et al 1991). Ultimately, a system-related ISI should be the objective but this will depend upon the improved standardization of performance of coagulometers.

It is advised that the MNPT should be based on the PT of 20 fresh plasmas obtained from healthy ambulant adults, tested individually. The geometric mean of these values should then be calculated from the anti-logarithm of the means of the logarithm of the individual PT. The British Society for Haematology Guidelines on Oral Anticoagulation (British Society for Haematology 1990) recommend that a locally determined geometric mean should be compared with the mean normal value provided by the manufacturer to confirm whether there is an acceptable degree of agreement between them.

Further multicentre evaluations are required to provide additional information which may be of assistance in resolving the problem of normal values in INR determination. The solution is not easy, given the multiplicity of reagent/instrument combinations in current use. In addition, manufacturers' MNPT may vary from batch to batch and this may not be appreciated. Such information is not necessarily recorded on package inserts. It is also conceivable that local MNPT are derived from plasma samples which have been affected by pre-test variables, e.g. activation, leading to acceleration of the PT. Strict control is required in subject selection, collection and handling of the samples before and during testing.

LOW ISI THROMBOPLASTINS

Reference has been made to the importance of a low ISI thromboplastin in maintaining good precision when PR are expressed as INR (p. 268). A major advantage of high sensitivity reagents, i.e. ISI ranging from 1.0 to 1.2 in terms of oral anticoagulant dosage, is shown in Fig. 9.10. It is now customary practice to recommend different dosage regimes of oral anticoagulants according to the clinical state of the patient (Hull et al 1982, Loeliger et al 1985a, Hirsh & Levine 1988, Hirsh et al 1989, British Society for Haematology 1990). PR equivalent to three dosage regimes of INR commonly used in clinical practice are illustrated in Fig. 9.10 (British Society for Haematology 1990). These have been related to increasing ISI of thromboplastins. It can be noted that as the ISI increases, the width of the therapeutic equivalents expressed in PR progressively diminish (Poller 1987c). Dosage control with a low sensitivity (high ISI) preparation spans a very narrow range compared with that observed with low-ISI reagents. Consequently, dosage adjustment based on a low ISI reagent which gives a wide therapeutic interval should be easier to achieve and therefore more safe. It will also be observed that the lower limit of the therapeutic range with the less sensitive (high ISI) reagents closely approaches the normal value. As a result, discrimination from the upper limit of the normal range is not easily apparent, whereas with high sensitivity thromboplastins there is a clear demarcation.

To facilitate the general application of the INR system a simple nomogram has been devised (Poller 1988) (Fig. 9.11). This enables an INR value to be obtained from the PR without the need for calculations. An amended version, to accommodate North American thromboplastins which are less responsive, i.e. high ISI reagents, is also available (Poller & Hirsh 1989). Approximately 90% of the thromboplastins used in North America (supplied by three manufacturers) have ISI values between 2.3 and 2.6 (Hirsh et al 1989). The nomogram has the advantage of a visual assessment of the global relationship between observed prothrombin ratios and the INR over a range of ISI values designated to thromboplastins currently marketed. INR values of PT ratios can be read directly from the

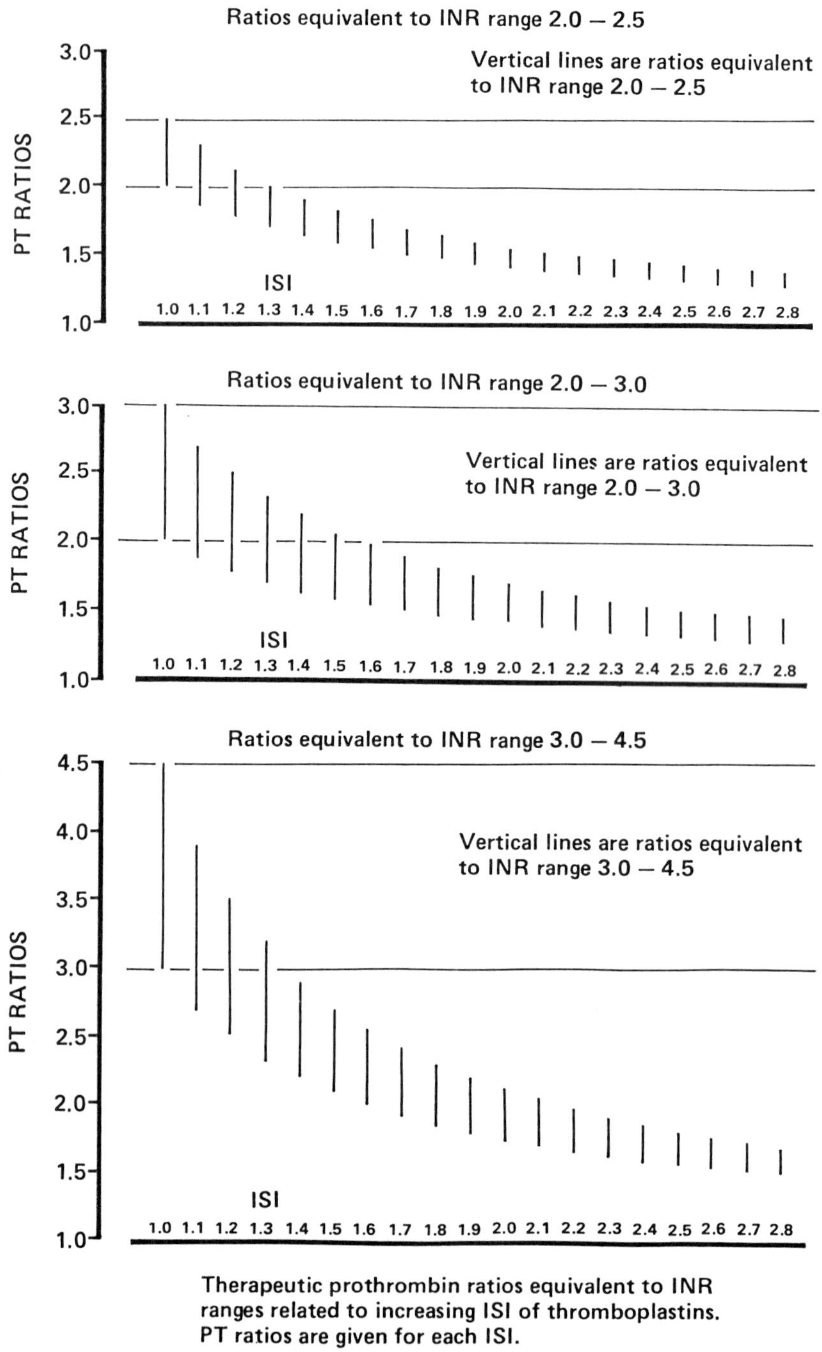

Fig. 9.10 Therapeutic PR equivalent to INR ranges related to increasing ISI of thromboplastins. PT ratios are given for each ISI. (From British Society for Haematology (1990), reproduced by permission of the publishers, British Medical Journal.)

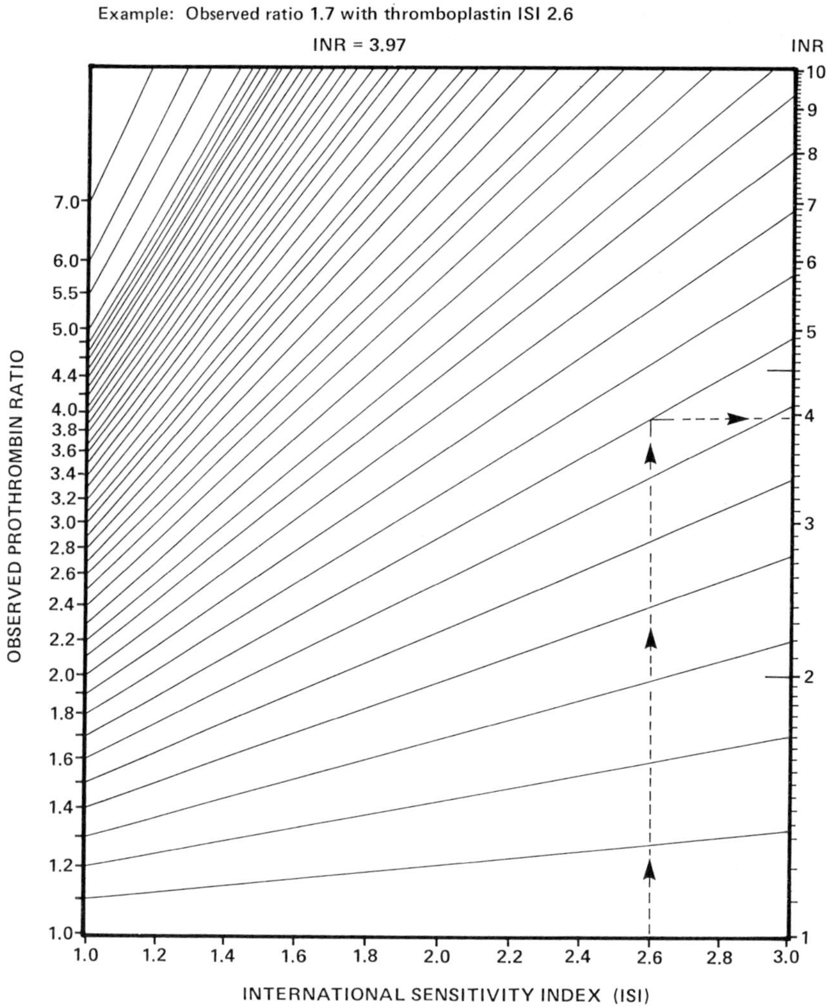

Fig. 9.11 Nomogram. (From Poller L (1988), reproduced by permission of the author and the publishers, F K Schattauer Verlag GmbH.)

nomogram, irrespective of the thromboplastin, thus dispensing with the need for statistical calculations and facilitating the application and understanding of the INR system.

In summary, the INR system has assisted in highlighting differences between the various methods of endpoint detection, allowed them to be quantified and also permitted measures to correct some of the problems. Certain fundamental issues nevertheless remain; for instance the distortion by some coagulometers of PR by disproportionate acceleration of normal PT compared with patient samples. Until rectified, this instrument effect may undermine the use of a simple PR and an INR derived from it, based on an ISI which has been calculated from manual PT.

REFERENCES

British Society for Haematology, British Committee for Standards in Haematology, Haemostasis and Thrombosis Task Force 1990 Guidelines on oral anticoagulation: second edition. Journal of Clinical Pathology 43: 177–183

Evatt B L, Brogan D, Triplett D A, Koepke J, Waters G 1981a Effect of thromboplastin and instrumentation on the prothrombin time test. Clinical Laboratory Haematology 3: 331–342

Evatt B L, Brogan D, Triplett D A, Koepke J A, Waters G 1981b Influences of thromboplastin and instrumentation upon prothrombin time tests: implications for standardization. In: Triplett D A (ed) Standardization of coagulation assays: an overview. Skokie, Illinois, College of American Pathologists p 39–49

Hermans J, van den Besselaar A M H P, Loeliger E A, van der Velde E A 1983 A collaborative calibration study of reference materials for thromboplastins. Thrombosis and Haemostasis 50: 712–717

Hirsh J, Levine M 1988 Confusion over the therapeutic range for monitoring oral anticoagulant therapy in North America. Thrombosis and Haemostasis 59: 129–132

Hirsh J, Poller L, Deykin D, Levine M, Dalen J 1989 Optimal therapeutic range for oral anticoagulants. Chest 95: 5S–11S (suppl)

Hull R, Hirsh J, Jay R 1982 Different intensities of anticoagulation in the long term treatment of proximal venous thrombosis. New England Journal of Medicine 307: 1676–1681

ICTH & ICSH (International Committee on Thrombosis and Haemostasis and International Committee for Standardization in Haematology) 1979 Prothrombin time standardization: report of the expert panel on oral anticoagulant control. Thrombosis and Haemostasis 42: 1073–1114

ICSH & ICTH (International Committee for Standardization in Haematology and International Committee for Thrombosis and Haemostasis) 1985 Recommendations for reporting prothrombin times in anticoagulant control. Thrombosis and Haemostasis 53: 155–156

Kirkwood T B L 1983 Calibration of reference thromboplastins and standardization of the prothrombin time ratio. Thrombosis and Haemostasis 49: 238–244

Lam Po Tang P R L C, Poller L 1975 Oral anticoagulant therapy and its control: an international survey. Thrombosis et Diathesis Haemorrhagica 34: 419–425

Loeliger E A 1979 The optimal therapeutic range in oral anticoagulation. History and proposal. Thrombosis and Haemostasis 42: 1141–1152

Loeliger E A 1984 Critical remarks from a clinician's point of view. In: van den Besselaar A M H P, Gralnick H R, Lewis S M (eds) Thromboplastin calibration and oral anticoagulant control. Martinus Nijhoff, Boston p 109–116

Loeliger E A, Lewis S M 1982 Progress in laboratory control of oral anticoagulants. Lancet ii: 318–320

Loeliger E A, van den Besselaar A M H P, Hermans J, van der Velde E A 1981 Certification of three reference materials for thromboplastin. BCR Information. Commission of the European Communities, Brussels

Loeliger E A, Poller L, Samama M, Thomson J M, Van den Besselaar A M H P, Vermylen J, Verstraete M 1985a Questions and answers on prothrombin time standardization in oral anticoagulant control. Thrombosis and Haemostasis 54: 515–517

Loeliger E A, van den Besselaar A M H P, Lewis S M 1985b Reliability and clinical impact of the normalization of the prothrombin times in oral anticoagulant control. Thrombosis and Haemostasis 53: 148–154

McKernan A, Thomson J M, Poller L 1988 The reliability of international normalised ratios during short-term oral anticoagulant treatment. Clinical Laboratory Haematology 10: 63–71

Peters R H M, van den Besselaar A M H P, Olthuis F M F G 1989 A multicentre study to evaluate method dependency of the international sensitivity index of bovine thromboplastin. Thrombosis and Haemostasis 61: 166–169

Poggio M, van den Besselaar A M H P, van der Velde E A, Bertina R M 1989 The effect of some instruments for prothrombin time testing on the International Sensitivity Index (ISI) of two rabbit tissue thromboplastin reagents. Thrombosis and Haemostasis 62: 868–874

Poller L 1987a Laboratory control of oral anticoagulants. British Medical Journal 294: 1184

Poller L 1987b INR — Calibration of therapeutic range. In: Wessler S, Becker C G, Nemerson Y (eds) The New Dimensions of Warfarin Prophylaxis. Plenum, New York.

Poller L 1987c INR and the therapeutic range. Biologia et Clinica Haematologica 9: 203–213

Poller L 1988 A simple nomogram for the derivation of international normalized ratios for the standardization of prothrombin times. Thrombosis and Haemostasis 60: 18–20

Poller L 1989 United Kingdom external quality assessment in blood coagulation: the first 21 years. Journal of Clinical Pathology 42: 1–3

Poller L, Hirsh J 1989 Special report: a simple system for the derivation of international normalised ratios for the reporting of prothrombin time results with North American thromboplastin reagents. American Journal of Clinical Pathology 92: 124–126

Poller L, Taberner D A 1982 Dosage of oral anticoagulants: an international survey. British Journal of Haematology 51: 479–485

Poller L, Thomson J M, Yee K F 1979 Quality control trials of prothrombin time: an assessment of the performance in serial studies. Journal of Clinical Pathology 32: 251–253

Poller L, Taberner D A, Thomson J M, Darby K V 1988 Survey of prothrombin time in National Quality Assessment Scheme exercises (1980–1987). Journal of Clinical Pathology 41: 361–364

Poller L, Thomson J M, Taberner D A 1989 Effect of automation on prothrombin time test in NEQAS surveys. Journal of Clinical Pathology 42: 97–100

Ray M J, Smith I R 1989 Instrument effect on the international sensitivity index. Thrombosis and Haemostasis 62: 529

Taberner D A, Poller L, Thomson J M, Darby K V 1989 Effect of international sensitivity index (ISI) of thromboplastins on precision of international normalised ratios (INR). Journal of Clinical Pathology 42: 92–96

Thomson J M 1980 Laboratory control of anticoagulant therapy. In: Thomson J M (ed) Blood coagulation and haemostasis: a practical guide, 2nd edn. Churchill Livingstone, Edinburgh p 279–330

Thomson J M, Tomenson J A, Poller L 1984 The calibration of the second international reference preparation for thromboplastin (thromboplastin human plain, coded BCT/253). Thrombosis and Haemostasis 52: 336–342

Thomson J M, Darby K V, Poller L 1986 Calibration of BCT/441, the ICSH reference preparation for thromboplastin. Thrombosis and Haemostasis 55: 379–382

Thomson J M, Taberner D A, Poller L 1990 Automation and the prothrombin time: a UK field study of two widely used coagulometers. Journal of Clinical Pathology 43: 679–684

Tomenson J A 1984 A statistician's independent evaluation. In: van den Besselaar A M H P, Gralnick H R, Lewis S M (eds) Thromboplastin calibration and oral anticoagulant control. Martinus Nijhoff, Boston p 87–108

Tomenson J A, Thomson J M 1985 Standardization of the prothrombin time. In: Thomson J M (ed) Blood coagulation and haemostasis: a practical guide, 3rd edn. Churchill Livingstone, Edinburgh p 370

Van Dijk-Wierda C A, Hermans J, Loeliger E A, Roos J 1977 Interlaboratory oral anticoagulant quality assessment by the Netherlands Foundation of Thrombosis services. Thrombosis and Haemostasis 37: 509–522

WHO Expert Committee on Biological Standardization 1983 33rd Report. WHO Technical Report Series 687: 81–105

WHO Expert Committee on Biological Standardization 1984 34th Report. WHO Technical Series 700: 18–19

Index